ANNUAL REVIEW OF NURSING RESEARCH

Volume 22, 2004

ANNUAL REVIEW OF NURSING RESEARCH

Volume 22, 2004

Eliminating Health Disparities Among Racial and Ethnic Minorities in the United States

Joyce J. Fitzpatrick, PhD, RN, FAAN
Series Editor

Antonia M. Villarruel, PhD, RN, FAAN
Cornelia P. Porter, PhD, RN, FAAN
Volume Editors

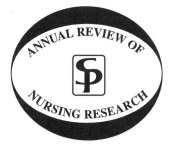

 SPRINGER PUBLISHING COMPANY

Order ANNUAL REVIEW OF NURSING RESEARCH, Volume 23, 2005, prior to publication and receive a 10% discount. See the last page of this volume for more information.

Springer Publishing Company, Inc.
536 Broadway
New York, NY 10012-3955

04 05 06 07 08 / 5 4 3 2 1

ISBN-0-8261-4134X
ISSN-0739-6686

ANNUAL REVIEW OF NURSING RESEARCH is indexed in *Cumulative Index to Nursing and Allied Health Literature* and *Index Medicus*.

Printed in the United States of America by Maple-Vail Book Manufacturing Group.

Contents

Part III: Special Conditions

Part IV: Intervention Approaches for Racial and Ethnic Minority Populations

Contributors

Evelyn Barbee PhD, RN, FAAN
Independent Consultant
Jamaica Plains, MA

Linda Burnes Bolton, DrPH, RN, FAAN
Vice President and Chief Nursing
    Officer
Cedars Sinai Medical Center
Los Angeles, CA

Linda Burton, PhD
Director, Center for Human
    Development and Family
    Research in Diverse Contexts
Pennsylvania State University
University Park, PA

Mary Canales, RN, PhD
Associate Professor
School of Nursing
University of Vermont
Burlington, VT

Constance Dallas, PhD, RN
Family Research Consortium III
    Postdoctoral Fellow
Assistant Professor, Department of
    Maternal-Child Nursing
University of Illinois at Chicago
Chicago, IL

M. Christina Esperat, RN, PhD, APRN-BC
Professor and Associate Dean for
    Research and Practice
Texas Tech University Health
    Sciences
School of Nursing
Lubbock, TX

Du Feng, PhD
Associate Professor
Texas Tech University College of
    Human Sciences
Lubbock, TX

C. Alicia Georges, EdD, RN, FAAN
Chair, Department of Nursing
Lehman College
Bronx, NY

Joyce Newman Giger, EdD, APRN, BC, FAAN
Professor, Graduate Studies
University of Alabama at
    Birmingham
Birmingham, AL

Elizabeth W. Gonzalez, RN, PhD, APRN-BC
Associate Professor
Drexel University
College of Nursing and Health Professions
Philadelphia, PA

Eun-Ok Im, PhD, MPH, RN, CNS
Associate Professor
School of Nursing
University of Texas at Austin
Austin, TX

Jillian Inouye, RN, PhD, APRN-BC
Professor and Graduate Chair,
Director, Office of Nursing Research
School of Nursing and Dental Hygiene
University of Hawaii at Manoa
Honolulu, HI

Bette Rusk Keltner, PhD, RN, FAAN
Professor and Dean
School of Nursing and Health Studies
Georgetown University
Washington, DC

Irene D. Lewis, APN, DNSc, FAAN
Professor
Department of Nursing, HB 411
San Jose State University
San Jose, CA

Melen R. McBride, PhD, RN
Social Science Research Associate and Associate Director for Curriculum, Technology, and Research
Stanford Geriatric Education Center
Stanford University
Palo Alto, CA

Cathy D. Meade, PhD, RN, FAAN
Professor, Department of Interdisciplinary Oncology, University of South Florida
Director, Education Program, H. Lee Moffitt Cancer Center and Research Institute
Tampa, FL

DeAnne K. Hilfinger Messias, PhD, RN
Associate Professor
University of South Carolina
Columbia, SC

Lee Anne Nichols, PhD, RN
Assistant Professor
The University of Tulsa School of Nursing
Tulsa, OK

Donna C. Owen, RN, PhD, AOCN
Professor
Texas Tech University Health Sciences
School of Nursing
Lubbock, TX

Carmen J. Portillo, PhD, RN, FAAN
Associate Professor
University of California, San Francisco
School of Nursing
San Francisco, CA

Barbara Powe, PhD, RN
Director, Special Populations Research
Behavioral Research Center
American Cancer Society
Atlanta, GA

Mercedes Rubio, PhD
Director, Minority Programs
American Sociological Association
Washington, DC

Mary Lou de Leon Siantz, PhD, RN, FAAN
Professor and Associate Dean for Research and Graduate Education
Georgetown University
Washington, DC

Roxanne Struthers, PhD, RN
Assistant Professor
University of Minnesota School of Nursing
Minneapolis, MN

Sandra Millon Underwood, RN, PhD, FAAN
American Cancer Society Oncology Nursing Professor
Northwestern Mutual Life Research Scholar
Professor, University of Wisconsin, Milwaukee
School of Nursing
Milwaukee, WI

Catherine Waters, PhD
Assistant Professor
University of California, San Francisco
San Francisco, CA

SeonAe Yeo, RNC, PhD
Associate Professor
University of Michigan
School of Nursing
Ann Arbor, MI

Preface

This 22nd volume in the *Annual Review of Nursing Research (ARNR)* series focuses on eliminating health disparities among racial and ethnic minorities in the United States. This topic is timely and important; it has been identified as a priority for several professional organizations and by key government funding agencies. Drs. Antonia Villarruel and Cornelia Porter, well-known scholars in this area, have served as the volume editors. They selected the content for the chapters and edited them into this comprehensive book.

The volume is comprised of four sections. In chapter 1, the volume introduction, Dr. Villarruel sets the tone for these sections. She not only captures the substance of the research themes, but also challenges future researchers to build on the work of the nurse leaders in the field, all of whom represent racial and ethnic minority groups.

Part I focuses on factors contributing to health disparities; it includes three chapters. Cornelia Porter and Evelyn Barbee address race and racism in nursing research in chapter 2. Linda Burnes Bolton, Joyce Newman Giger, and Alicia Georges present structural and racial barriers to health care in chapter 3. And, in chapter 4, SeonAe Yeo reviews research on language barriers and access to care.

In Part II the focus is on special populations; four chapters are included. Constance Miles Dallas and Linda Burton address health disparities among men from racial and ethnic minority populations in chapter 5. DeAnne Hilfinger Messias and Mercedes Rubio review research on immigration and health in chapter 6. Research on health disparities among Asian Americans and Pacific Islanders is reviewed by Christina Esperat, Jillian Inouye, Elizabeth Gonzalez, Donna Owen, and Du Feng in chapter 7. And in chapter 8, Melen McBride and Irene Lewis delineate an ethnographic perspective on the research on African American and Asian American elders.

Part III includes two chapters concerned with research on special conditions among racial and ethnic minorities. Sandra Millon Underwood, Barbara Powe, Mary Canales, Cathy Meade, and Eun-Ok Im focus chapter 9 on a review of the research on cancer among and between racial and ethnic minorities in the United States. In chapter 10 Mary Lou Siantz and Bette Keltner review research on mental health and disabilities in children.

The final section is focused on intervention approaches for racial and ethnic minority populations. In chapter 11 Roxanne Struthers and Lee Ann Nichols discuss research on use of complementary and alternative medicine among racial and ethnic minorities; and in chapter 12 Carmen Portillo and Catherine Waters address research on community partnerships.

As with previous volumes, it is important to acknowledge the contributions of the nurse scholars who contributed the chapters for this volume. In addition, we would like to acknowledge the *ARNR* Advisory Board members who have supported this effort over the past several years. And, most important, recognition is due to the volume editors for their special efforts to engage minority researchers in writing the chapters and for involving the national community of nurse scholars who study health disparities among ethnic and minority groups.

JOYCE J. FITZPATRICK, PHD, RN, FAAN
Series Editor

Chapter 1

Introduction:
Eliminating Health Disparities Among Racial and Ethnic Minorities in the United States

ANTONIA M. VILLARRUEL

ABSTRACT

Numerous policy, research, and practice recommendations have been developed to address the persistent disparities among racial and ethnic groups in the United States. Although nurse researchers have made significant contributions in addressing health disparities, there are significant gaps that remain to be addressed. Racial and ethnic minority nurses and nurse researchers have played a significant role in addressing health disparities. The individual and collective contributions of this group of nurses in addressing health disparities is included in this Introduction. Recommendations from chapters presented in this volume of the *Annual Review of Nursing Research* are highlighted.

Keywords: health disparities, racial and ethnic minority nurses

Health disparities can be viewed as inequalities or inequities signified by differences in environment, access, utilization, and quality of care, health status, or particular health outcomes (Carter-Pokras & Baquet, 2002). In the past three decades, there have been numerous national policy initiatives addressing the persistence of health disparities among racial and ethnic minorities. These include the *Report of the Secretary's Task Force on Black and Minority Health* (U.S. Department of Health and Human Ser-

1

vices, 1985), *Healthy People 2010* (U.S. Department of Health and Human Services, 1999), and most recently the report *Unequal Treatment: Confronting Racial and Ethnic Disparities in Healthcare* by the Institute of Medicine (2002). Critical recommendations in each of these reports have included specific and targeted areas of research to both understand and address health disparities.

Although there is ample evidence that documents health disparities in conditions such as HIV/AIDS, diabetes, and cancer among racial and ethnic minority groups, the reasons that disparities exist are not clear. Paradoxically, among some racial and ethnic minority groups, health outcomes are good, despite suboptimal living contexts. Further, less is known about successful interventions to address health disparities. The purpose of this volume of the *Annual Review of Nursing Research* is to critically examine the research base on health disparities among racial and ethnic minorities in order to inform and advance nursing science in this area.

HEALTH DISPARITIES AND NURSING RESEARCH

Nurse researchers have made significant and important contributions in addressing health disparities. For example, Villarruel (1999) reviewed nursing research conducted with African American, Hispanic, Asian/Pacific Islander, and Native American children and families from 1994 through 1998. Important research areas addressed during that time included instrument development, the effects of exposure to environmental hazards and health, health behaviors (including sexual risk behavior, condom use, alcohol use, substance use, and help-seeking behaviors), and access to preventive care such as immunizations. Although the majority of research was descriptive, it was evident that some nurse researchers were engaged in programs of research with racial and ethnic minority populations that could subsequently lead to interventions.

Similarly, Flaskerud et al. (2002) reviewed the contributions in *Nursing Research* related to health disparities in vulnerable populations between 1952 and 2000. Vulnerable populations were not restricted to racial and ethnic minority populations but included people living in poverty and those marginalized by sexual preference, immigrant status, and religion. Results of the review indicate that nursing has evolved in its focus and methods. The number of reports increased in the 1990s and moved from the documentation of disparities through comparison methods to the development of intervention studies. Further, the focus of intervention studies was broadened to consider the effect of providing resources (e.g., facilitating access to care, education programs) with a decrease in health disparities among adolescents, low-income women, the elderly, and various ethnic groups.

These reviews, although highlighting the progress and contribution of nurse researchers, also indicated areas for further study and development. Flaskerud and Nyamanthi (2002) state, "If our goal is to reduce health disparities—and not just study them, nursing research must include a major focus on resources—income, education, access to care, social and political power and human rights" (p. 139). Villarruel (1999) questioned whether nurse researchers are prepared to conduct research with racial and ethnic minority populations and presented guidelines for the conduct and critique of culturally competent research. These guidelines were first proposed by Porter and Villarruel (1993) and were revised subsequently by Villarruel (1995).

CONTRIBUTIONS OF RACIAL AND ETHNIC MINORITY NURSES IN ADDRESSING HEALTH DISPARITIES

An important element in addressing the research gap related to racial and ethnic minority populations is the contribution of nurse researchers from those respective groups. Despite the lack of a critical mass, there have been significant contributions by racial and ethnic minority nurse researchers in addressing health disparities in children's health, in women's health, and in specific areas such as mental health, cancer, and HIV/AIDS. This *Annual Review* volume incorporates the expertise of this group in conjunction with the National Coalition of Ethnic Minority Nurse Associations (NCEMNA).

The idea for NCEMNA was born in 1997 during the Third Invitational Minority Nursing Congress, "Caring for the Emerging Majority: A Blueprint for Action," sponsored by the Division of Nursing. Presidents of the Asian Pacific/Island, Black, Hispanic, and Native American/Alaska Native Nursing Associations met to discuss the possibilities, issues, opportunities, and advantages of forming a unified entity. The presidents left with a commitment to develop a coalition that would be beneficial, on both an individual and collective level, to member associations and to the communities that they served.

According to the NCEMNA (2003) mission, the coalition is a unified force advocating for equity and justice in nursing and health care for ethnic minority populations. A leading voice of professional nursing, it is the driving force to realize a healthy society of ethnic minority populations. Membership is open to any national ethnic minority nursing association. Efforts to find such entities led to the invitation to the Philippine Nurses Association of North America. There are five existing member associations to date, and the respective boards of each association have approved membership in the coalition.

The initial and continued activities of NCEMNA have been focused on eliminating racial and ethnic disparities and also on increasing the number of minority nurse researchers. Association members have demonstrated leadership within each of their respective ethnic/minority groups. Nursing has been well represented by these associations in research and policy initiatives such as the Black Health Brain Trust, the Hispanic Health Agenda, the Asian/Pacific Islander Health Initiative, and the Native American Health Initiative.

The NCEMNA partnered with the National Institute of Nursing Research (NINR) to develop recommendations for the nursing research agenda for minority health and to discuss strategies for developing minority nurse researchers. An invitational meeting, "Minority Health Research Development for Nurse Investigators" (NINR, 2000), was sponsored by the NINR, the Office of Research on Minority Health, and NCEMNA. As part of this meeting, each association developed a white paper presenting important demographic background and historical perspectives, a broad summary on the state of the science for nursing research with respective racial and ethnic minority populations, and recommendations for future nursing research. Each of the five white papers was subsequently published in *Nursing Outlook*.

Although the NINR had already developed a strategic plan to address racial and ethnic disparities, this conference resulted in the identification of priority areas from racial and ethnic minority nurse researchers. Further, in discussing issues within each racial and ethnic minority group, it was evident that there were many similarities across groups. Crosscutting opportunities for nursing research related to minority health were identified collectively for all groups in the areas of health promotion and illness management, and for special populations across the lifespan.

OVERVIEW OF THIS VOLUME

This volume focuses on the health disparities experienced by racial and ethnic minority groups in the United States. These major groups include African American, Hispanic, American Indian/Alaska Native, and Asian/Pacific groups. Although gender, socioeconomic and immigration status, and age are also important considerations, the major focus is on these underrepresented groups because of the persistence of health disparities by race and ethnicity.

Consistent with the definition of health disparities proposed by Carter-Pokras and Baquet (2002), this volume addresses differences in environment; access, utilization, and quality of care; and health status. A lifespan approach was used to address disparities affecting children through older adults. Chapters were selected not only to describe health disparities but also to highlight the strengths of racial and ethnic minority groups in promoting health and managing illness within the current social and political contexts. Chapters also were selected to address crosscutting issues such as access to care, language use, and immigration. Authors were not limited to reviews of nursing research, although that is the focus of some chapters (e.g., chapters 2 and 9).

This volume was compiled with the support and input of the NCEMNA regarding potential themes or content areas, and each member association proposed potential authors. A unique aspect of this volume is that the editors and contributors are accomplished and promising researchers as well as members of racial and ethnic minority groups.

Despite the diversity of topics and populations addressed in this volume, there are many similarities in the "state of the science." First, there are important areas that have not been extensively studied. For example, Underwood et al. noted the lack of research on prostate and lung cancer; Bolton, Giger, and Georges, as well as Porter and Barbee, pointed to the lack of research on discrimination in health care and nursing education and practice. Second, there was limited research on racial and ethnic minority groups in nearly all substantive areas, and certain populations and subpopulations have been minimally included in research. Finally, nearly all authors indicated the need for more well-constructed intervention studies to address health disparities.

It is hoped that the research reviews in this volume will illuminate some of the contributing factors related to health disparities, good health outcomes despite social and economic adversity, and evidence-based practices that can be used to eliminate disparities. Further, it is hoped that the identification of the gaps related to health disparities in nursing science will influence nurse researchers to address these important areas. Finally, it is hoped that the unique scientific and leadership contributions of racial and ethnic minority nurse researchers will be recognized and affirmed.

REFERENCES

Carter-Pokras, O., & Baquet, C. (2002). What is a "health disparity"? *Public Health Reports, 17*, 426–434.

Flaskerud, J. H., Lesser, J., Dixon, E., Anderson, N., Conde, F., Kim, S., Koniak-Griffin, D., Strehlow, A., Tullman, D., & Verzemnieks, I. (2002). Health disparities among vulnerable populations: Evolution of knowledge over five decades in *Nursing Research* publications. *Nursing Research, 51*(2), 74–85.

Flaskerud, J. H., & Nyamanthi, A. M. (2002). New paradigm for health disparities needed. *Nursing Research, 51*(3), 139.

Institute of Medicine. (2002). *Unequal treatment: Confronting racial and ethnic disparities in health care.* Washington, DC: National Academies Press.

National Coalition of Ethnic Minority Nurse Associations (2003). *Mission and vision.* Retrieved August 29, 2003, from http://www.NCEMNA.org

National Institute of Nursing Research. (2000). *Minority health research development for nurse investigators. Executive Summary.* Retrieved August 29, 2003, from http://www.nih.gov/ninr/research/diversity/exec_sum_mhrdni.pdf

Porter, C. P., & Villarruel, A. M. (1993). Nursing research with African-American and Hispanic people: Guidelines for action. *Nursing Outlook, 41*(2), 59–67.

United States Department of Health and Human Services. (1999). *Healthy people 2010.* Retrieved August 29, 2003, from http://web.health.gov/healthypeople/

United States Department of Health and Human Services. (1985). *Report of the Secretary's Task Force on Black and Minority Health.* Washington, DC: Government Printing Office.

Villarruel, A. M. (1995). Moving towards cultural competence? *Capsules and Comments in Pediatric Nursing, 1*(4), 18–25.

Villarruel, A. M. (1999). Culturally competent nursing research: Are we there yet? Reprint with a new commentary by the author, Dr. Antonia Villarruel. *Journal of Child and Family Nursing, 2*(2), 82–92.

PART I

Factors Contributing to Health Disparities

Chapter 2

Race and Racism in Nursing Research: Past, Present, and Future

CORNELIA P. PORTER AND EVELYN BARBEE

ABSTRACT

Nursing research on race and racism began in the 1970s. However, because these concepts were seen as cultural attitudes, race and racism were obscured. The evidence on the presence of negative attitudes, biases, and stereotypes about different racial and ethnic groups is inconsistent. During the past two decades, research on race and racism has grown, but there is still an urgent need for more high-quality research on this subject. The major recommendations from this review are to conduct observational research on racism in clinical and practice settings, not as an intellectual end in itself; to assist in eliminating of the historically based disparities among members of racial and ethnic groups; and to conduct research about racism as it affects mobility in educational and practice settings.

Keywords: biases, nursing education, racism

> The problem of the twentieth century is the problem of the color line; the relation of the darker to the lighter races of men in Asia and Africa, in America and the islands of the sea . . .
>
> —DuBois (1901)

Regrettably, DuBois's challenge resonates with the "color problem" of the twenty-first century. Race, "the color line," matters in the American

9

health and medical care system (Thomas, 2001). Race matters despite the biological fact that only one human race exists. Race matters whether viewed from the perspective of racism adversely affecting health professionals' clinical decisions and quality of service (e.g., Schulman et al., 1999; VanRyn & Burke, 2000); the history and legacy of racial segregation of medical care (e.g., Byrd & Clayton, 2002; Cobb, 2002); scientific racism (e.g., Tucker, 1994); discriminatory barriers to entry into nursing (e.g., Carnegie, 1995; Hine, 1989) and other health professions, or unfair and biased treatment after becoming a health professional (Byrd & Clayton, 2002; IOM, 2002). Since race as a sociopolitical concept continues to matter (Thomas, 2001), the historical race-based pattern of health disparities will not change in the near future. The immutability of health disparities has far-reaching implications for the world, the nation, and particularly for the largest group of health professionals, nurses, and in turn, for nursing education, practice, and research.

As we move into the new millennium, nurses have the responsibility to become more knowledgeable about the health disparities among racial and ethnic groups in the United States. Although health disparities among dominant and subordinate groups have existed for centuries (Byrd & Clayton, 2002), they were not highlighted publicly until the *Report of the Secretary's Task Force on Black and Minority Health* (USDHHS, 1985) and most recently by *Healthy People 2010* (USDHHS, 2001). The findings of these national reports imply that we in nursing can no longer ignore the disproportionate burdens of morbidity and mortality that members of racial and ethnic groups carry. Nor can we afford ignorance about one of the major factors that contribute to the multiple health disparities—racism (e.g., Browne, Johnson, Bottoroff, Grewal, & Hilton, 2002; IOM, 2002). Although nurses in the United States have not frequently recognized and discussed the broader societal problems of individual and institutional racism, both continue to influence access to services and the quality of services received by various people. Nurses, in order to actively participant in eliminating disparities, must consider critically the issue of how race and racism within the broader contexts of power relations and social inequality influence the quality of their services.

The purposes of this chapter are to review how race and racism have been conceptualized, investigated, and discussed in nursing research and to stimulate critical discourse about nursing's future investigative approaches. Using literature on race and racism from anthropology, philosophy, and sociology, we begin with a brief review of the basic concepts.

RACE

Race is a category that has far-reaching social effects. As the meaning of the concept of race changes historically, so does what constitutes racism (Goldberg, 1990). Harrison, an anthropologist, describes race as

> a historically specific social and sometimes legal classification applied in populations presumed to share common physical and biological traits or in the absence of anatomical and physiognomic homogeneity, to those presumed to share at least in part socially and politically salient ancestry. Race is an ideologically charged cluster of contradictory and contested meanings that change over time. (Harrison, 1997, p. 392)

The contested meanings of race are exemplified by the British sociologist Gilroy's (1990) extension of the description to include social class, politics, and economics. Gilroy contends: "Races are not, then, simple expressions of either biological or cultural sameness. They are imagined—socially and politically constructed. . . . Thus ideas about race may articulate political and economic relations in a particular society" (p. 264).

RACISM

Common features of racism are described as inclusionary and exclusionary undertakings (Goldberg, 1990), the reduction of the cultural to the biological (Delacampagne, 1990), and a transformative nature (Harrison, 1998; Ignatiev, 1995). Although it is beyond the scope of this chapter to discuss the historical dimensions of racism, we do need to understand its transformative nature, that is, its change over time. Because of historical changes, Goldberg (1990, p. xiii) points out: "The presumption of a single monolithic racism is being displaced by a mapping of the multifarious historical formulations of *racisms*" (emphasis in original).

According to Appiah, a philosopher (1990), at least three distinct doctrines express the theoretical content of racism. One is "racialism," the doctrine that there are heritable characteristics that allow us to divide people into races, each of which has certain traits and tendencies that it does not share with other races. Racialism is a presupposition of the other two doctrines, "extrinsic racism" and "intrinsic racism." "Extrinsic racists make moral distinctions between members of different races because they believe that racial essence entails certain morally relevant qualities. . . . Intrinsic racists are people who differentiate morally between members of different races because they believe that each race has a different moral status. . . . " (Appiah, 1990, pp. 5–6). Individuals can be both intrinsic and extrinsic racists (Appiah, 1990). In one sense, Appiah's doctrines are related to Delacampagne's (1990) statement that "racism is the reduction of the cultural to the biological, the attempt to make the first dependent on the second" (p. 85).

Racism's transformative nature means that it is persistent and has an ability to reinvent itself in new forms, including those that disguise or deny its existence (Harrison, 1998). Essed (1991) expands our understanding of the perpetuation of racism, regardless of its form, with the point that racism is both a system of structural inequalities and a historical process that is created and maintained through routine practices. "In other words, structures of racism do not exist external to agents—they are made by agents—but specific practices are by definition racist only when they activate existing structural racial inequalities in the system" (Essed, 1991, p. 39).

These descriptions suggest the complex and multidimensional nature of race as a category and concept and the transformative nature of racism. The descriptions indicate that "race is formed and fashioned and racism operates in relation to and through other systems of exclusion, marginalization, abuse, and repression" (Goldberg & Essed, 2002, p. 3).

The transformative, sociopolitical fluidity of racism is apparent today. In the United States, we are in an era in which race (color) is being redefined (e.g., Census Bureau classifications). People raise questions about who we are, what we call ourselves, and how we deal with one another. Despite the redefinition and the heightened awareness of the nuances of color, racism with all of its insidiousness and complexity continues to exist. Race still matters (Thomas, 2001).

METHOD

Several methods were used to obtain the sample of studies. A search of the literature was conducted using the Cumulative Index to Nursing and Allied Health Literature (CINAHL) and Medical Literature, Analysis and Retrieval System Online (MEDLINE) databases. The keywords *race, racism, discrimination, prejudice, minority groups, racial discrimination*, and various permutations of keywords were used to search the databases from 1980 to 2003. The total number of citations varied with keywords. For example, in CINAHL the keywords and their permutations revealed a total of 935 citations and in MEDLINE a total of 82 citations. However, of the total CINAHL citations, only 340 (36%) were classified as research reports. Because few of these citations were in nursing journals, we expanded the search by combining the keywords with the terms *education* and *practice* to locate other citations and detect any evolving patterns. In order to include all possible sources, we expanded the search further with an exploration of specific databases such as Sigma Theta Tau International and pertinent bibliographic references on the citations from the computerized databases.

The exclusion criteria included reports not in nursing journals, research about the use of race and ethnicity as variables in nursing research (see Drevdahl, Taylor, & Phillips, 2001; Flaskerud et al., 2002 for reviews), research with racial and ethnic samples, and contributions such as essays, editorials, and theoretical articles and the many research reports published in international nursing journals. The latter were included only if they provided insights that were significantly different from those in United States reports.

To identify the research reports fitting the keywords, we read the titles and abstracts and mutually agreed on the thematic categorization of education ($N = 8$) and clinical practice ($N = 14$). The category of education included reports that focused on students, curriculum, and faculty-student relationships. The category of clinical practice included reports related to attitudes and nursing practice. The review is composed of English-language research reports published primarily in the United States, leaving a total of 22 citations published from 1970 to 2003.

CLINICAL PRACTICE

Despite the oft-quoted gap, nursing education and practice *are* interwoven. Nursing education exists to prepare students for professional practice in which either the individual or various-size groups are the focus. The individual's or group's need for services is the reason for the profession's existence. Thus, the quality of services provided has been of paramount importance to nursing's existence and societal mandate (American Nurses Association, 2003). Since nursing was and continues to be a predominantly White profession and White nursing students have had little or no experience with people from backgrounds other than their own (Eliason, 1998), the focus on cultural attitudes (e.g., feelings and beliefs about people who are different from themselves) as an early stream of research is not astounding.

Richek's (1970) study is an exemplar of early comparative explorations about attitudes. Its purpose was to explore relationships among demographic variables and prejudice toward two minority groups (Negroes and Indians) among preprofessional "female nursing and social work students at a large state university in the Southwest." The preprofessional sample of 195 (163 nursing and 63 social work) female undergraduate students (11 male students were excluded) completed a short attitude scale. Interestingly, when the prejudice scores were aggregated, the mean scores indicated that the prospective professional groups held "essentially nonprejudicial attitudes toward Negroes and Indians." However, when the scores were disaggregated and compared, nursing students held significantly more prejudicial attitudes toward "Negroes" than their social work counterparts. Four demographic variables (i.e., age, religious affiliation, urban/rural backgrounds, state of residence) were related to prejudicial attitudes among nursing students but not social work students. The reasons for these differences could not be explained because the demographic characteristics of the two groups were not controlled. Despite the caveat, implications for educators were discussed.

LaFargue (1972), motivated by a local report that revealed mothers were not using maternal and infant care centers, explored the amount of prejudice among White nurses who worked in prenatal and child health clinics and the degree to which these attitudes influenced Black families' decisions to return for services. Prejudice was very broadly described as "an attitude of the reference group, both past and present, taken on by individual members" (p. 54). A Black graduate student interviewed 10 low-income Black families from the high-risk program at the pediatric clinics of a large Seattle hospital. The families, divided into those that did keep ($n = 5$) and those that did not keep appointments ($n = 5$), were questioned about their experiences with discriminatory behaviors. All families believed they had been personally discriminated against at some time by all health professionals and clerks, simply because they were Black. More families who had not kept appointments believed they had been discriminated against than those who had kept appointments. A larger number of families knew of discriminatory incidents than had actually experienced them. No families believed that White public health nurses and the Black nutritionist had discriminated against them. However, the families who had kept appointments reported discriminatory behaviors by clinic nurses and hospital clerks. Families who had not kept appointments reported discriminatory behaviors of all health professionals and clinic staff.

Twenty-three White nurses were administered a questionnaire specifically constructed to measure "emotional acceptance, rationality and justice." Much like in Richek's (1970) study, the findings indicated that 77.7% ($n = 18$) of the nurses had little or no prejudice and demonstrated "an ability to sympathize with the underdog." Low prejudicial scores were expected because nurses were aware that prejudicial attitudes were not accepted by society. Despite this admission, validity issues were not discussed. The results may have represented expressions of unreported prejudicial attitudes. For example, 48% of the nurses agreed that "Negroes were moving too slowly," yet 82% opposed giving Blacks special considerations in employment.

This early mixed design study had several obvious limitations. First, neither the training of the interviewer, the interview format, nor the approaches to the interpretive analyses of the narrative data were described. Second, the demographic characteristics of the family and nurse samples were not described. Third, the extremely small number of families from a narrow income stratum of African American families rendered the findings inconclusive and nongeneralizable. The study's significant contribution is to raise our awareness of the contributions of clinic staff (clinic nurses and clerks) to the ambience in service settings.

Bonaparte's (1979) study was another broad exploration of how attitudes influence nursing practice. Bonaparte investigated how nurses' personality variables (i.e., open- or closed-mindedness or ego defensiveness) affected nurse-patient relationships with culturally different patients. Three hundred female registered nurses who were actively employed in various hospitals and health care agencies in New York City participated in the study. From the 338 returned questionnaires a convenience sample of 75 nurses who represented four cultural groups (Anglo-Saxon White, Black, Jewish, and Hispanic) were administered the *Cultural Attitude Scale* (CAS). It was a 34-item Likert-type, forced-choice questionnaire that consisted of four patient vignettes that matched the race and ethnicity of the nurses.

The findings revealed that both positive and negative attitudes were associated with the personality characteristics. That is, when caring for patients whose cultural health beliefs and practices were different from their own, open-minded nurses would be more likely to seek information about patients that would enhance their quality of care than close-minded nurses. Close-minded nurses would more likely have a negative attitude toward, be more anxious about, and attempt to avoid patients that were unfamiliar to them or had beliefs incongruent with their own. Although there were no statistical differences in nurses' responses to patient vignettes based on their racial and ethnic self-identity, there were clear differences in responses to each patient group by all nurses. Bonaparte contended that providing students with information about and contact with different patients would foster positive attitudes.

Frenkel, Greden, Robinson, Guyden, and Miller's (1980) study was different from the previous because the notion of interracial contact and its effects was explicit. They used an interracial contact hypothesis to explore the question of whether patient contact with different others changed racial perceptions. Similar to LaFargue (1972), Frenkel and colleagues were interested in how racial perceptions influenced minority patients' utilization of services and cooperative behaviors with medical directives. To determine the effect of interracial contact, a survey was administered to 114 White, female, young (19 to 22 years of age) student nurses before patient contact (i.e., their first day of clinical nursing experience) and after clinical contact (i.e., 11 months later). These upper-division students were completing clinical rotations at a large army hospital in Washington, DC. The small number of males and non-Whites were excluded from analyses. Between survey administrations all students participated in "two mandatory four-hour race relations discussion groups." A comparison of the before and after survey findings about direct nurse-patient contact revealed both "favorable" and "unfavorable" shifts in responses to all items. The increase in disagreement over items such as "young Black male patients are frequently sexually provocative with White nurses" was classified as a favorable shift. The higher percentage of students that disagreed with statements such as "Black patients are more reliable in keeping appointments, have better personal hygiene" was classified as an unfavorable shift. A notable result was students' reactions to attending race relations classes. Specifically, 80% disagreed with the premise that race relations classes successfully decreased racial prejudice. Consistent with the previous percentage, 73% disagreed that White nurses should take a Black history course. Students rejected these courses as approaches to changing racial attitudes and stereotypes. The major finding was that direct nurse-patient contact did change racial perceptions—albeit not all favorably. The authors concluded that some of the unfavorable shifts in attitudes could be detrimental to nurse-patient relationships and recommended that nurse educators work with students when the actual interracial contact occurred. The inability to measure the independent effect of the race relations classes on attitudes was acknowledged.

Ruiz (1981) extended Bonaparte's (1979) research about relationships among personality characteristics and attitudes toward culturally different patients with a sample of predominantly White ($n = 137$, 86%) female nursing faculty, (mid-20s to over 50 years of age) from 19 East Coast baccalaureate schools of nursing. Bonaparte's (1979) *Cultural Attitude Scale* (CAS) was adapted. The results revealed that faculty had both positive and negative attitudes toward patients from different cultural backgrounds. Patient ethnicity influenced faculty's negative perceptions. Characteristics such as open- or closed-mindedness and intolerance of ambiguity (i.e., ethnocentrism) influenced the direction of the attitude (e.g., close-minded faculty had more negative attitudes than faculty who were more open-minded). Ruiz concluded, "Closed-minded faculty might be more likely to resist teaching cultural differences and/or conveying a positive attitude while supervising students who were caring for heterogeneous populations" (p. 181). The major recommendations for research were to observe whether closed-minded faculty in clinical settings actually taught cultural differences and to identify ways to facilitate change in dogmatic faculty members. To our knowledge, there have been few observational studies about the influence of race on the quality of services provided.

Morgan (1983) explored relationships among White nursing students' attitudes toward Black American patients with selected personality characteristics, attitudes of significant others, and selected interracial contact variables within a theoretical framework of prejudice. Questionnaires were administered to 252 White female (96%) senior nursing students enrolled in baccalaureate ($n = 57$, 28%), associate degree ($n = 99$, 49%), and diploma ($n = 45$, 22.5%) nursing programs in Rhode Island. Students who were non-White, who held previous degrees, or who were licensed practical nurses or registered nurses were deleted from the sample. Attitudes toward Black American patients were measured with a semantic differential scale constructed specifically to measure attitudes toward Black Americans. The findings suggested that prejudice was learned during socialization processes and was neither the result of underlying personality characteristics nor interracial contact. Peer attitudes toward Black Americans, as the best single predictor of directionality and maintenance of attitudes, lent credence to the finding. The inferences for nursing education were to foster positive attitudes through discussion groups that sensitized students to problems inherent in stereotyping, prejudice, and discriminatory practices.

Since attitudes of nurses toward Black Americans generally and Black American patients specifically had been not been compared, Morgan (1984) investigated whether White registered nurses' and nursing students' attitudes toward Black Americans as a generic category and Black Americans patients as a specific category differed. Morgan's novel study questioned the necessity for race-specific instruments for attitude measurement. To answer the question, the attitudes of 242 White senior nursing students enrolled in one diploma, one associate, and three baccalaureate programs in the Northeast were measured with Morgan's (1983) semantic differential scale. Students who were non-White, who held previous degrees, or who were registered nurses were excluded. The findings were mixed. White students had more favorable attitudes toward White Americans. Surprisingly, White students perceived Black American patients more favorably than Black Americans generally. Students' responses to the evaluative factor of the scale for Black American patients were neutral. Morgan speculated that "while neutral attitudes may be interpreted as reluctance to disclose true feelings, an alternative explanation is that students prefer to judge others on an individual basis rather than respond to a group stereotype" (p. 161). No rationale for the speculation was presented. Recommendations were to consider nurses' differential responses to items when selecting an instrument to measure attitudes and to conduct workshops to assist nurses to explore their feelings. The recommendations implied a relationship between attitudes and "feelings" but failed to extend the discussion to how attitudes might motivate behaviors and, in turn, influence services.

Felder (1990) used an attitude theory framework to investigate the effect of cultural diversity education on baccalaureate and associate degree students' cultural knowledge of and attitudes toward Black American clients. The sample consisted of 110 baccalaureate ($n = 57$, 52%) and associate degree ($n = 53$, 48%) freshman and senior female students from four schools of nursing (two baccalaureate and two associate degree) located in a region of southeastern Wisconsin with a large population of Black Americans. The sample was significantly different by educational program (e.g., larger numbers of non-White, older, and separated or divorced students in associate degree programs). Unfortunately, there were no disaggregated descriptions of the sample. Each school reported that its curriculum included cultural diversity content and experiences. An instrument composed of 43 multiple-choice items measured four categories of knowledge (e.g., sociocultural characteristics, common diseases) of Black Americans. Morgan's (1984) semantic differential scale (i.e., evaluative factor scale) and Bonaparte's (1979) *Cultural Attitude Scale* (i.e., vignette of Black patient) were adapted and combined to measure attitudes. The findings indicated that the majority of students had average cultural knowledge that increased between the freshman and senior year of the baccalaureate programs. Although associate degree program students possessed more cultural knowledge than baccalaureate students, attitudes toward Black Americans were neutral across program and class levels. Felder contended that the neutral attitudes toward Black American clients were consistent with Morgan's (1984) findings. Notably absent was any discussion of alternative explanations, for instance, how sample characteristics might have influenced the findings.

Rooda (1992) used social contact theory to explore the extent to which level of exposure to culturally different patients affected White nurses' attitudes toward such patients in acute care hospitals in a racial and ethnically diverse urban area in the Midwest. This study was an extension of Rooda's earlier research, whose findings indicated that White nurses expressed the most positive attitudes and least cultural bias toward African American patients if they were the largest minority population in the setting. The sample consisted of 329 nurses ($N = 265$ White) who were employed by the same institution but located at either the inner city or suburban hospital. Each differed significantly in the racial and ethnic makeup of their patient populations. In keeping with the research tradition of the theory, only data about the attitudes of White nurses were analyzed. A self-administered questionnaire (*Ethnic Attitude Survey*) was an adaptation of Bonaparte's (1979) CAS and included two scenarios describing Anglo and African American patient care situations. The findings indicated that White nurses working at the inner-city hospital expressed less bias toward African American patients than those nurses working at the suburban hospital. The findings generated many unanswered questions, such as, how does bias affect nursing practice? Again, the recommendation was to conduct observational research. Despite the inherent methodological and ethical difficulties, an observational design would document actual behaviors that White nurses exhibited toward non-White patients in clinical settings. Recommendations for nurse educators included, but were not limited to, increased student contact with African American and other patients from different backgrounds.

Rooda (1993) extended her research about attitudes with members of other racial and ethnic groups. This study explored the level of basic knowledge and attitudes of nurses toward Black American, Asian American, and Hispanic patients. It was "based on the premise that concepts of cultural diversity related to health care must be cognitively and affectively understood, and incorporated into nursing practice on a systematic basis, if the multicultural dimension of nursing is to become a reality" (p. 209). A random sample (N = 274) of White female baccalaureate (16.9%), associate (61%), and diploma (21.6%) program registered nurses practicing in nine acute care hospitals located in one urban midwestern county participated. A small number of non-Whites were excluded from the analyses. The participants were fairly evenly distributed as to the inclusion of cultural diversity content in their nursing programs. Data about knowledge and attitudes were collected with a self-administered questionnaire that measured level of cultural diversity knowledge and an adaptation of Bonaparte's (1979) CAS that included four racial and ethnic patient vignettes. Notably, White female registered nurses had more knowledge about the culture and health care practices of Asian Americans than of Hispanics and Black Americans, and their level of knowledge was directly related to their educational preparation. Associate degree and diploma educated nurses had more knowledge of Black cultural content than did baccalaureate educated nurses. The most insightful finding was that these White female registered nurses possessed hierarchically ranked attitudes toward the three groups. That is, rankings from most to least positive attitudes were assigned to Whites, Black Americans, Asian Americans, and Hispanics, respectively. Consistent with previous findings, White nurses had the most positive attitudes toward members of their own group. For this sample, cultural bias and attitudes were related. Rooda recommended that nurse educators explore how differences in curricular content resulted in distinctive attitudes and biases among nurses with different academic preparation.

McDonald's (1994) study was an attempt to measure how patient characteristics influenced nursing practice. The retrospective study about the effect of gender and ethnic stereotyping on the administration of pain medication provided an example of how bias influenced nurses' behaviors. The sample consisted of medical record reviews of 180 individuals (2% Asian, 12% Black, 8% Hispanic, 78% White) who had a diagnosis of nonperforated appendicitis that resulted in an uncomplicated appendectomy. The findings revealed modest support for gender differences in analgesic dose administration in the initial postoperative period but not in the total postoperative period ($M = 3.5$ days). In contrast, there were large unexplainable differences between total doses received by Asian, Black, and Hispanic Americans compared to White patients. The small total analgesic doses suggested that regardless of gender, undermedication in the initial and total postoperative periods might be very serious for members of racial and ethnic groups. "The differences in narcotic analgesic administration lend further support to the hypothesis that irrelevant cues may be used by nurses in their medication decisions" (p. 48). Despite the study's limitations, which influenced the internal and external validity, it provided a *first* glimpse of how the quality of nursing care might be influenced by phenotypic characteristics.

Greipp (1996) used the construct of "ethnocentrism" to investigate nurses' predictions of their own and colleagues' reactions to clients of different age, gender, and cultural backgrounds. The study was based on the frameworks of Aversive Insidious Racism and Ingroup Favoritism and was designed to test the fourth assumption of Greipp's ethical model. Survey data were collected from 268 predominantly White (91%) female nurses employed on all units and in all specialties in one urban teaching hospital. Nine percent of the respondents self-identified as minority group members. Notably absent was a statement about their inclusion or exclusion from analyses. The questionnaire was composed of three mini-client situations (Black, Caucasian, and Latino) that measured four dimensions for potential nurse bias: culture, age, gender, and overt behavior. Amazingly, the researcher reported "the clients' cultures are implied in the clients' given names" (p. 86). The statement may be construed as stereotypical thinking and raises questions about the researcher's biases. That is, how can an individual's "given name" be a valid indicator of self-identified racial and ethnic group membership? The findings indicated (a) the presence of biases, prejudices, and stereotyping in relation to age, gender, and culture in nurse-client interactions (e.g., reactions were most positive toward young, male, Latino clients and least positive toward old male Latino clients); (b) responses consistent with the Aversive Insidious Racism Theory (i.e., "prejudice expressed in ways that protect and perpetuate a non-prejudiced non-discriminating self image"); (c) mixed responses for the Ingroup Favoritism Theory (i.e., favoritism toward White clients); and (d) validation of the fourth assumption of the model.

> In clinical practice, observations of staff demonstrate that certain clients receive more and quicker attention than others. Hopefully, those in the greatest need for care and attention receive it. But, this may not be the

> case . . . is credible. However, the researcher does not want to imply that subjects' responses are necessarily a reflection of the quality of care that would be delivered. The presence of feelings and biases (positive or negative) does not mean that the person acts on them. (p. 94)

This statement was troublesome in view of the findings that supported the Aversive Insidious Racism Theory. The recommendations, consistent with earlier ones, included the need for direct observations of and interviews with nurses to document the effect of bias on the quality of services provided.

The relationships among social justice, ethical behavior, biases, and discriminatory behavior are relevant to nursing's Social Policy Statement and Code of Ethics. However, the lack of a clear conceptualization and operationalization of the term *ethnocentrism* was problematic. Without this, the sections of the research were not consistently and conceptually linked. That is, the study was grounded in a current theory of racism; the literature review consisted of investigations classified under the rubric of cultural attitudes, bias, and stereotyping; and the findings were related to ethical decision making. This study attempted to examine the relationships between attitudes and selected patient characteristics in relation to self and others' perceptions. Although flawed, it was one of the few attempts at a multidimensional investigation of attitudes in nursing.

Kirkham (1998) extended the qualitative work of Murphy and Clark (1993) (as cited in Kirkham) that described British nurses' feelings of frustration, stress, and helplessness precipitated by their lack of knowledge about cultural differences. Kirkham's interpretive descriptive design described recently graduated nurses' perceptions of caring for diverse clients in a variety of hospital units. The participants consisted of eight female nurses who had recently graduated from a Canadian diploma or baccalaureate program. The nurses' narratives about their experiences were "conceptualized as a continuum of levels of commitment to caring for culturally diverse clients." The fluid, theoretical continuum ranged from being "resistant" to "generalist" to "impassioned" about caring for patients different from themselves. As expected, strategies used for providing equitable care for culturally diverse clients differed across the continuum. These findings provide support for the commonly acknowledged fact that not all nurses are committed to providing culturally competent care, regardless of institutional expectation.

Kirkham declared, "The most disturbing finding of this study was the pervasive racism . . . present at both individual and institutional levels"

(p. 140). Examples of both overt and covert and individual and institutional racism were cited and were associated with interpersonal conflict between and inner turmoil within nurses with various levels of commitment. The nurses' descriptions highlighted the intersection of level of commitment and personal and contextual factors. Kirkham argued eloquently for a nonlinear, nonsequential developmental model of progression toward and commitment to culturally competent care. Nurses in the United States must begin to create a new paradigm that enhances our understanding of the barriers to equitable nursing services. Individual and institutional racism is just as impregnable in the United States as it is in Canada. There is no reason to believe that the Canadian findings would not be duplicated in this country.

A Canadian study by Browne, Johnson, Bottorff, Grewal, and Hilton (2002) described how discriminatory attitudes were manifested in clinical encounters between South Asian women and health professionals in hospital and community settings in British Columbia. Data were obtained from interviews and focus groups conducted with 80 South Asian immigrant women from various religious backgrounds and 42 health professionals, 23 of whom were nurses. The findings revealed that the women wondered if their health care experiences differed from those of non-Asian women. "Sometimes they blamed themselves for what was perceived to be inadequate health care" (p. 25). The most discomfiting description was about the women's expectations. They did not have unrealistic expectations about the encounters; they simply wanted the usual amenities, such as for practitioners "to listen carefully," "to be polite," and "to take time."

Discriminatory attitudes of health professionals were not unusual. They included, but were not limited to, negative stereotypes, victim blaming, and beliefs based on racial characteristics. Several strategies for recognizing discriminatory practices were recommended for health professionals, such as developing critical consciousness, monitoring the language used to refer to people who are different from self, exploring approaches to naming and discussing racism and other forms of discriminatory behaviors, and attending to patients' claims of discriminatory and racist experiences (p. 27).

Another Canadian investigation, by Hagey, Choudhry, Guruge, Turruttin, Collins, and Lee (2001), had no counterpart in the United States literature base. It described how the social dynamics created by race and racism resulted in conflict in a diverse workforce. The sample consisted of nine non-White immigrant nurses from seven different countries. Five nurses did not participate because of feelings of vulnerability and fear of retaliatory behaviors. The study documented and described their personal experiences with filing formal grievances for racial discriminatory practices or complaints of racism against their Canadian employers. One of the purposes of the study was to "raise awareness about racial discrimination within the nursing profession" (p. 390). Data were collected through face-to-face interviews, from focus group discussions, and from the nurses' legal documents. The interpretive analysis revealed recurring themes: "(a) being marginalized and acknowledging and naming racism; (b) experiencing physical stress (e.g., cardiovascular problems) and emotional pain (e.g., depression); (c) strategizing to cope and survive (e.g., support from families and friends and seeking legal redress); and (d) recommending policy changes and interventions to dismantle racism and gain inclusion."

The fact that these nurses experienced daily messages of being "lesser than" in institutions that had implemented diversity programs raised several questions. First, how are nurses sensitized to the issue of racism in their profession? Second, what are the long-term benefits of diversity programs? Third, how are nurses helped to apply the information presented in diversity programs? A significant contribution of the study is that the findings could be used for legal and administrative reforms and policy recommendations.

Turrittin, Hagey, Guruge, Collins, and Mitchell (2002) expanded the previous exploratory study with an interpretive analysis of discourses of the previously described nine non-White immigrant registered nurses who had migrated to Canada and experienced racism. One of the exciting focuses of the study was "the problem of how to make racism visible among those who have a vested interest in denying its existence" (p. 655). The methodology for interpreting the pattern of the discourse was based on a tradition of interpretive methodologies. Data were collected through individual and focus group interviews. Two theoretical perspectives, "democratic racism" (i.e., "coexistence of both democratic values and practices that discount non-White people advertently or inadvertently," p. 655) and "cosmopolitan citizenship" (i.e., "a mode of political identity in a global post-modern society . . . which has a universalist interest in human rights and the person as a human being," p. 660) were introduced. The language the nurses used was consistent with the mental and emotional approaches of cosmopolitan citizenship (e.g., astuteness to being marginalized or problematized, irony). The authors argued that a cosmopolitan citizenship ethic would facilitate the move toward racial integration in nursing through a sharing of power and privilege. Given that the United States's history of racism has left a lasting legacy of inequality that continues today, the theoretical perspectives used to interpret Canadian nurses' discourse would be pertinent in the United States. The findings stimulated questions such as the following: Is the U.S. nursing profession mired in democratic racism? What are some of the reasons U.S. researchers have not conducted similar research about the workforce?

SUMMARY

Although the majority of the research has been about attitudes toward African Americans, these findings relate to members of other racial and ethnic groups who experience discriminatory behaviors and practices grounded in racist ideologies. The prevalent research paradigm for these studies was cultural attitudes. Strangely, no conceptualization matched the operationalization of the phrase. The topics of race and racism were not named explicitly. They were addressed with proxy terms such as *cultural attitudes*, *prejudice*, and *interracial contact*. Regardless of the label, at the heart of the studies was the underappreciated truth about racism and discriminatory practices in nursing and how some researchers attempted to explore and explain the phenomenon.

The results documented inconsistent evidence of biases, stereotyping, and discriminatory attitudes among White nurses and nursing students. The early studies were a product of their times and unfortunately possessed methodological and theoretical limitations. Their findings were descriptive and so fragmented; little could be concluded about the content of the nurses' attitudes. The studies differed in geographical region, sample size and composition, and approaches to measuring cultural (read as "racial") attitudes. In addition, terms used to describe the samples' ethnic and racial group memberships were used differently (e.g., *ethnically diverse* implied racial, national, and ethnic membership). These sample characteristics led to variations in perceptions and responses that influenced the results. Despite the limitations, measurement consistency was obvious. That is, Bonaparte's (1979) Cultural Attitude Scale was adapted by researchers until 1993 (i.e., Rooda). However, the consistent use of the same instrument did not override limitations. For example, were the vignettes created to tap implicit or explicit attitudes? Each kind of attitude influences different types of race-relevant behaviors in Whites (Dovidio, Gaertner, Kawakami, & Hodson, 2002).

In concert with Ganong, Bzdek, and Manderino's (1987) critical review of research about stereotyping by nurses and nursing students, the glaring limitation among the studies was their rudimentary theoretical nature. This limitation prevented the exploration of the multidimensional aspects of race and racism. For instance, Rooda (1992, 1993) and Morgan (1983, 1984) continued to explore cultural attitudes at the same descriptive, exploratory level with different samples. Researchers were unable to expand their studies without a framework that permitted multidimensional approaches and alternative explanations.

Consequently, the evidence has not contributed to nurses' understanding of themselves in relation to different others, whether patients or colleagues. Why would we expect nurses *not* to harbor racist ideologies? Asked another way, where is the evidence that documents nurses as antiracists? Sadly, the limited published research is incapable of responding to these questions. However, they are important for a reflective profession.

Although blatant forms of discriminatory practices in the medical or health care system are no longer socially acceptable, they do occur (IOM, 2002). This fact raises many questions about nurses and their roles. Why would nurses *not* be implicated in these discriminatory clinical practices? But the more important question for this chapter is: Why did the research stream about so-called cultural attitudes dry up? In other words, why did researchers stop studying White nurses' attitudes toward different others? Another unanswered question! Despite the fact that only one study (i.e., McDonald, 1994) addressed directly whether nurses act upon their biases and stereotypes in the clinical setting, a frequent statement in many studies implied that attitudes may not motivate behavior (see Greipp, 1996). An odd disjunction existed between the implication and persistent recommendations for observational research in clinical practice settings. That is, the recommendations for observational studies implied a tacit belief in a relationship between attitude and behavior.

EDUCATION

In nursing education, race as a category is most frequently included in terms such as *multiculturalism, transculturalism,* and *diversity.* Diversity or cultural diversity has been described broadly as characteristics of the individual that render them identifiably different from the accepted norm (e.g., sexual identity, age, physical ability, economic status, religion) (Eliason & Raheim, 2000). Nursing has a long history of transposing the category of race into the category of "minorities." Consequently, in nursing education two streams of research have emerged. One has focused on the experiences of non-White nurses in academic institutions and the other on the education of White students about cultural diversity, race, and racism.

Non-White Individuals in Nursing

The first stream was related to the consistently small numbers of non-White individuals in nursing. The findings were consistent across the few studies. Racism, negative stereotyping, and discriminatory assumptions and practices have been cited as major barriers to Black students for many years (e.g., Carnegie, 1995; Hine, 1989; Tucker-Allen, 1991, 1992). According to Tucker-Allen (1991), Black nursing students reported having experienced discriminatory behaviors throughout their academic programs. Discriminatory behaviors by White faculty have been described as having lower expectations, attributing exemplary performance to luck or factors other than abilities, and giving minimal guidance compared to their White counterparts. Despite the consistent findings, both historical and anecdotal evidence has suggested that not all White nurses hold negative attitudes toward and biases about Black nurses (e.g., Hine, 1989).

In an early attempt to identify the determinants of the retention of Black nursing students in predominantly White and Black institutions, Allen, Nunley, and Scott-Warner (1988) studied students, faculty, and administrators from one public and private institution in four regions of the United States. The convenience sample consisted of Black female nursing students ($n = 41$, 30%), Black faculty and administrators ($n = 16$, 12%), and White faculty and administrators ($n = 79$, 57%). A questionnaire that measured barriers to admission, retention, and possible remedies for the barriers was administered. The study, completed in 1984, identified barriers to the admission and retention of Black students. Barriers to admission included indifferent recruitment and a hostile university. White administrators' comments revealed their inability to believe that the university was hostile. Barriers to retention included, but were not limited to, inadequate financial aid, feelings of alienation and loneliness, and inadequate secondary school preparation. Despite the identification of barriers, the descriptive level of analyses (percentages) prohibited an in-depth understanding of how important the barriers were to the total sample. The study failed to answer the question of what and which barriers influence retention. A multisite, longitudinal design with a large stratified representative sample would be necessary to understand the issue of barriers.

The findings of Langston-Moss's (1997) study suggested the occurrence of discriminatory behaviors in academic institutions. The study was a phenomenological exploration of the personal experiences and perceptions of 9 Black American female senior nursing students ($n = 1$ BSN [Bachelor of Science in Nursing]; $n = 8$ ADN [Associate Degree in Nursing]) who attended predominantly White associate degree ($n = 3$) and baccalaureate ($n = 1$) programs. Eight themes emerged from the data. The theme about student experiences was reflected by statements such as "racial offensive comments," "greater expectation of errors," "different consequences for similar situations," and "prejudicial treatment of Black students" (p. 23). Sadly, as demonstrated by their statements, discriminatory behaviors (called racism) were common experiences for most Black students. The small sample and lack of generalizability were major limitations. However, these consistent findings enhance our understanding of how phenotypic characteristics inform and structure interactions between non-White students and White faculty.

A more recent qualitative study by Hassouneh-Phillips and Beckett (2003) described the perceptions of students in doctoral programs. The nine participants, predominantly African American ($N = 8$) had been enrolled for at least one year in nursing doctoral programs in the western United States. Unstructured group and individual interviews were conducted during which participants commented about selected aspects of their experiences. "The pervasive influence of racism on the participants' lives at personal/interpersonal, institutional, and cultural levels was evident in their narratives" (p. 261). The interpretive analyses yielded four major categories that all related to the presence and consequences of racism in their lives. One such category, "maintaining the status quo," included statements about White faculty and students' lack of interest in cultural issues, a racist assumption that non-White women want and need to be like their White counterparts, and personalizing disapproval of difference. One significant contribution of this exploratory study was the documentation that "women of color . . . were grappling with the effects of racism, while shouldering the work of doctoral study" (p. 264). The findings indicated that non-White women in doctoral programs have to face many challenges. The authors challenged nurse educators to strive toward a new and more equitable vision.

Villarruel, Canales, and Torres (2001) used a focus group format to explore the barriers and bridges experienced by Hispanic nurses during their academic programs. A total of 37 nurses participated in six same-academic-degree focus groups (4 to 9 participants in each group) in six sites that ensured geographic diversity and broad representation of Hispanic subgroups. A number of barriers were identified by participants at both the baccalaureate and master's levels. The institutional barriers included "unsupportive faculty, perceived discrimination by faculty and peers and lack of advisement" (p. 248). The perceived discrimination of faculty was particularly problematic and directly contributed to unsupportive relationships and learning environments. Discriminatory practices, a frequent, strong, and resonant theme, were described affectively as "horrific" and "painful" and were discussed with varying degrees of "anger, sadness, and pain."

The findings of the single study in which the relationship between faculty behavior and "ethnic minority" students' perceptions was described lend credence to the previously described perceptions of barriers by Hispanic nurses' and Black nursing students. Yoder (1996) used a grounded theory methodology to explore (a) nurse educators' and "ethnic minority" nurses' perceptions of problems and issues involved in teaching ethnic students and (b) "ethnic minority" nurses' perceptions of the problems experienced during their educational experiences. The purposive sample consisted of 26 nurse educators from nine nursing programs in California (15 community college and 11 university), and 46% were from "ethnic minority" backgrounds. Seventeen African American, Asian-Pacific Islander, and Mexican American nurses either had baccalaureate and master's degrees or were enrolled in master's programs. The central organizing social process was the interactive responding between educators and students mediated by faculty's cultural awareness. Five different teaching patterns, grounded in lower to higher levels of faculty cultural awareness and responding, resulted in positive and negative consequences for faculty and students. For instance, the lower the level of faculty cultural awareness and responding, the more students perceived barriers. The study generated a beginning substantive theory. Although the theory increased the knowledge base about how differences influence interactions, it possessed some limitations. Most important, as Yoder noted, it did not describe other broad structural linkages (e.g., the philosophy and mission of the school and its practices, the percentages of racially and ethnically diverse students) that influenced faculty's level of cultural awareness. In addition, the demographic characteristics of the faculty sample were not described in enough detail to determine how they (e.g., faculty group membership) might have influenced faculty cultural awareness and response.

Discriminatory behaviors grounded in racist ideology create many barriers and additional burdens for non-White nurses throughout their academic and workforce experiences. One of the many consequences of the individual and institutional barriers has been the struggle of non-White nurses to remain in the center, not on the margins. According to Hagey, Choudhry, Guruge, Turruttin, Collins, and Lee (2001), being perceived as marginal at entry means that the non-White nurse is "someone who can be subordinated, disadvantaged, restricted, silenced, not told about opportunities nor given cooperation for control" (p. 390). The authors argued that interpersonal issues with nurses from racial and ethnic backgrounds cannot be effectively dealt with without examining racism and inequity in professional and educational institutions.

Education of White Nursing Students

The second stream of research was concerned with educating White students about race and other differences under the rubric of cultural competence. This investigative approach suggested that nursing was beginning to ease out of its traditional position of colorblindness and "politically correct cultural diversity agendas without substance" (Hassouneh-Phillips & Beckett, 2003, p. 262) and perhaps was beginning to move toward a paradigm of antiracism. The slow movement is exciting, principally because in the past the impact of racism in people's daily lives had been discussed infrequently with students at any level, in any academic program. Abrums and Leppa (2001) have argued that "culturally competent" care could not be provided "unless underlying issues of discrimination and oppression are examined and confronted" (p. 270). Despite nurse educators' slow movement away from the traditional paradigm of silence, researchers have continued to study attitudes toward different others.

Eliason (1998) explored the correlates of prejudice with 116 (87 females; 29 males) undergraduate nursing students who ranged in age from 19 to 49 years and were enrolled in a midwestern university. Non-White and nonheterosexual students were omitted from the analyses. Students responded to a racial consciousness scale. The most noteworthy finding was that low levels of racial awareness were associated with higher levels of comfort and more positive attitudes toward non-White than people from "sexual minorities." In view of these findings, the authors pointed out that students might think they were capable of treating everyone the same, but this false sense of security in conjunction with lack of awareness might constitute a barrier to effective communication with different others. Socially desirable responses were discussed as a plausible explanation for the contradictory findings. Nurse educators should begin to attend to the facts that the United States is both race and class segregated and that in all likelihood undergraduate students have had minimal contact and feeling of comfort with different others.

In a similar study, Eliason and Raheim (2000) examined experience and levels of comfort working with diverse clients with White undergraduate students. Working on the premise that these students "have had little or no exposure to or education about people from cultures different from their own" (p. 161), they surveyed 196 students (n = 173 females, 23 males) between 18 and 24 years of age enrolled in a midwestern university. Thirteen non-White students were excluded from the analyses. The results were consistent with their premise: that is, lack of experience and feeling uncomfortable were strongly related. Interestingly, despite lack of experience, students reported little discomfort with members of racial and ethnic groups. In response to these results, the authors questioned if the results reflected a decrease in racist attitudes or whether political correctness merely inhibited people from expressing them (p. 164). Interestingly, students possessed no inhibitions about exposing their considerable discomfort with working with lesbian, gay, or bisexual people and people who were HIV positive. Apparently, students' inconsistent responses were not based solely on lack of experience, political correctness, or social desirability. The notion that political correctness may silence student biases, stereotypes, and myths is one that should be seriously considered by all nurse educators. Unfortunately, few, if any, researchers have examined the outcomes of cultural diversity education.

An international study that had no known counterpart in the U.S. literature was Hagey and MacKay's (2000) report of the first phase in a university school to begin to integrate culture and antiracism into the undergraduate curriculum. The qualitative study was precipitated by a need to identify issues and perceptions that could be used both in faculty development and in the construction of an evaluation tool for measuring change after the integration of culture and antiracism in the curriculum (p. 46). Data were collected with open-ended interviews with 40 students and one staff person and small focus groups with eight students ($n = 40$) with one faculty member and one preceptor. The findings were related to racialist social cognitions and practices as reflected in discourse (p. 47). A dominant paradigm emerged and was named "whiteness/otherness," which indicated groups segmented into in-group/out-group. Additional analyses indicated how the reality of this paradigm was activated and conveyed by students' and instructors' use of language and denial of racism in the profession. The authors speculated about how the paradigm remained entrenched in the everyday practices of people engaged in nursing. A noteworthy finding was how the uncomfortableness of faculty with this qualitative phase resulted in their relinquishing the idea of constructing an instrument for measuring change. A significant contribution of this study was to highlight how faculty development might be essential prior to curricular changes about cultural diversity. Nurse educators are faced with the dual challenges of enhancing their own and students' cultural competence and its corollary, a diverse and sensitive workforce.

SUMMARY

The predominant and consistent finding in the research about retention of non-Whites in nursing was the struggle to deal with racist behaviors and discriminatory practices regardless of academic level. The qualitative designs permitted the expression of personal experiences and perceptions. The evidence from these studies has been commonly acknowledged for many years. The question is, why has so very little changed? How does nursing get beyond the research findings to modeling some approaches and racist and antidiscriminatory for faculty and students?

The stream of research about White nursing students suggested that the measurement of attitudes remains the predominant paradigm among researchers. However, the fact that "cultural attitudes" are no longer the focus is an indication of growth. As in earlier studies, the relationship between attitude and behavior has not been determined for nurses because there have been no studies to determine if the relationship exists. We must begin to ask how the study of individual attitudes will increase our understanding of the profession and the quality of services delivered. Nurses must begin to examine the underlying values and attitudes that pervade the provision of health and medical care. The focus on attitudes diverts us from a critical examination of multidimensional, theoretically based models for the study of clinical practice.

FUTURE DIRECTIONS

There is a dire need for systematic investigations of how the category of race (phenotypes) and the concept of racism influence nursing education and practice. The paucity of studies and the magnitude of health disparities demand a greater knowledge base about racial attitudes and discriminatory behaviors grounded in racist ideologies. We need to move beyond attitudinal studies with convenience samples to multisite observational studies with large samples of nurses from different academic backgrounds in a variety of urban, rural, and community settings. The ethical and logistical aspects of the design can be surmounted.

Simultaneously, research designs for the investigation of racism demand serious consideration. Much of the nursing research about racism uses qualitative methodologies. These data, analyzed using various interpretive frameworks, enhance our awareness of perceptions and perspectives that are necessary to the provision of quality services. However, these isolated studies are not enough. What comes after the studies?

Currently, research about racism and nursing practice remains the domain of Canada and Great Britain. In terms of method, there are differences between U.S. and Canadian research. For example, in the United States the participants in nursing education research were non-White students, seldom White faculty. Generally, the Canadian researchers were much more exact in their definition of concepts. Consistent with Drevdahl, Taylor, and Phillips (2001), U.S. researchers tended not to define race or used dated or questionable materials when they did. Also, by default, the objects of racism were African Americans/Blacks, American Indian/First Nations, Asians, and Hispanics/Latinos. The importance of racism in everyday life is increasing (Shaha, 1998), but researchers, although paying more attention than in the past, remain selective about what aspects of racism they will study. Future research should include the effects of racism on mobility in both clinical and educational settings and the effects of racism on client/patient care. Most important, because there are no nursing theories that deal with racism, the theoretical basis of research about the effects of racism needs to be well grounded in the social science literature.

Furthermore, there is a need for clear conceptual distinctions among *race, racism,* and *culture.* This means that the notion of "cultural diversity" needs to be carefully scrutinized and operationalized for inclusion in studies. Nurse educators have a responsibility to prepare graduates to function with others different from themselves. However, a growing body of evidence indicates that nursing's multicultural and transcultural approaches to "cultural diversity" exclude racism (e.g., Hagey et al., 2001). Consequently, researchers must interject the concept of racism into these frameworks. How do nurse educators effectively discuss socioecological context if the concept of racism is excluded? How does the exclusion of the concept fit with nursing's purported holism ideology? Despite nursing's focus on cultural diversity and cultural competence, few formal evaluations of such programs exist. Thus nurse educators have minimal evidence about their effectiveness, regardless of the participants. Investigations that examine how nurses and nursing students apply cultural diversity content are imperative.

In the future, nursing needs to reflect upon its own. The fact that nurses "care" is not enough if they are to become active participants in the struggle to eliminate disparities among dominant and subordinate groups. In concert with Richek (1970), "it would indeed be a naïve psychological and sociological stance to maintain that career commitment to a helping profession perforce leads to relinquishment of prejudicial attitudes" (p. 173). Nursing must continue its struggle to name and acknowledge race and racism.

> After all if we pretend racism does not exist, that we do not know what it is or how to change it—it never has to go away. (hooks, 1995, p. 4)

REFERENCES

Abrums, M. E., & Leppa, C. (2001). Beyond cultural competence: Teaching about race, gender, class, and sexual orientation. *Journal of Nursing Education, 40*, 270–275.

Allen, M. E., Nunley, J. C., & Scott-Warner, M. (1988). Recruitment and retention of Black students in baccalaureate nursing programs. *Journal of Nursing Education, 27*, 107–116.

American Nurses Association. (2003). Nursing's Social Policy Statement 2003. Washington, DC: Author (Public Comment draft, February 2003).

Appiah, K. A. (1990). Racisms. In D. Goldberg (Ed.), *Anatomy of racism* (pp. 3–17). Minneapolis: University of Minnesota Press.

Bonaparte, B. (1979). Ego-defensiveness, open-closed mindedness, and nurses' attitudes toward culturally different patients. *Nursing Research, 28*, 166–172.

Browne, A. J., Johnson, J. L., Bottorff, J. L., Grewal, S., & Hilton, B. A. (2002). Recognizing discrimination in nursing practice. *Canadian Nurse, 98*(5), 24–27.

Byrd, W. M., & Clayton, L. A. (2002). *An American health dilemma: Race, medicine, and health care in the United States 1900–2000* (Vol. 2). New York: Routledge.

Carnegie, M. E. (1995). *The path we tread* (3rd ed.). New York: National League for Nursing Press.

Cobb, W. J. (2002). Medical progress and African Americans. *American Journal of Public Health, 92*, 191–194.

Delacampagne, C. (1990). Racism and the west: From praxis to logos. Translated by Michael Edwards. In D. Goldberg (Ed.), *Anatomy of racism* (pp. 83–88). Minneapolis: University of Minnesota Press.

Dovidio, J. F., Gaertner, S. L., Kawakami, K., & Hodson, G. (2002). Why can't we just get along? Interpersonal biases and interracial distrust. *Cultural Diversity and Ethnic Minority Psychology, 8*(2), 88–102.

Drevdahl, D., Taylor, J. Y., & Phillips, D. A. (2001). Race and ethnicity as variables in *Nursing Research*, 1952–2000. *Nursing Research, 50*, 305–313.

DuBois, W. E. B. (1901). The Freedman's Bureau. *Atlantic Monthly, 87*, 354–365.

Eliason, M. J. (1998). Correlates of prejudice in nursing students. *Journal of Nursing Education, 37*(1), 27–29.

Eliason, M. J., & Raheim, S. (2000). Experiences and comfort with culturally diverse groups in undergraduate pre-nursing students. *Journal of Nursing Education, 39*, 161–165.

Essed, P. (1991). *Everyday racism.* Newport, CA: Sage Publications.

Felder, E. (1990). Baccalaureate and associate degree student nurses' cultural knowledge of and attitudes toward Black American clients. *Journal of Nursing Education, 29*, 276–282.

Flaskerud, J. H., Lesser, J., Dixon, E., Anderson, N., Conde, F., Kim, et al. (2002). Health disparities among vulnerable populations. *Nursing Research, 51*(2), 74–85.

Frenkel, S. I., Greden, J. F., Robinson, J. A., Guyden, T. E., & Miller, R. (1980). Does patient contact change racial perceptions? *American Journal of Nursing, 80*, 1340–1342.

Ganong, L. H., Bzdek, V., & Manderino, M. A. (1987). Stereotyping by nurses and nursing students: A critical review of research. *Research in Nursing and Health, 10*(1), 49–70.

Gilroy, P. (1990). One nation under a groove: The cultural politics of "race" and racism in Britain. In D. Goldberg (Ed.), *Anatomy of racism* (pp. 263–282). Minneapolis: University of Minnesota Press.

Goldberg, D. (Ed.). (1990). *Anatomy of racism.* Minneapolis: University of Minnesota Press.

Goldberg, D. T., & Essed, P. (2002). Introduction: From racial demarcations to multiple identifications. In P. Essed & D. T. Goldberg (Eds.), *Race critical theories: Text and context* (pp. 1–11). Oxford, UK: Blackwell Publishers.

Greipp, M. E. (1996). Culture, age and gender: Effects on quality of predicted self and colleague reaction. *International Journal of Nursing Studies, 33*(1), 83–97.

Hagey, R., Choudhry, U., Guruge, S., Turruttin, J., Collins, E., & Lee, R. (2001). Immigrant nurses' experience of racism. *Journal of Nursing Scholarship, 33*, 389–394.

Hagey, R., & McKay, R. W. (2000). Qualitative research to identify racialist discourse towards equity in nursing curricula. *International Journal of Nursing Studies, 37*(1), 45–46.

Harrison, F. (1997). Race and racism. In T. Barfield (Ed.), *The dictionary of anthropology* (pp. 392–396). Oxford, UK: Blackwell Publishers.

Harrison, F. V. (1998). Introduction: Expanding the discourse on "race." *American Anthropologist, 100,* 609–631.

Hassouneh-Phillips, D., & Beckett, A. (2003). An education in racism. *Journal of Nursing Education, 42,* 258–265.

Hine, D. (1989). *Black women in White.* Bloomington: Indiana University Press.

hooks, b. (1995). *Killing rage: Ending racism.* New York: Henry Holt & Co.

Ignatiev, N. (1995). *How the Irish became White.* New York: Routledge.

Institute of Medicine. (2002). *Unequal treatment: Confronting racial and ethnic disparities in healthcare.* Washington, DC: National Academy Press.

Kirkham, S. R. (1998). Nurses' descriptions of caring for culturally diverse clients. *Clinical Nursing Research, 7,* 125–146.

LaFargue, J. P. (1972). Role of prejudice in rejection of health care. *Nursing Research, 21*(1), 53–58.

Langston-Moss, R. (1997). Experiences and perceptions of Black American female nursing students attending predominantly White nursing programs. *Journal of the National Black Nurses Association, 9*(2), 21–30.

McDonald, D. D. (1994). Gender and ethnic stereotyping and narcotic analgesic administration. *Research in Nursing and Health, 17,* 45–49.

Morgan, B. S. (1983). Selected correlates of White nursing students' attitudes toward Black American patients. *International Journal of Nursing Studies, 20,* 109–121.

Morgan, B. S. (1984). A semantic differential measure of attitudes toward Black patients. *Research in Nursing and Health, 7,* 155–162.

Richek, H. G. (1970). A note on prejudice in prospective professional helpers. *Nursing Research, 19,* 172–175.

Rooda, L. A. (1992). Attitudes of nurses toward culturally diverse patients: An examination of the social contact theory. *Journal of the National Black Nurses Association, 6*(1), 48–56.

Rooda, L. A. (1993). Knowledge and attitudes of nurses toward culturally different patients: Implications for nursing education. *Journal of Nursing Education, 32,* 209–213.

Ruiz, M. C. J. (1981). Open-closed mindedness, intolerance of ambiguity and nursing faculty attitudes toward culturally different patients. *Nursing Research, 30,* 177–181.

Schulman, K. A., Berlin, J. A., Harless, W., Kerner, J. F., Sistrunk, S., Gersh, B. J., et al. (1999). The effects of race and sex on physicians' recommendations for cardiac catheterization. *New England Journal of Medicine, 340,* 618–625.

Shaha, M. (1998). Racism and its implications in ethical-moral reasoning in nursing practice: A tentative approach to a largely unexplored topic. *Nursing Ethics, 5,* 139–146.

Thomas, S. B. (2001). The color line: Race matters in the elimination of health disparities. *American Journal of Public Health, 91,* 1046–1048.

Tucker, W. H. (1994). *The science and politics of racial research.* Chicago: University of Illinois Press.

Tucker-Allen, S. (1991). Minority student nurses' perceptions of their educational programs. *ABNF Journal, 2*(3), 50–63.

Tucker-Allen, S. (1992). Diversity in nursing faculty hinges on diversity in nursing students in NLN. In *Perspectives in nursing 1991–1993* (pp. 35–42). New York: National League for Nursing Press.

Turrittin, J., Hagey, R., Guruge, S., Collins, E., & Mitchell, M. (2002). The experience of professional nurses who have migrated to Canada: Cosmopolitan citizenship or democratic racism? *International Journal of Nursing Studies, 39,* 655–667.

U.S. Department of Health and Human Services. (2001). *Healthy people 2010: Understanding and improving health* (Superintendent of Documents Stock No. 017-001-00550-9). Washington, DC: U.S. Government Printing Office.

U.S. Department of Health and Human Services. (1985). *Report of the Secretary's Task Force on Black and Minority Health, Vol. 1. Executive Summary.* Washington, DC: U.S. Government Printing Office.

VanRyn, M., & Burke, J. (2000). The effect of patient race and socio-economic status on physician's perceptions of patients. *Social Science and Medicine, 50,* 813–828.

Villarruel, A. M., Canales, M., & Torres, S. (2001). Bridges and barriers: Educational mobility of Hispanic nurses. *Journal of Nursing Education, 40,* 245–251.

Yoder, M. K. (1996). Instructional responses to ethnically diverse nursing students. *Journal of Nursing Education, 35,* 315–321.

Chapter 3

Structural and Racial Barriers to Health Care

LINDA BURNES BOLTON, JOYCE NEWMAN GIGER, AND C. ALICIA GEORGES

ABSTRACT

Limited access to health care and a system fraught with discriminatory practices inhibit some racial and ethnic minorities from gaining access to health care and assurance of equal treatment once they enter the health care system. The purpose of this chapter is to critically and systematically analyze the research literature to determine what impact individual and institutional racism has had on the prevailing health disparities across racial and ethnic minority groups. The chapter includes the following: (1) a review of the term *racism* and a brief overview of the history of racism in health care; (2) a review of the research literature analyzing the impact of racism on health disparities; and (3) recommendations to end the systematic institutional racism in scientific research, which is necessary to end health disparities.

Keywords: access, racism, structural barriers

The education of health care practitioners has been primarily based on the biopsychosocial characteristics of the dominant White culture (Giger & Davidhizar, 1999). A profound lack of understanding of biological and genetic differences, cultural beliefs, attitudes, and cultural health-seeking behaviors has resulted in less than optimum health care for persons who are not members of the dominant culture. According to Braithwaite and Taylor (2001), this lack of knowledge on the part of health care providers has often resulted in "culturally incompetent care."

Some experts in transcultural health care, such as Giger and Davidhi-zar (1999), contend that where ethnic minorities are concerned there appear to be three intervening and reinforcing variables that either hinder access to health care or perpetuate culturally inappropriate care. These variables include poverty, discrimination, and social and psychological barriers that occur as a result of racism—both institutional and individual. In fact, these three reemerging variables usually impact racial and ethnic minority populations so profoundly that these groups are often unlikely to use the health care services that are available.

It is also plausible that poverty, discrimination, and psychological barriers, as a result of institutional or individual racism, may also explain why morbidity and mortality rates are higher among most racial and ethnic minorities as compared with their White counterparts (Giger & Davidhizar, 1999). Although underrepresented in the general U.S. population, most racial and ethnic minorities, including African Americans, Hispanics, Asians, and American Indians, remain overrepresented among the health statistics for life-threatening illnesses.

Cohall and Bannister (2001) noted that although poverty and limited access to health care undoubtedly are key factors affecting the health status of most racial and ethnic minorities, these factors do not explain the health care utilization and often the culturally incompetent care experienced by these groups. They further contend that racial and ethnic minorities, regardless of educational attainment, socioeconomic status, and level of viable medical insurance, often experience personal frustration stemming from perceived racism and lack of cultural competency on the part of health care providers.

In a highly industrial society such as a United States, it is difficult to conceive why race and ethnicity are factors in the life expectancies of its citizens and also in access to and quality of health care. In 2002, a committee under the auspices of the Institute of Medicine (2002) released the landmark report *Unequal Treatment: Confronting Racial and Ethnic Disparities in Health Care*. The committee unequivocally stated that evidence of racial and ethnic disparities in health care is, for the most part, consistent and persistent, regardless of the nature of the illness or the type of health care services rendered. Braithwaite and Taylor (2001) noted that even if income levels were standardized and all impediments regarding access to care were eliminated, disparities in health outcomes might still exist. It is plausible to conclude that limited access and a system fraught with racism and discriminatory practices hinder some racial and ethnic minorities from gaining access to health care and assurance of equal treatment once they enter the health care system.

UNDERSTANDING RACISM

According to Bobo (2001), throughout the 1990s we as a nation became increasingly racially polarized. Racism is a complex belief system that prescribes and often legitimizes an ethnic or other minority group's subordination by claiming that that particular group is either biogenetically or culturally inferior (See & Wilson, 1989). There are two essential components that differentiate racism from prejudice. The first component is an ideology that justifies, for individuals who actually are racist, social avoidance and ultimately domination because of the unaltered characteristics (e.g., skin color) of a particular minority group. The second component of racism is a set of norms that prescribe differential treatment for these groups (See & Wilson, 1989).

Historical Incidences of Racism in Health Care

Health care services in the United States have not been exempt from "Jim Crow" laws, which were legally sanctioned until the mid-1960s throughout the South. However, the northern regions of the United States also were not exempt from such discriminatory practices in health care. This is evident in the passage of the Hill-Burton Act in 1946, which was not abolished until 1966 with the passage of the Federal Medicare Act (Bullough & Bullough, 1982). The Hill-Burton Act, also known as the Hospital Construction Survey Act, provided federal grants for hospitals, both private and public, that admittedly did not service African Americans. Under this law, hospitals, whether private or public, were allowed to discriminately service populations based on race. In addition, these same hospitals were allowed to extend these discriminatory practices in regard to hiring and staffing patterns. From such practices were born the all-African American hospitals, which were found not only in the South but also in the North.

Proprietors of the hospitals were able to establish inclusions and exclusions for purposes of rendering health care services to those persons in need. Thus patterns of admission and service to African Americans, in particular, varied throughout the country without regard to region. In some northern and western states, admission to and service by some hospitals remained theoretically open to all races on equal terms, whereas in other states the courts upheld the rights of hospital proprietors to segregate as they saw fit.

INSTITUTIONAL RACISM: CONTRIBUTIONS TO HEALTH DISPARITIES

Though legislation now prohibits institutions from withholding services to persons because of their race, religion, or gender, the patterns of discrimination (institutional racism) remain embedded in the organizational structure of health care and other institutions in this country. Institutional racism prevents ethnic and racial minorities from access to the goods, services, and opportunities provided to others. This differential access may occur even when the group may be in need of services (Jones, 2000).

To understand the dynamics of individual and institutional racism and their potential contributions to health disparities, a literature search was done using CINAHL, MEDLINE, and Behavioral and Social Sciences electronic databases. The search focused on the years 1991–2003. The descriptors used to initiate the search were "minority health and research," "ethnic minority health disparities," and "health and institutional racism and health care."

Over 200 articles were identified from the search. A number of articles were deemed relevant for this chapter if they included African Americans and or other minorities in the sample, identified racial variations as a factor in health outcomes, addressed access to care issues, and centered on certain diseases or health problems, such as cardiovascular diseases, which included stroke, or cardiovascular risk factors such as hypertension, dyslipidemias, and infant mortality. Particular attention was given to studies that utilized large databases that provided appropriate numbers of African Americans and other racial and ethnic minorities in the sample. Excluded were articles that were not data based. The articles were descriptive studies and population studies. No experimental studies were found that met the inclusion criteria. The research articles containing the inclusion criteria were in the following areas: prenatal care, preterm birth, cardiovascular disease, hypertension, diabetes, and HIV/AIDS.

REVIEW OF THE LITERATURE

Prenatal Care

Infant mortality remains a significant problem among African Americans and also in some other ethnic and racial minorities in the United States. Infant mortality rates are related to the type of prenatal care and its timeliness. Using data from the National Center for Health Statistics 1981–1998 natality files on singleton births, Alexander, Kogan, and Nabukera (2002) examined racial differences in prenatal care between White and African American women. They examined the trends and racial disparities in the use of prenatal care of U.S. White and African American women, including those in special at-risk groups: young unmarried or less-educated mothers. Available for analysis were 60 million birth certificates. Records of singleton births of White and African American women were scrutinized to determine the trimester in which prenatal care began. The Revised Graduated Index of Prenatal Care Utilization and the Adequacy of Prenatal Care Index were used to determine the number of visits and the adequacy of the prenatal care visits. The results indicated that both White and African American women had an increase in adequate use of prenatal care. There was a 50% improvement for Whites and a 64% increase for African Americans. There was also an increase in first-trimester visits for prenatal care for both groups. The study noted that African American women had more intensive use of care during the study period.

The outcome of this study indicates that White and African American women tend to have few disparities in early prenatal care and adequate use of this care. It was clear that there has been a great improvement over time in the United States in access to prenatal care and the types of care available. The researchers cautioned that although this pattern existed during the period of time studied, there is no guarantee that the then *Healthy People 2000* objective of 90% of pregnant women starting care in the first trimester would be realized for White or African American women. What is the implication of this study? Since no data were available about birth outcomes, the relation of prenatal care to infant or maternal mortality is not clear. Perceptions of the African American women about the quality of care they received would be an area that could benefit from further study.

In other studies, racial and ethnic differences in prenatal care have been reported. Brett, Schoendorf, and Kiely (1994) assessed the use of prenatal care technologies, including ultrasonography, tocolysis, and amniocentesis, among African American, Hispanic, and White women. There were appreciable and inconsistent racial differences in the utilization of these various services, even when maternal age, education, marital status, location of residence, birth order, and timing of first prenatal birth were all statistically controlled. Likewise, Barfield and colleagues (1996) found that prenatal care utilization was generally lower for African Americans than for their White counterparts in both civilian and military populations. In concert with these findings, Komaromy et al. (1996) studied 8,300 African and White women to assess their self-reports of prenatal advice from health care providers. Researchers controlled for age, martial status, education, income, site of prenatal care, type of payment, maternal health behaviors, when trimester began, and prior adverse pregnancy outcomes. Findings indicated that White women were more likely to receive positive health advice about such topics as smoking and alcohol cessation than their African American counterparts.

Preterm births are a contributing factor in infant mortality. Rosenberg, Palmer, Wise, Horton, and Corwin (2002) used data from the Black Women's Health Study, a longitudinal study of African American women ages 21–69 begun in 1995 to assess the experiences of racism in relation to preterm birth among African American women. A group of 422 mothers of babies born three weeks or more early were compared with mothers of 4,544 babies of longer gestation. The 1997 and 1999 questionnaires had nine questions regarding job, housing, and police discrimination. The other questions on race dealt with the frequency in daily life of other people's discriminatory behavior toward them. The analyses were limited to those women who had answered the 1997 questionnaire and who reported on the 1997 or 1999 questionnaire that they had a singleton birth. Generalized equation models were used to estimate odds ratios for preterm birth. The researchers controlled for potential confounds.

The results of the study indicated that women who perceived that they were being treated unfairly at work or that people acted afraid of them had a high incidence of preterm births. The results of this study, though not surprising, have provided us with some evidence of the potential impact of racial discrimination on birth outcomes. African American high school and college educated women recounted unfair treatment on the job and had a statistically higher number of preterm births when compared to White women. The researchers felt that this was not a chance occurrence. They surmised that the racism or the perception of racism experienced by the women in the study contributed to this finding.

The data about racism and its effects on the health of African Americans have long been debated. Evidence in this area has been scanty. Though only addressing birth outcomes, this study adds to the emerging database about racism and health outcomes. Since preterm birth is the major cause of perinatal death, eliminating racism should be a primary goal of health care providers. Further study of other health outcomes using the discrimination questions presented in this study would contribute to a needed database.

Another study used the 1989–1997 U.S. live birth, fetal death, and infant death databases from the National Center for Health Statistics to investigate the trends in preterm birth and neonatal mortality among Blacks and Whites. Demissie et al. (2001) found that the pattern for preterm birthrates was fairly consistent for singleton births for Blacks and Whites. Preterm births decreased for Blacks but increased for Whites over the time period. The researchers found that reduction of risk factors such as cigarette smoking and late prenatal care, though not explicitly examined, may have been contributing factors to the decrease in preterm births. However, the higher number of neonatal deaths and infant mortalities for Blacks negates these accomplishments. What is needed is further investigation of potential factors suggested by the researchers, such as access to neonatal intensive care services, use of new pharmacologic interventions, and the impact of race in the specific interventions.

Management of Chronic Diseases

Cardiovascular disease is the leading cause of death for all Americans. The impact of cardiovascular disease on African American communities has been widely discussed in health and medical literature. Ayala et al. (2001) examined the disparities in mortality by stroke subtype using National Vital Statistics data for death certificates for persons over 25 years of age during 1995–1998. They found that African Americans and American Indians/Alaska Natives have higher mortality rates for all types of stroke. They also observed that Hispanics and Asian Pacific Islanders have a greater risk of stroke deaths from intracerebral hemorrhage. Using data from previous studies, they surmised that risks factors such as hypertension, smoking, alcohol abuse, obesity, diabetes, and genetic and environmental factors may contribute to stroke mortality. Since African American, Hispanic, and other racial and ethnic minority populations will continue to grow, the researchers believe that more emphasis should be placed on public health programs to decrease the incidence of strokes and stroke mortality.

Since decreasing risk factors is crucial in reducing the incidence of stroke, further research is needed to determine what types of programs decrease risk factors. Studies are needed on lifestyle modification programs for decreasing cardiovascular risk factors. Is the behavior of the person the overriding factor in modifying lifestyle, or do the barriers to care (individual and or institutional racism), late intervention, and lack of access to new treatment regimes contribute to the incidence and prevalence of stroke? However, no studies were found that addressed these critical questions.

After experiencing a near fatal event such as a cardiac arrest out of the hospital, is race an independent predictor of survival? Chu et al. (1998) collected data for four years (1991–1994) from a convenience sample of out-of-hospital cardiac arrest patients transported to nine hospitals to answer this question. All known cardiac arrests were included in the study. The primary outcome measured was survival until hospital discharge. This study included 1,690 patients, of whom 223 were Blacks and 1,467 Whites. Though income varied between Blacks and Whites, the groups were considered affluent by national standards. Blacks were younger, and there were more females in the group. Though more Blacks than Whites experienced witnessed cardiac arrest outside of their homes, bystanders did not resuscitate Blacks. These findings were consistent with previous studies. Even in light of these findings, those in the sample who were in ventricular fibrillation/ventricular tachycardia had similar survival rates to hospital discharge.

In a similar study, Becker et al. (1993) found that there are other plausible reasons for the differences between the rates and lethality of sudden cardiac arrest in some ethnic minority groups such as African Americans as compared with their White counterparts. These differences might clearly indicate lack of knowledge and racial differences in treatment. Data from this study suggested that there are reasons for nonsurvivability following cardiac arrest. These included (1) inexperience and lack of familiarity with basic CPR techniques of the persons at the site; (2) slow response time of the emergency ambulance to the site, particularly in "African-American neighborhoods"; and (3) slow response time of the hospital emergency team to the African American client in full cardiac arrest (Becker et al., 1993).

The outcome of these and similar studies prompts one to ask the following questions: Who are the bystanders? Do they share the same racial group? Is the failure to resuscitate because of lack of skills in CPR by persons in the Black community? Further research in these areas is warranted.

Research findings are controversial as to why there is a higher incidence of hypertension among some racial groups and not others. In what is viewed as one of the most controversial studies on the subject, Klag et al. (1991) found that there was a positive association between skin color (darker) and systolic and diastolic blood pressures (higher). In the study, 457 African Americans were surveyed in three United States cities by use of a reflectometer to note the intensity of skin color and the correlation with blood pressure. The findings from the study indicate that both systolic and diastolic blood pressures may be higher in darker persons than in lighter ones and increase by 2 mm Hg for every 1-SD (standard deviation) increase in skin darkness. However, the data indicated that the association was dependent on socioeconomic status, whether measured by education or on another index consisting of education, occupation, and ethnicity. Significant findings were present only in persons on the lower level of either index, education only or education ethnicity and occupation (Klag et al., 1991). Using multiple linear regressions, the researchers found that both systolic and diastolic blood pressures remained significantly associated with darker skin in the lower socioeconomic status, independent of age–body mass index and concentration of blood glucose. The researchers concluded that the findings may be attributed to two factors:

1. Either the inability to deal with psychosocial stress associated with darker skin or
2. The findings may be consistent with an interaction between the environmental factors associated with low socioeconomic status and a susceptible gene that has a higher prevalence in persons with darker skin (Klag et al., 1991).

While there is a prevalence of hypertension among racial and ethnic minorities, there also exist differences in regard to treatment for hypertension. In fact, Stewart and Silverstein (2002) found that Mexican Americans are more likely to have high blood pressure than non-Hispanic Whites (29% vs. 27%). In addition, according to the findings, Mexican Americans are also less likely to have high-risk cholesterol than their non-Hispanic White counterparts (18% vs. 21%). Yet Nelson, Norris, and Mangione (2002) found that even when Mexican Americans were diagnosed with high cholesterol that required medication, they were less likely than their White counterparts to take cholesterol-lowering agents or to be offered medication treatment by their health care provider.

Although African Americans, Hispanics, and American Indians experience a 50% to 100% greater burden of diabetes and higher mortality from this disease than White Americans, the disease appears to be treated very poorly. Chinn, Zang, and Merril (1998) conducted a study of 1,400 Medicare beneficiaries with a diagnosis of diabetes. These researchers found that the health care providers did not have African Americans undergo routine diabetes maintenance such as HBA1C, lipid testing, ophthalmologist visits, and influenza vaccine, even after controlling for gender, education, and age. Reporting similar findings, Cowie and Harris (1997) noted that African Americans with type 2 diabetics were more likely to be treated with insulin as compared with Whites or Mexican Americans. Insulin therapy is not the first step in the care of patients with type 2 diabetes. Why was this intervention used?

HIV and AIDS continue to plague racial and ethnic minority groups, particularly African Americans. This is happening at the same time that treatment options have increased and persons with AIDS are living longer with this chronic disease. Moore, Stanton, Gopalan, and Chaisson (1994), researchers at Johns Hopkins University School of Medicine, conducted a study on HIV-positive individuals to determine if there were notable differences in the administration of antiretroviral drugs among Black and White clients. Findings from this study suggest that Black HIV-positive individuals are less likely than their White counterparts to be given antiretroviral drugs, including medication to prevent *Pneumocystis carinii* pneumonia (PCP). Of the number of Blacks surveyed, only 58% of those medically eligible received drug therapy, compared with 82% of their White counterparts.

Researchers found no significant differences in receipt of drug therapy with respect to such moderating variables as age, gender, and mode of HIV transmission, type of insurance, income, education, or place of residence. Similarly, Shapiro et al. (1999) noted that even when adjusting for insurance status, CD4 cell count, sex, age, methods of exposure to HIV, and region of country, African Americans, along with their Hispanic counterparts, were 24% less likely than their White counterparts to receive protease inhibitors or nonnucleoside reverse transcriptase inhibitors at the initial assessment by their health care providers.

Structural Barriers to Health Care

Structural barriers in health care are ingrained within the fabric of the health care delivery system. Barriers have been identified since 1950. The most commonly reported barriers have included lower rates of health insurance for ethnic and racial minority populations, lower socioeconomic status, lower rates of health literacy, lower English fluency, certain cultural and spiritual beliefs, and lack of confidence in health care providers compared with White persons (Celano, Geller, Phillips, & Ziman, 1998; Cohen, Bloom, Simpson, & Parsons, 1997; Decklebaum et al., 1999; Luder, Melnick, & DiMaio, 1998; National Cancer Institute, 2001; Resnick, Valsania, Halter, & Lin, 1998; Winkleby, Robinson, Sundquist, & Kraemer, 1999). The effect of these barriers on access to health services, quality of health care services, and cost of services will be discussed in the review of the literature in these areas.

Racial and ethnic differences in access and utilization of services have been related to education and income differences more than to any other factors (Esser-Stuart & Lyons, 2002). Descriptive and correlational studies have suggested that the differences continue to exist within the same socioeconomic and education group. Explanations for these differences, which result in disparities in health care indices among ethnic and racial groups, have not been fully explained. Therefore, race and ethnicity should be considered as variables in health outcomes.

Esser-Stuart and Lyons (2002) conducted a study to (1) describe perceived barriers to seeking health care; (2) determine perceptions of confidence in health practitioners; and finally, (3) explore strategies to enhance, promote, and improve early health care intervention among low-income minority women. These researchers used a convenience sample of low-income elderly women ($N = 24$) who actively participated in a foster grandparent program (FGP) that was sponsored by Focus on Senior Citizens (FOCUS). These subjects were 62 to 84 years of age, with a mean age of 68 years. By race, 21 participants were African American, 2 were White, and 1 was American Indian. Using focus group methodology, researchers identified lack of confidence in the delivery system as a key barrier to accessing and utilizing health services. Notable among these findings was the perception of minority women that practitioners were unable to recognize their spiritual and cultural needs. The health care delivery system was perceived as uncaring. The women indicated that, as a result, they limited their interaction with providers and were less likely to follow their instructions.

Not all studies have found interethnic or racial difference in care, particularly for racial and ethnic minority women. It is essential to examine these studies to determine what variables were included that would necessitate differences in the findings. To determine factors that hindered racial and ethnic minority women from obtaining preventive health care, a probability Commonwealth Minority Health Survey (CMHS) was conducted in 1994. The intent of the study design was to ensure the CMHS would reflect the distribution by race of the general U.S. population. The sample consisted of 3,789 adults who were 18 years of age or older and who were African American, Hispanic, Native American or Alaskan Native, White, and Asian Pacific Islander (as cited in Cornelius, Smith, & Simpson, 2002).

Findings from the CMHS revealed intra racial and ethnic differences in access and utilization of health services. These differences were associated with the educational level of the women and their perceived need for care. Neither perceived discrimination nor residence was associated with the amount of care women received (Cornelius, Smith, & Simpson, 2002). Although others have not supported these findings, these findings do support recommendations that include equitable access to health care providers, care that is culturally sensitive, and differentiation of groups by socioeconomic status in future research.

Kataoka, Zhang, and Wells (2002) conducted a secondary analysis of National Health and Nutrition Examination Survey (NHANES) data fielded in 1996–1998. The findings indicated that nearly 80% of children and adolescents between the ages of 6 and 17 years did not receive needed mental health services. The unmet need was greatest among Latino children. This finding was both troubling and unexplainable. The researchers concluded that Latino adolescents have higher rates of suicidal thoughts, depression, and anxiety symptoms. In addition, these vulnerable adolescents tended to have higher dropout rates from high school than their White counterparts.

The Department of Veterans Affairs ambulatory care system was examined to determine if racial and ethnic variations existed in utilization of health services. Washington and colleagues (2002) found that removing the financial barrier to health care alone (i.e., because health care is free to veterans) did not lead to improved utilization rates among racially and ethnically diverse populations. Black, Hispanic, and American Indian veterans were 4.4, 2.5, and 1.9 times more likely, respectively, to report inability to receive care than White veterans (Washington et al., 2002).

In another study that examined access to care, Musey et al. (1995) found that lack of self-management skills, lack of funds to purchase insulin, and lack of transportation to be significant factors contributing to the observed differences in the occurrence of diabetic ketoacidosis among African Americans. The authors also reported that African Americans in this study failed to recognize symptoms of metabolic decomposition. The failure to recognize danger signals and to take action contributes to higher incidence of mortality among ethnic people of color. One plausible explanation for these findings is that African American diabetics may not have been taught appropriate preventive techniques, thereby suggesting racial differences in the care of ethnic minorities. It has been noted prior to this that racial and ethnic minority type 2 diabetics is frequently treated less efficaciously (i.e., with appropriate treatment regimes).

In a related study, the level of professionalism exhibited by a health care agency was associated with decreased use of health services by minority women. Jennings-Dozier, Simpson, Howard, and Marquez (2001) conducted focus group interviews in a public housing project. Women in these focus groups were asked open-ended questions about their feelings, attitudes, and perceptions of biases from health care providers. Findings from the interviews suggested that women in public housing were reluctant to use health services because of perceived racism and bias. Waiting time and the manner in which they were approached and addressed by health care professionals dissuaded the women from using the health care services. Gee (2002) found similar findings in a study of 1,503 individuals. Institutional and individual racial discrimination was reported as a barrier to the utilization of health services and was associated with poor health status as expressed by the respondents. The findings from these studies are consistent with findings of perceived discrimination reported by Rosenberg et al. (2002).

A RAND study of 83,000 people with the HIV virus found that going without needed care was associated with lack of funding, lack of transportation, feeling too ill, and inability to get out of work (Cunningham, 1999). These results are similar to those of studies seeking to explain the variation in health care indices reported in Secretary Heckler's report for the U.S. Department of Health and Human Services in 1985. However, little progress in changing the barriers to care, in changing access to care, and in developing culturally competent models of care has been observed, as noted in the report of Healthy People 2000 (Cunningham, 1999).

INTERVENTIONS AND APPROACHES TO REDUCE STRUCTURAL BARRIERS

Some successful strategies have been developed to increase access to health care. For example, Haas, Phillips, Sonneborn, McCulloch, and Liang (2002) found that managed care enabled Hispanic women to participate in health screening and detection programs. Hispanic women with managed care participated in mammography, papanicolau smear, and breast exams at higher rates than Hispanic women with fee-for-service insurance. Women in the managed care system may have felt more comfortable with an organized system that publicized the availability of the services and required no out-of-pocket costs. This factor may have contributed to the differences in health screening and detection.

In another study, the Community Hypertension Improvement Project improved treatment adherence in high-risk, underserved, ethnically diverse populations by utilizing a variety of interventions. Both African Americans and Hispanics exhibited significant and sustained improvement in the management of their hypertension at 12-month follow-up from individualized counseling provided by racially and ethnically matched community health workers and from home visits. This and other studies have demonstrated that health disparities can be eliminated by the development and implementation of culturally and racially competent interventions (Morrisky, Lees, Sharif, Liu, & Ward, 2002). The inclusion of community workers from the same racial group was an important variable in the success of the interventional strategies. Similarly, Earp and colleagues (2002) in their North Carolina Breast Screening program observed increased use of preventive health screening and detection programs. The authors utilized African American lay health advisors to provide education and motivation to African American women in rural settings.

Finally, Burnes-Bolton and Georges (1996) developed the National Black Nurses Association Community Collaboration Model in 1992–1993 to teach ethnic and racially diverse populations preventive care techniques and methods for these individuals to recognize racially different care. Between 1994 and 1996 the model was used to address specific health care disparity issues in 100 communities in the United States. Working with community action groups, faith-based programs, public health departments, and ethnic health professional organizations, the researchers identified health care needs, quantified gaps in health care access and quality, and developed specific programs.

Since 1996, the model has been used in communities throughout the United States, the eastern Caribbean, and South Africa. Subsequent studies have used the model to launch health literacy screening projects. The inability to read and comprehend health messages and instructions contributes to the gap in health disparities among ethnic people of color. Launching projects to improve health literacy has led to improvement in the utilization of health services, personal health behavior improvement, and a decrease in risky health behavior.

A review of the literature points out a glaring gap in the research on racial and ethnic minority groups and health disparities. For example, there were no intervention studies found that addressed structural barriers, such as institutional racism, that contribute to health disparities. More rigor in these types of studies is needed. Nurse researchers should be encouraged and supported to do this research. Further, this should be a priority area for the Center on Health Disparities and the National Institute for Nursing Research.

Research studies continue to use small samples of African Americans, Latinos, and other racial and ethnic minorities. Researchers must make more concerted efforts to increase the number of racial and ethnic minorities in their samples. This must be part of the criteria used by funding sources and must monitored by funders. Further, African Americans and other racial and ethnic minority groups must also be encouraged to participate in these types of studies.

National databases such as NHANES give us descriptive information but do not scrutinize the variables of racism and discrimination. Other studies with small sample size reduce the ability to generalize to a larger population. Follow-up studies are needed to further investigate the findings from smaller descriptive studies. Nurse researchers and other researchers interested in health disparities research should be encouraged to replicate studies related to racism and discrimination.

RECOMMENDATIONS TO REMOVE BARRIERS TO HEALTH CARE AND CLOSE THE GAP IN HEALTH DISPARITIES

The studies reported in this chapter illustrate the existence of structural barriers and the relation of these barriers to health outcomes among African

American, Hispanic, Asian Pacific Islander, Native American, and Alaskan Native populations. The gaps in health disparities continue to widen despite national policy efforts launched at the federal, state, and local level. It is critical that concerted and sustained initiatives be launched to remove the barriers, including the observed racial bias and discrimination in the delivery of primary and tertiary health care services.

A summary of the recommendations based on a critique and analysis of published research follows.

1. Use collaboration and empowerment models such as the National Black Nurses Association Community Collaboration model to reach ethnic and racially diverse populations and to teach preventive care techniques and methods for these individuals to recognize racially different care.
2. Implement the recommendations of the National Advisory Council on Nursing Education and Practice, the Division of Nursing, and the Health Resource Service Administration Racial and Ethnic Populations Agenda. The recommendations call for an increase in the number of providers from ethnic and racial populations. Because consumers have noted concern specifically regarding provider behavior, it is essential that the health care team complement the demographic population of those they serve.
3. Conduct more research to determine whether ethnically and racially diverse populations are more likely to utilize health services and have more confidence in professionals from their ethnic and racial group.
4. Expand the work on perception of racism and birth outcomes and other disease entities.
5. Work with professional associations to set and implement standards for developing and disseminating self-care health messages that are culturally relevant. Using culturally relevant and appropriate messages increases the likelihood of acceptance and initiation of actions to address the specific health problem experienced by the ethnically and racially diverse individual.
6. Develop health professional curricula that are gender- and culturally sensitive. The curricula should factor in the biogenetic differences by race and the implications to rendering culturally competent care to diverse populations.
7. Develop and financially support a federal health policy agenda beyond *Healthy People 2010*: identify of the health problems

facing Americans, articulate the gaps in health disparities, and delineate the most effective interventions and preventive health care practices at the individual and population level. While obvious health disparities have been identified, many of these disparities have not been linked with specific actions for funding the necessary programs to ensure access to quality, culturally relevant health care services.

REFERENCES

Alexander, G., Kogan, M., & Nabukera, S. (2002) Racial differences in prenatal care use in the United States: Are disparities decreasing? *American Journal of Public Health, 92,* 1970–1975.

Ayala, C., Greenlund, K., Croft, J., Keenan, N., Donehoo, R., Giles, W., Kittner, S., & Marks, J. (2001). Racial/ethnic disparities in mortality by stroke subtype in the United States, 1995–1998. *American Journal of Epidemiology, 154,* 1057–1063.

Barfield, W. D., Wise, P. H., Rust, F. P., Rust, K. J., Gould, J. B., & Gortmaker, S. L. (1996). Racial disparities in outcomes of military and civilian births in California. *Archives of Pediatrics & Adolescent Medicine, 15,* 1062–1067.

Becker, L., Han, B., Meyer, P., et al., & CPR Chicago Project. (1993). Racial difference in the incidence of cardiac arrest and subsequent survival. *New England Journal of Medicine, 329,* 600–607.

Bobo, L. (2001). Racial attitudes and relations at the close of the twentieth century. In N. J. Smelser, W. J. Wilson, & F. Mitchell (Eds.), *America becoming: Racial trends and their social consequences* (Vol. 1, pp. 273–301). Washington, DC: National Research Council.

Braithwaite, R., & Taylor, S. (2001). *Health issues in the Black community* (2nd ed.). San Francisco: Jossey-Bass.

Brett, K., Schoendorf, K., Kiely, J. (1994). Differences between Black and White women in the use of prenatal care technologies. *American Journal of Obstetrics and Gynecology, 170*(1), 41–46.

Bullough, V. L., & Bullough, B. (1982). *Health care for the other Americans.* East Norwalk, CT: Appleton-Century-Crofts.

Burnes-Bolton, L., & Georges, C. A. (1996). National Black Nurses Association Community Collaboration Model. *Journal of the National Black Nurses Association, 8*(2), 48–67.

Celano, M., Geller, R. J., Phillips, K. M., & Ziman, R. (1998). Treatment adherence among low-income children with asthma. *Journal of Pediatric Psychology, 23,* 345–349.

Chinn, M., Zang, J., & Merrell, K. (1998). Diabetes in African-American Medicare populations: Morbidity, quality of care, and resource utilization. *Diabetes Care, 21,* 1090–1095.

Chu, K., Swor, R., Jackson, R., Domier, R., Sadler, E., Basse, E., Zaleznak, H., & Gitlin, J. (1998). Race and survival after out-of-hospital cardiac arrest in a suburban community. *Annals of Emergency Medicine, 31*, 478–482.

Cohall, A., & Bannister, H. (2001). The health status of children. In R. Braithwaite & S. Taylor (Eds.), *Health issues in the Black community* (pp. 13–43). San Francisco: Jossey-Bass.

Cohen, R. A., Bloom, B., Simpson, G., & Parsons, P. E. (1997). Access to health care, part 3: Older adults. *Vital Health Statistics, 10* (198).

Cornelius, L., Smith, P., & Simpson, G. (2002, April). What factors hinder women of color from obtaining prenatal care? *American Journal of Public Health, 92*, 535–534.

Cowie, C., & Harris, M. (1997). Ambulatory medical care for Non-Hispanic Whites, African-Americans, and Mexican Americans with NIDDM in the U.S. *Diabetes Care, 20,* 142–147.

Cunningham, W. (1999). The impact of competing subsidence and barriers on access to medical care. *Medicare, 37*, 1270–1281.

Decklebaum, R. J., Fisher, E. A., & Winston, M., et al. (1999). Summary of a scientific conference on preventive nutrition: Pediatrics to geriatrics. *Circulation, 100*, 450–456.

Demissie, K., Rhoads, G., Ananth, C., Alexander, G., Kramer, M., Kogan, M., & Joseph, K. (2001). Trends in preterm birth and neonatal mortality among Blacks and Whites in the United States from 1989 to 1997. *American Journal of Epidemiology, 154,* 307–315.

Earp, J., Eng, E., O'Malley, M., Altpeter, M., Rauscher, G., Mayne, L., Mathews, H., Lynch, K., & Qaqish, B. (2002, April). Increasing use of mammography among older, rural African-American women: Results from a community trial. *American Journal of Public Health, 92*, 646–654.

Esser-Stuart, L., & Lyons, N. (2002). Barriers and influences in seeking health care among lower income minority women. *Social Work in Health Care, 35*, 85–99.

Gee, G. (2002). A multi-level analysis of the relationship between institutional and individual racial discrimination and health status. *American Journal of Public Health, 92*, 615–623.

Giger, J. N., & Davidhizar, R. (1999). *Transcultural nursing: Assessment and intervention.* St. Louis: Mosby.

Haas, J., Phillips, K., Sonneborn, D., McCulloch, C., & Liang, S. (2002, September). Effect of managed care insurance on the use of preventive care for specific ethnic groups in the US. *Medical Care, 40*, 743–751.

Institute of Medicine. (2002). *Unequal treatment: Confronting racial and ethnic disparities in health care.* Washington, DC: National Academy Press.

Jennings-Dozier, K., Simpson, E., Howard, M., & Marquez, M. (2001). Health and healthcare barriers among minority women in public housing. *Journal of the National Black Nurse Association, 12*(1), 18–24.

Jones, C. P. (2000). Levels of racism: A theoretical framework of a gardener's tale. *American Journal of Public Health, 90,* 1212–1215.

Kataoka, S., Zhang, L., & Wells, K. (2002, September). Unmet needs for mental health care among U.S. children: Variation by ethnicity and insurance status. *American Journal of Psychiatry, 159*, 1548–1555.

Klag, M., Whelton, P., Coresh, J., et al. (1991, February 6). The association of skin color with blood pressure in U.S. Blacks with low socioeconomic status. *Journal of the American Medical Association, 265*, 599–602.

Komaromy, M., Grumbach, K., Drake, M., Vranizan, K., Lurie, N., Keane, D., & Bindman, A. (1996). The role of Black and Hispanic physicians in providing healthcare for underserved populations. *New England Journal of Medicine, 334*, 1305–1310.

Luder, E., Melnick, T., & DiMaio, M. (1998). Association of being overweight with greater asthma symptoms in inner city Black and Hispanic children. *Journal of Pediatrics, 132*, 699–703.

Moore, R., Stanton, D., Gopalan, R., & Chaisson, R. (1994). Racial differences in the use of drug therapy for HIV disease in the urban community. *New England Journal of Medicine, 330*, 763–768.

Morrisky, D., Lees, N., Sharif, B., Liu, K., & Ward, H. (2002). Reducing health disparities in hypertension control: A community based hypertension control project for an ethnically diverse population. *Health Promotions Practice, 3*, 264–275.

Musey, V., Crawford, R., Klatkat, M., McAdams, D., & Phillips, L. (1995). Diabetes in urban African-Americans: Cessation of insulin therapy is the major precipitating cause of diabetic ketoacidosis. *Diabetes, 18*, 1483–1489.

National Cancer Institute. (2001). Highlights of NCI's cancer prevention and control programs. Available at: *http://cis.nci.nih.gov//fact4_5htm*. Accessed July 24, 2001.

Nelson, K., Norris, K., & Mangione, C. (2002, April 22). Disparities in the diagnosis and pharmacologic treatment of high serum cholesterol by race and ethnicity: Data from the Third National Health and Nutrition Examination Survey. *Archives of Internal Medicine, 162*, 929–935.

Resnick, H. E., Valsania, P., Halter, J. B., & Lin, X. (1998). Differential effects of BMI on diabetes risk among Black and White Americans. *Diabetes Care, 21*, 1828–1835.

Rosenberg, L., Palmer, J., Wise, L., Horton, N., & Corwin, M. (2002). Perceptions of racial discrimination and the risk of preterm birth. *Epidemiology, 13*, 646–652.

See, K., & Wilson, W. (1989). Race and ethnicity. In N. J. Smelser (Ed.), *Handbook of sociology* (pp. 223–242). Beverly Hills, CA: Sage.

Shapiro, M., Morton, S., McCafferty, D., Senterfitt, J., Fleishman, J., Perlman, J., Athey, L., Keesey, J., Goldma, D., Berry, S., & Bozette, S. (1999). Variations in the care of HIV-infected adults in the United States: Results from the HIV VOST and Service Utilization Study. *Journal of the American Medical Association, 265*, 3255–3264.

Stewart, S. H., & Silverstein, M. D. (2002). Racial and ethnic disparity in blood pressure and cholesterol measurement. *Journal of General Internal Medicine, 17*, 405–411.

U.S. Department of Health and Human Services. (1985). *Report of the Secretary's Task Force on Black and Minority Health, Vol. 1 Executive summary.* Washington, DC: U.S. Government Printing Office.

Washington, D., Harada, D., Villa, V., Damron-Rodriguez, J., Dhanani, S., Shon, H., & Makinodan, T. (2002, March). Racial variations in Department of Veteran Affairs ambulatory care use and unmet health care needs. *Military Medicine, 167,* 235–241.

Winkleby, M., Robinson, T., Sundquist, J., & Kraemer, H. (1999). Ethnic variation in cardiovascular disease risk factors among children and young adults: Findings from the Third National Health and Nutrition Examination Survey, 1988–1994. *Journal of the American Medical Association, 281,* 1006–1013.

Chapter 4

Language Barriers and Access to Care

SeonAe Yeo

ABSTRACT

The purpose of this chapter is to examine how language barriers contribute to health disparities among ethnic and racial minorities in the United States. A literature search was systematically conducted using selected computer databases (MEDLINE and CINAHL). Searches were limited to English-language-published research in the years from 1985 to 2003. A total of 47 published articles were included in this review. Overall these studies indicate that language barriers are associated with longer visit time per clinic visit, less frequent clinic visits, less understanding of physician's explanation, more lab tests, more emergency room visits, less follow-up, and less satisfaction with health services. The results also indicate that people who are older, poorer, and female tend to have severe language barriers compared to those who are younger, wealthier, and male. Improvement of communication between patients and providers in relation to health disparity consists of cultural competency and communication skills. Implications of these studies for practice and further research are outlined.

Keywords: access to care, cultural and linguistic competency, language barriers

Language is the means by which a patient accesses the health care system, learns about services, and makes decisions about her or his health behavior (Woloshin, Schwartz, Katz, & Welch, 1997). Language is also the means by which the health care provider accesses a patient's beliefs about health

59

and illness, and thus creates an opportunity to address and reconcile different belief systems. In essence, communication between nurses and patients is the heart of nursing care.

In the last twenty years, the United States has experienced a dramatic increase in the number of people who speak a language other than English as their primary language (U.S. Census Bureau, 2002). This is mainly because during this time the United States has experienced a rapid increase in the number of immigrants from Mexico and various countries from Latin America and Asia. In the 1990s, the foreign-born population nearly doubled to 31 million, or 11% of the 281 million that constitute the U.S. population (Morse, 2002). Of the total foreign-born population, 51% were born in Latin America and 25.5% were born in Asia. When both citizens and noncitizens are combined, it is estimated that nearly 25 million adults experience language barriers when they receive health care.

Within the broad Hispanic or Asian categories, the ethnic minority groups in the United States are quite diverse. Within the 35 million counted as Hispanic or Latino, more than half are Mexican; the remainder are Puerto Rican, Cuban, Dominican, Costa Rican, Guatemalan, Honduran, Nicaraguan, Panamanian, Salvadoran, Argentinean, Bolivian, Chilean, Colombian, Ecuadorian, Paraguayan, Peruvian, and Venezuelan. Though they share a common language, Spanish, they differ vastly in their health beliefs, behaviors, and lifestyles. Asian and Pacific Islander Americans (APIAs) are estimated at 11 million (or 4% of the U.S. population), with almost 60 different national and ethnic origins, including such groups as Chinese, Japanese, Korean, Mon-Khmer/Cambodian, Mian/Hmong, Thai, Laotian, Vietnamese, and Tagalog. Each APIA possesses at least one unique language and usually multiple distinctively different cultures. Hispanics or Asians who perceive language barriers when they access health care tend to be new to the United States (D'Avanzo, 1992) and often do not have commercial health insurance (Hampers, Cha, Gutglass, Binns, & Krug, 1999; Schur & Albers, 1996).

Differences in language between health care providers and patients increasingly impose barriers to health care. The purpose of this critical research review is to describe the relation of language barriers among racial and ethnic minorities and to examine how language barriers may contribute to health disparities among these populations. The Health Resources and Service Administration (HRSA) defines health disparity as a population-specific difference in the presence of disease, health outcomes, or access to care (*Eliminating Health Disparities in the United States,*

2001). Language barriers between patients and health care providers may affect all three outcomes (i.e., disease incidence, health outcomes, or access to care). This review focuses specifically on published studies that address language barriers and access to care in an effort to address health disparities in racial and ethnic minorities.

METHODS

A literature search was systematically conducted using selected computer databases (MEDLINE and CINAHL). The databases were searched using the following keywords with various logical connections: *language, communication barrier, access to care, health service accessibility, health disparity,* and *health outcome.* Searches were limited to English-language published research from 1985 to 2003.

RESULTS

A total of 47 articles were included in this review. Research studies accounted for 28 of the articles (16 quantitative and 12 qualitative studies); 8 were review articles, and the others consisted of reports, consensus statements, or position papers. Data-based articles conducted in the United States form the basis for this review. Of these 16 quantitative studies, 11 studies were conducted in the United States, 3 were in Australia, 1 in England, and 1 in Canada. Twelve articles report the results of qualitative studies. Four of these studies were conducted in the United States, four were in Australia, three in England, and one in Canada.

Only one study used a randomized trial method (Hornberger et al., 1996). The other 10 quantitative studies included 4 cross-sectional studies (Derose & Baker, 2000; David & Rhee, 1998; Feinberg, Swartz, Zaslavsky, Gardner, & Walker, 2002; Meredith, Stewart, & Brown, 2001); 3 cohort studies—1 retrospective (Jacobs et al., 2001) and 2 prospective (Hampers et al., 1999; Kravitz, Helms, Azari, Antonius, & Melnikow, 2000); and 1 chart review (Heilemann, Lee, Stinson, Koshar, & Goss, 2000).

Overall, these studies indicate that language barriers are associated with lack of awareness about health care benefits (such as Medicaid eligibility) (Feinberg et al., 2002), less insured status (Hampers et al., 1999), longer visit time per clinic visit (Kravitz et al., 2000), less frequent clinic visits (Derose & Baker, 2000), less understanding of the physician's explanations (David & Rhee, 1998; Gerrish, 2001), more lab tests (Hampers et al., 1999), more emergency room visits (Hampers et al., 1999), less follow-up (Kravitz et al., 2000), and less satisfaction with health services (Meredith et al., 2001; Morales, Cunningham, Brown, Liu, & Hays, 1999). Because these are observational studies (i.e., descriptive study design), no causal relations can be established between a language barrier and these negative consequences. Furthermore, none of the studies address how these negative experiences are related to actual health outcomes or disease incidences. In the following discussion section, the content of 47 articles is discussed in an attempt to answer the research question: How do language barriers contribute to health disparities among ethnic and racial minorities in the United States?

DISCUSSION

A limited number of database studies provide a platform from which to analyze possible relationships between language barrier, access to care, and health outcomes. In order to examine these relationships, the characteristics of people with language barriers in the United States are summarized from other sources so that potential spurious relationships can be identified. Various translation services have been used to facilitate communication in daily clinical settings, and the effectiveness of these translation services is discussed. Lastly, research directions are suggested based on the results of this review.

Characteristics of People with Language Barriers

In the reviewed articles, only a few studies conducted in the United States concur that certain demographic factors are associated with the level of English proficiency across races and ethnicities. Jacobs and colleagues (2001) studied a total of 4,380 adults continuously enrolled in a health maintenance organization for two years. Their descriptive data indicate that those who did not speak English well enough were significantly older ($p < .01$) and poorer ($p < .01$). In addition, more women than men tended to have severe language barriers. Derose and Baker's (2000) study of Latinos ($N = 724$) also revealed that Latinos with limited English proficiency (LEP) were older than Latinos with better English proficiency. Further, Latinos with LEP were more likely to be female and to be less literate than English speakers of all ethnicities.

Some groups of Asians, such as Japanese, are an exception to the characteristics of persons with LEP previously described. Japanese are often excluded from underserved populations because of their greater similarity to non-Hispanic Whites in socioeconomic status. Yet Japanese clients also identify language as the most difficult and obvious obstacle to access to health care in the United States (Yeo, Fetters, & Maeda, 2000). Many Asians share similar disadvantages as Latinos when it comes to language barriers (Carey Jackson et al., 2000; D'Avanzo, 1992; Gerrish, 2001; Meredith et al., 2001). Thus a language barrier, regardless of socioeconomic status, may be an independent factor that negatively affects access to care.

Language Barriers and Access to Care

The consequences of language barriers range from miscommunication (David & Rhee, 1998) to inefficient use of health care services (Hampers et al., 1999; Kravitz et al., 2000). Some studies describe behavior due to cultural beliefs without clearly differentiating it from behavior due to language barriers (Carey Jackson et al., 2000; Derose & Baker, 2000; Feinberg et al., 2002; Meredith et al., 2001). Culturally specific health beliefs and behaviors must be considered separately from barriers related to language. In other words, the use of translators does not in itself decrease barriers to care.

As an example, one study (David & Rhee, 1998) compared the understanding of side effects of two groups (those who had good English skills and those who either had poor English skills or brought translators) using a written survey of yes/no questions. In this study, Spanish-speaking people who had poor English skills regardless of having a translator had significantly less understanding of the side effects explained to them than those with good English skills (41% vs. 16%). Researchers did not examine whether language barriers or culturally specific health beliefs were the reason for the lack of understanding. Both groups showed similar responses regarding (1) how the understanding of side effects corresponded to *compliance* with medication; (2) the feeling that they had enough time to communicate with doctors; and (3) whether they received enough explanation about preventive tests. Both groups also demonstrated a similar proportion of people who took preventive tests in last 2 years.

Differences exist in the proportions of people who say (1) that they understand the side effects of medication; (2) that they are satisfied with medical care; and (3) that they feel that their doctor understands how they feel. If the language was the only barrier, why did the translator fail to explain the side effects of medication? Why are they less satisfied with medical care? And why do they feel the doctor does not understand how they feel? It is possible, though caution must be applied because of overinterpretation, that side effects of medication, medical care, and doctor's responses are difficult to comprehend because of the differences in the health beliefs of patients and the health care system.

Language barriers have been linked to limited access to health services. For example, several studies have reported negative associations between the presence of language barriers and the number of health care visits (Derose & Baker, 2000; Feinberg et al., 2002; Jacobs et al., 2001). Feinberg and others examined Medicaid enrollment of children in non-English-speaking families. They report that those who did not speak English at home were less likely to be aware of Medicaid eligibility for their children. The study did not indicate the effect on health outcomes; further studies are necessary to determine this effect.

In contrast, some studies do not present a clear relationship between the patient's perception of health services (e.g., satisfaction with or acceptance of health service) and a language barrier (Carey Jackson et al., 2000; Meredith et al., 2001; Morales et al., 1999). For example, the association between adherence to various regimens and language barriers is not well delineated. Brach and Fraser (2000), in their review article, attribute the mixed findings to the literature's failure to find a clear relationship between general clinician-patient communication and adherence. Regardless of language barrier, communications between health care providers and patients often involve misunderstanding, and thus poor compliance. Morales and colleagues (1999) studied English- and Spanish-speaking Latinos in a cross-sectional study ($N = 7,093$). They report that Latinos who responded in Spanish were significantly more dissatisfied than Latinos who spoke in English. Dissatisfaction was measured by five observations about medical staff: (1) they listen to what patients say; (2) they give answers to questions; (3) they explain about prescribed medications; (4) they explain about medical procedures and test results; and (5) they give reassurance and support. It is important to note that dissatisfaction indicates the poor quality of communication—but this may or may not be related to language barriers.

According to a national survey, 33% of Hispanics and 27% of Asians, as compared to 16% of Whites and 23% of African Americans, reported communication problems similar to the study's results. Similarities included failing to understand their physician, feeling that their physician did not listen to them, or declining to ask the physician questions about their care. These statistics included both English- and non-English-speaking people. The study further reported that, among Hispanics, 43% of non-English speakers had communication problems compared to 26% of English-speaking Hispanics. Among Asians, these percentages were 39 and 25, respectively (Anonymous, 2002). It should be pointed out that one in four minority patients who speak English have communication problems with their doctors, compared to 16% of Whites. In sum, both language barrier and minority status are associated with poor communication with care providers. The causal relationships among minority status, language barriers, and perceived barriers to care are not well examined.

A few more insights into this relationship are provided by small-scale ethnographic studies. Focus group studies with content and semantic analyses were conducted by Cave, Maharaj, Gibson, and Jackson (1995) to improve cross-cultural communication in Edmonton, Canada. The results of this study provide rich qualitative information applicable to the United States. The study involved recent immigrants from various countries and a group of physicians who treated them. Patients were from Chile, India, East Africa, and Jamaica. They had lived in Canada from 9 months to 7 years. Both physicians and patients raised the problem of compliance; however, the physicians questioned the patients' compliance with prescribed medications, while the patients insisted they complied until the point where they thought the treatment failed. The doctors felt that understanding the patients' culture better would help achieve better diagnosis and more effective management. The patients did not understand the intent of the physicians' questions about their culture and habits and sometimes found such inquiries intrusive or irrelevant. Thus they did not disclose personal information about themselves. At the same time, patients sometimes expected physicians to inherently know their perspective with little or no explanation. These cultural differences can be viewed as barriers to care, but they are not necessarily language barriers.

In efforts to understand the relation between language and health outcomes, Heilemann and colleagues (2000) conducted a chart review in rural northern California hospitals. The investigators compared perinatal outcomes of 773 women of Mexican descent. They measured acculturation in three different ways: by place of birth, by language spoken, and by the two factors combined as on the acculturation index. The results indicated that language spoken was a less useful indicator of perinatal outcome complications than place of birth or the acculturation index. This study intended to demonstrate that negative health outcomes are the result of culturally determined health behaviors, not a language barrier. In this study, language was not correlated with the degree of acculturation among Latinos. A study by Meredith and colleagues (2001) comparing health perspectives among different ethnic groups may give further insight into the issue of language, culture, and health behaviors. In this study, Asian and Pacific Islanders had better self-reported health, but they were less satisfied and perceived less sharing in physician-patient relationships as compared to Whites. A limitation of this study is that findings were not analyzed by language proficiency, but only by ethnicity and race. Although there is a significant percentage of Asians and Hispanics with LEP, it is unclear how language barriers contributed to negative perceptions of health encounters.

Thompson and others (2002) reported that Hispanics were much less likely than non-Hispanic Whites to ever have had cancer screening. Socio-economic status was explored as a predictor of differences between Hispanics and non-Hispanic Whites in cancer prevention behavior. In a cross-sectional study, in-person interviews ($N = 1,795$) were conducted in a population-based random sample of adults in 20 communities with a high proportion of Hispanics. Hispanics were significantly less likely than non-Hispanic Whites to ever have had cervical ($p < 0.001$), breast ($p = 0.007$) or colorectal cancer screening (FOBT $p = 0.008$; sigmoidoscopy/colonoscopy $p < 0.002$). After adjusting for socioeconomic status (education and having health insurance), only differences in cervical cancer remained significant ($p = 0.024$). After adjusting for socioeconomic status, Hispanics had a significantly higher intake of fruits and vegetables per day (4.84 servings) than non-Hispanic Whites (3.84 servings) ($p < 0.001$); and the fat behavior score was marginally significant after adjustment for socioeconomic status ($p = 0.053$). Significantly fewer Hispanics were current smokers than non-Hispanic Whites ($p < 0.001$). The researchers concluded that there is only limited support for the hypothesis that socioeconomic status is a major determinant of some cancer-related behaviors. Specifically, in this study, socioeconomic status was related to mammography and colorectal screening, but not to cervical cancer, dietary behavior, or smoking. Cancer screenings were lower in Hispanics regardless of the existence of language barriers. The study did not assess health beliefs related to screening. This may have been a factor in the low rates of screening.

In addition, several studies demonstrate that language barriers result in both inefficiency and potential increases in costs (Hampers et al., 1999; Kravitz et al., 2000). For instance, Hampers indicates that patients with language barriers have significantly higher test costs ($145 vs. $105) and longer emergency department stays (165 minutes vs. 137 minutes) than their English-speaking counterparts. Kravitz also demonstrated that Spanish- and Russian-speaking patients averaged 9.1 and 5.6 minutes longer for visits, respectively, than English-speaking patients. Clearly, health services must be made more effective and efficient for non-English-speaking patients.

Translation Services as a Solution

When a language barrier is identified between patient and care provider, provision of various interpreter services is an obvious and frequently proposed solution (Baker, Hayes, & Fortier, 1998; Poss & Beeman, 1999; Tang, 1999; Woloshin, Bickell, Schwartz, Gany, & Welch, 1995; Zimmermann, 1997). Various approaches to interpretation exist, including on-site professional interpreters, ad hoc interpreters (e.g., staff pulled away from other duties to interpret, friends and family members, strangers from the waiting room), and simultaneous remote interpretations using earphones and microphones with off-site professional interpreters (Brach & Fraser, 2000).

The quality of interpretation depends on the adequacy of interpretation, the bilingual ability of staff, and the accuracy and content of a competent medical interpretation (Woloshin et al., 1995). For example, when patients have to rely on family members for interpretation, the content of medical advice is often not fully understood (Gerrish, 2001) and patients are less satisfied with the health service (Lee, Batal, Maselli, & Kutner, 2002). Lee surveyed the satisfaction of English- and Spanish-speaking patients receiving acute care. Spanish speakers who had to rely on family members or ad hoc interpreters were 54% and 49% less satisfied than those who were provided AT&T telephone interpreters. Only a few studies have examined the effect of translation service and access to health care (Baker et al., 1998; Derose & Baker, 2000; Feinberg et al., 2002; Jacobs et al., 2001; Lee et al., 2002). But no study in this review examined the relationship between quality of interpretation service and disease incidence or improvement in compliance and health outcomes. Rather, the studies assessed satisfaction and perception of care. These studies reasonably demonstrated, however, that translation services may improve access to care, satisfaction with health care, and possibly adherence (Brach & Fraser, 2000).

The current evidence indicates that simultaneous translation service is an effective and satisfactory mode of translation (Hornberger et al., 1996; Lee et al., 2002). According to Lee et al., patients who were provided access to AT& T telephone interpretation services reported identical satisfaction to English-speaking patients. As a result, both patient and care provider maintained higher-quality communication and perceived less disruption and more privacy. For example, Hornberger and others examined the effectiveness of a remote-simultaneous interpretation system on the communication between patients and physicians during routine postpartum checkups on women who spoke only Spanish. They measured the quality of communications by the outcome variables (i.e., satisfaction, number of physician-mother utterances, and accuracy of translation) using tape-recorded visits coded by trained native Spanish speakers who were fluent in English. The results indicated that, compared to traditional translators (control group), the number of utterances increased significantly among patients and physicians (23% and 10%, respectively). In terms of accuracy of translation, there were 12% fewer inaccuracies with the remote system than with on-site translation with a translator. Both physicians and patients preferred remote systems, giving reasons such as "feels more private" or "less disruption by a third party."

One study also evaluated the effectiveness of professionally trained translators. Jacobs et al. (2001) studied the effects of a systematic professional interpretation service on access to health care. The study revealed a significant increase in the number of office visits as well as the number of prescriptions written and filled among patients who received a systematic professional interpreter service on all occasions, including appointment desk and lab visits. On-site provision of a comprehensive interpretation service may be available at large facilities, but remote systems may be more a realistic solution for many community-based clinics. A few available studies examined different types of translation services (Hornberger et al., 1996; Lee et al., 2002). However, these studies were interested in patient satisfaction. Further research is needed to examine the effect of translation services on different health outcomes.

In summary, this critical research review found that language barriers are more pronounced among older, poorer, less educated, and newer immigrants. Addressing language barriers is an obvious means to improve access to health care among LEP persons. However, as these studies indicated, this will not be sufficient. Research is needed to further determine the effect of language on access to care, adherence to the regimens, quality of health care, satisfaction, disease incidences, and health outcomes.

Future Research Directions

Based on this review, the following areas are identified as future research needs. Among the three components that constitute a health disparity, access to care has been most studied and thus is the focus of this review. Access to care is analyzed from two aspects: exploration of interpretation services and improvement of communication between patients and providers. The former may require relatively straightforward research methodologies when the outcomes are patient satisfaction. Currently only one randomized control trial has been identified for this review. Similar studies are needed to evaluate and support policy changes.

For example, national standards for culturally and linguistically appropriate services in health care (CLAS, 2001) are a means to correct the inequities that currently exist in the provision of health services and to make these services more responsive to the individual needs of all patients. Further elaboration in designs and methodologies are required to determine the causal relationship between choice of interpretation service and health outcomes. Clinical trials need to be conducted to determine which interpretation services lead to better communication (i.e., access to care), change behaviors (i.e., health outcomes), and ultimately reduce diseases. With these reports, state and national health service policies must incorporate the optimal interpretation services. When systems such as a telephone translation service become widely available subsequent to policy changes, large-scale epidemiological studies may address these relationships.

Improvement of communication between patients and providers involves more complex and daunting tasks, since this is a more pervasive medical problem than language barriers alone. This issue involves cultural competency and communication skills. We need qualitative studies in cultural competency to develop more efficient models. Existing health belief and behavior models in the United States must be scrutinized for their cultural appropriateness before they are applied. A language barrier, a component of cultural appropriateness, then is clearly identified and analyzed in relation to other factors, which are closely related to it (Brach & Fraser, 2000). These factors include the role of bilingual care providers and an understanding of other health belief models.

Culture, defined as an "integrated pattern of human behavior that includes thoughts, communications, actions, religious or social group" (Cross et al., 1989), and language go hand-in-hand. Therefore, it is probably necessary to view the language barrier through a cultural competency model such as that of Brach and Fraser (2000). They propose a conceptual model of how interpreter services could reduce health disparities, based on their understanding of cultural competency. This model is by far the most developed and detailed. There is a merit to examining the direct link between language barriers and racial and ethnic health disparities because provision of interpretation is a tangible yet costly hypothesized solution. Other conceptual models, such as Anderson's access-to-care model, can be also used (Andersen, 1995; Andersen, Rice, & Kominski, 2001).

Historically, a language barrier was considered a disability, according to the expansion of the Civil Rights Act of 1964 (Woloshin et al., 1995). A language that has unique and fundamental characteristics of national origin should thus be protected rather than punished. This view was upheld by the Supreme Court in 1974; it thus enforced health programs funded by the Department of Health and Human Services (DHHS) to provide translation services to people with LEP. According to Woloshin, however, this law had three problems: (1) the regulation was vague; (2) funds were inadequate; and (3) enforcement was complaint-driven and ad hoc.

In 1997, the Office of Minority Health (OMH) undertook the development of more comprehensive national standards to provide culturally and linguistically appropriate services (CLAS, 2001). The CLAS standards were published in final form in the *Federal Register* on December 22, 2000, as recommended national standards for adoption or adaptation by various organizations and agencies.

Although it is clear that adequate funding is needed to provide high-quality translation services, currently only a handful of states reimburse for outpatient use of interpreters via a Medicaid mechanism. Health care providers in other states still put themselves at risk because they are obligated to perform a proper health assessment without adequate resources. The failure to do so can constitute negligence for which nurses and other health care providers may be held liable if the patient suffers some subsequent injury attributable to this failure (CLAS, 2001). In order to implement and evaluate the latest national standards (i.e., CLAS), evidence should be generated by studies with sound research designs and methodologies.

ACKNOWLEDGMENT

The author thanks Ms. Katherine Roberts for her assistance in the literature review.

REFERENCES

Andersen, R. M. (1995). Revisiting the behavioral model and access to medical care: Does it matter? *Journal of Health and Social Behavior, 36*(1), 1–10.

Andersen, R. M., Rice, T. M., & Kominski, G. F. (2001). *Changing the U.S. health care system: Key issues in health services, policy, and management.* San Francisco: Jossey-Bass.

Anonymous. (2002). Poor communications, cultural barriers impacting quality of health care for minorities. *Quality Letter for Healthcare Leaders, 14*(4), 11–13.

Baker, D. W., Hayes, R., & Fortier, J. P. (1998). Interpreter use and satisfaction with interpersonal aspects of care for Spanish-speaking patients. *Medical Care, 36,* 1461–1470.

Brach, C., & Fraser, I. (2000). Can cultural competency reduce racial and ethnic health disparities? A review and conceptual model. *Medical Care Research and Review, 57*(Suppl 1), 181–217.

Carey Jackson, J., Taylor, V. M., Chitnarong, K., Mahloch, J., Fischer, M., Sam, R., & Seng, P. (2000). Development of a cervical cancer control intervention program for Cambodian American women. *Journal of Community Health, 25,* 359–375.

Cave, A., Maharaj, U., Gibson, N., & Jackson, E. (1995). Physicians and immigrant patients. Cross-cultural communication. *Canadian Family Physician, 41,* 1685–1690.

CLAS. (2001). *National standards for culturally and linguistically appropriate services in health care: Final report* (Report). Washington, DC: U.S. Department of Health and Human Services, OPHS, Office of Minority Health.

Cross, T. L., Bazron, B. J., Dennis, K. W., & Isaacs, M. R. (1998). *Towards a culturally competent system of care: A monograph on effective services for minority children who are severely emotionally disturbed.* Washington, DC: CASSP Technical Assistance Center, Georgetown University Child Development Center.

D'Avanzo, C. E. (1992). Barriers to health care for Vietnamese refugees. *Journal of Professional Nursing, 8,* 245–253.

David, R. A., & Rhee, M. (1998). The impact of language as a barrier to effective health care in an underserved urban Hispanic community. *Mount Sinai Journal of Medicine, 65,* 393–397.

Derose, K. P., & Baker, D. W. (2000). Limited English proficiency and Latinos' use of physician services. *Medical Care Research and Review, 57*(1), 76–91.

Eliminating health disparities in the United States. (2001). Rockville: Health Resources and Service Administration.

Feinberg, E., Swartz, K., Zaslavsky, A. M., Gardner, J., & Walker, D. K. (2002). Language proficiency and the enrollment of Medicaid-eligible children in publicly funded health insurance programs. *Maternal and Child Health Journal, 6*(1), 5–18.

Gerrish, K. (2001). The nature and effect of communication difficulties arising from interactions between district nurses and South Asian patients and their carers. *Journal of Advanced Nursing, 33,* 566–574.

Hampers, L. C., Cha, S., Gutglass, D. J., Binns, H. J., & Krug, S. E. (1999). Language barriers and resource utilization in a pediatric emergency department. *Pediatrics, 103*(6 Pt 1), 1253–1256.

Heilemann, M. V., Lee, K. A., Stinson, J., Koshar, J. H., & Goss, G. (2000). Acculturation and perinatal health outcomes among rural women of Mexican descent. *Research in Nursing and Health, 23,* 118–125.

Hornberger, J. C., Gibson, C. D., Jr., Wood, W., Dequeldre, C., Corso, I., Palla, B., & Bloch, D. A. (1996). Eliminating language barriers for non-English-speaking patients. *Medical Care, 34,* 845–856.

Jacobs, E. A., Lauderdale, D. S., Meltzer, D., Shorey, J. M., Levinson, W., & Thisted, R. A. (2001). Impact of interpreter services on delivery of health care to limited-English-proficient patients. *Journal of General Internal Medicine, 16,* 468–474.

Kravitz, R. L., Helms, L. J., Azari, R., Antonius, D., & Melnikow, J. (2000). Comparing the use of physician time and health care resources among patients speaking English, Spanish, and Russian. *Medical Care, 38,* 728–738.

Lee, L. J., Batal, H. A., Maselli, J. H., & Kutner, J. S. (2002). Effect of Spanish interpretation method on patient satisfaction in an urban walk-in clinic. *Journal of General Internal Medicine, 17,* 641–645.

Meredith, L., Stewart, M., & Brown, J. B. (2001). Patient-centered communication scoring method report on nine coded interviews [Comment]. *Health Communication, 13*(1), 19–31.

Morales, L. S., Cunningham, W. E., Brown, J. A., Liu, H., & Hays, R. D. (1999). Are Latinos less satisfied with communication by health care providers? *Journal of General Internal Medicine, 14,* 409–417.

Poss, J. E., & Beeman, T. (1999). Effective use of interpreters in health care: Guidelines for nurse managers and clinicians. *Seminars for Nurse Managers, 7,* 166–171.

Schur, C. L., & Albers, L. A. (1996). Language, sociodemographics, and health care use of Hispanic adults. *Journal of Health Care for the Poor and Underserved, 7,* 140–158.

Tang, S. Y. (1999). Interpreter services in healthcare. Policy recommendations for healthcare agencies. *Journal of Nursing Administration, 29*(6), 23–29.

Thompson, B., Coronado, G. D., Solomon, C. C., McClerran, D. F., Neuhouser, M. L., & Feng, Z. (2002). Cancer prevention behaviors and socioeconomic status among Hispanics and non-Hispanic Whites in a rural population in the United States. *Cancer Causes & Control, 13,* 719–728.

U.S. Census Bureau. (2000). *Coming to America: A profile of the Nation's Foreign Born Census Brief: Current population survey.* Washington, DC: U.S. Department of Commerce, Economics and Statistics Administration.

Woloshin, S., Bickell, N. A., Schwartz, L. M., Gany, F., & Welch, H. G. (1995). Language barriers in medicine in the United States. *Journal of the American Medical Association, 273,* 724–728.

Woloshin, S., Schwartz, L. M., Katz, S. J., & Welch, H. G. (1997). Is language a barrier to the use of preventive services? *Journal of General Internal Medicine, 12,* 472–477.

Yeo, S., Fetters, M., & Maeda, Y. (2000). Japanese couples' childbirth experiences in Michigan: Implications for care. *Birth, 27,* 191–198.

Zimmermann, P. G. (1997). Enhancing your use of interpreters. *Nursing Spectrum (D.C./Baltimore Metro Edition), 7*(12), 12.

PART II

Special Populations

Chapter 5

Health Disparities Among Men from Racial and Ethnic Minority Populations

CONSTANCE DALLAS AND LINDA BURTON

ABSTRACT

The purpose of this chapter is to review empirical nursing literature on the health care of racial and ethnic minority men, specifically African American/ Black, Hispanic/Latino, American Indian/Alaskan Native, and Asian/Pacific Islander men. CINAHL and MEDLINE computer databases were searched from their earliest online date until 2003 using a combination of manual and computer-based methods to identify the nursing literature with samples that included minority men. Articles were selected according to their relevance to the four areas of adult health disparities targeted by the Department of Health and Human Services (DHHS): heart disease, malignant neoplasms (cancer), diabetes, and HIV/AIDS.

A total of 52 empirical articles were selected. Findings were categorized as addressing disease prevention, disease screening, or disease management of the targeted conditions. This review demonstrates that some important work has already been accomplished in nursing research to address the four adult health disparities targeted by DHHS. Future research should be based on gaps identified in existing literature and should be guided by culturally appropriate theories and constructs.

Keywords: health disparities, men's health

REVIEW OF NURSING LITERATURE ON MINORITY MEN

Racial and ethnic minority men face special health risks in addition to those faced by all men in the United States. The Secretary's Task Force

77

on Black and Minority Health of the Department of Health and Human Services (DHHS) reported that 60,000 excess or preventable deaths occur each year in minority populations (Centers for Disease Control (CDC), 1986). Heart disease and cancer, leading causes of death for all racial and ethnic groups and both sexes in the United States, kill Black men 45 to 64 years of age at 50% higher rates than White men of the same age (National Center for Health Statistics, 2002). Additionally, homicides and accidents (unintentional injuries) account for 60% of excess mortality among Latino males less than 65 years of age. Unintentional injuries account for 44% of excess mortality among American Indian males and 38% among Black males under age 45. Cirrhosis of the liver, secondary to excessive alcohol use, accounts for 13% of excess mortality among American Indian males less than 70 years of age. The purpose of this chapter is to review nursing literature on the health care of racial and ethnic minority men, specifically those men belonging to the DHHS targeted racial and ethnic minority groups: African American/Black, Hispanic/Latino, American Indian/Alaskan Native, and Asian/Pacific Islander.

The nursing profession has the potential to contribute significantly to the reduction of health disparities and to decrease the number of preventable deaths in vulnerable populations through research, education, and clinical practice. Nursing research provides the foundation for future research, education, and clinical practice, but it has traditionally limited its focus to the health issues of women and children. DHHS is committed to achieving significant reductions of racial and ethnic health disparities for adults by 2010 in cardiovascular disease, cancer screening and management, diabetes, and HIV infection/AIDS. Minority men face health disparities in life expectancy, cancer prevention and control, heart disease, diabetes, and mental health disorders (Smedley, Stith, & Nelson, 2002).

To promote quality research, education, and clinical care of minority populations targeted by DHHS, nursing research must provide adequate and appropriate knowledge to prevent, assess, and manage the leading causes of morbidity and mortality for minority men. The 10 leading causes of mortality in the United States vary both by gender and by race and ethnicity (CDC, 2002). Men from all racial and ethnic groups constitute 49.1% of the U.S. population. Including sex as a research variable could improve the overall quality of medical science and benefit the health of both men and women (Doyal, 2001). Although cancer mortality is the second leading cause of death for both genders, prostate and lung cancer are the leading causes of cancer mortality for men, who smoke more than women (American Cancer Society, 2003).

Being born non-White in the United States all too often means living a significantly less healthy life (Rich & Ro, 2002). All men in the United States have a lower life expectancy than women (74.1 versus 79.4 years), but the rate is even worse for minority men. The life expectancy of most minority men is lower than that for White men and for both White and ethnic women. American Indian men (66.1 years) and African American men (67.6 years) have the lowest life expectancies of any group (Hoyert, Arias, Smith, Murphy, & Kochanek, 2001). The expected lifespans for Native Hawaiian men (71.5 years), Puerto Rican men (70.8 years), and Latino men (69.6 years) are also lower than for White men. There many reasons for these disparities, but some are related to the quality of services received.

For example, when researchers controlled for socioeconomic factors such as financial status, symptom acuity, and patient preference, African American men still received lower-quality care and were less likely than their White counterparts to undergo invasive diagnostic cardiac procedures (Schulman et al., 1999). In addition, almost two thirds of African American patients and more than half of Hispanic patients believe that they receive lower-quality health care than do White patients (Lillie-Blanton, Brodie, Rowland, Altman, & McIntosh, 2000; Weinrich, Weinrich, Priest, Fodi, & Talley, 2001). How much of the difference in life expectancy is related to these and other reasons needs to be examined critically.

The increasing racial and ethnic diversity of the U.S. population and growing evidence of significant racial and ethnic health disparities make having adequate knowledge of racial and ethnic minority men a critical priority for quality nursing care. This review provides an important foundation for understanding these health disparities, and the other National Institutes of Health (NIH) have designated this as a research priority. This review also provides an important foundation for future nursing research that will be consistent with the NINR's (National Institute of Nursing Research) Strategic Plan to address health disparities.

METHODS

CINAHL and MEDLINE computer databases were searched from their first online year (1983 for CINAHL, 1966 for MEDLINE) to the present, using a combination of manual and computer-based methods to identify the nursing literature that included any racial and ethnic minority men in the sample and that addressed any of the four areas of adult health disparities targeted by DHHS: heart disease, malignant neoplasms (cancer), diabetes, and human immunodeficiency virus (HIV)/AIDS. CINAHL and MEDLINE databases were selected because of their long-standing reputations as the principal databases of English-language scholarly nursing literature.

Keywords used included *Hispanic men/Latino men, African American men/Black men/Negro men, Asian men/Oriental men, Pacific Islander men/ Hawaiian men/Samoan men, American Indian men/Alaskan men/Eskimo men,* and *colored men/men of color.* The search was then expanded to combine the keywords above with one or more of the following terms: *heart disease, cardiovascular disease, cancer, diabetes, HIV, AIDS, acculturation,* and *immigrants.* Articles were included if they were English-language articles published in a U.S. nursing journal after 1983 for CINAHL and 1966 for MEDLINE, and if they involved at least one adult Hispanic/Latino, African American/Black, American Indian/Alaskan Native, or Asian/Pacific Islander man and addressed one of the four areas of health disparities targeted by NIH. Articles with a primary focus on culturally competent care, theoretical or conceptual articles, reviews, editorials, commentaries, letters, research reports, dissertations, articles written for the lay public, and clinical articles such as drug reports were excluded.

FINDINGS

Despite the high morbidity and mortality rates for heart disease, cancer, diabetes, and HIV/AIDS among minority men, nursing research published from 1983 to the present rarely included racial and ethnic minority men in study samples. Only 52 empirical articles met the inclusion criteria, and most of those included African Americans and Whites rather than members of other racial and ethnic groups. The 52 citations included at least one minority man in the sample and addressed heart disease (9), cancer (29), diabetes (4), and/or HIV/AIDS (10). These 52 articles were published in 18 nursing journals. Approximately 78% of the 52 studies were quantitative, 11% were qualitative, and 11% were mixed method. Researchers overwhelmingly favored cross-sectional, correlational designs. Thus intervention studies (8%) and experimental studies (8%) were rare, and only 18% included either a randomized sample or a control group.

Ideally, empirical studies lead to the validation or refinement of theoretical or conceptual frameworks (LoBiondo-Wood & Haber, 1998); however, validation and refinement are best when investigators incorporate theory into their studies. Less than half of these 52 studies (34%) used a theoretical or conceptual framework, and approximately half used the Health Belief Model (47%). None of the investigators used conceptual frameworks specifically developed for the populations they studied. Many of the studies included small convenience samples, but 38% of the articles used sample sizes of at least 100 persons, and a few included sample sizes of over 1,000 men. Despite using samples composed of persons from mixed subgroups, only Jemmott, Jemmott, and Villarruel (2002) separately discussed racial and ethnic subgroups.

The selected studies addressed disease prevention and screening or treatment for a disease condition within the health care system. The 52 articles were conceptualized as a continuum, with disease prevention and disease management at the poles and disease screening at the midpoint. The disease prevention category included articles that addressed risk factors for developing heart disease, cancer, diabetes, and HIV/AIDS for minority men. The disease screening category included articles that addressed factors that influence health-promoting behaviors such as screening procedures to identify prevalence rates in high-risk populations. This category also included studies that described health promotion behaviors to decrease the severity of a disease or to prevent disease complications. Lastly, the disease management category addressed issues related to the health care management of men already diagnosed with the targeted disease conditions.

Disease Prevention

Differences in social, historical, and cultural experiences and variations in acculturation and socioeconomic class may influence health service utilization and responses to interventions (Porter & Villarruel, 1993). These differences are related to communication and comprehension of the English language. For instance, when instruments to measure knowledge and behaviors for HIV/AIDS prevention are translated into Spanish, they are not effective because additional cultural translation is required. Those that are effective with persons whose primary language is English may require additional cultural translation. Latino and African American persons accounted for approximately 55% of the adult AIDS cases reported in the United States in 1999 (Hoyert, Arias, Smith, Murphy, & Kochanek, 2001).

One study explored the issue of translation and comprehension with a sample of 18 recently arrived Mexican immigrants who reported that the wording of the questions, the two-part instructions, and the differences in translation of the National Center for Health Statistics Scale were confusing (McQuiston, Larson, Parrado, & Flaskerud, 2002). A mixed methods approach examined whether the narrative responses matched responses to the Likert scale items. During the focus group interviews, subjects reported that the choices offered on the Likert scale items were confusing. They reported choosing the more extreme responses, such as "very likely," rather than the more subtle choices, such as "somewhat likely." Respondents felt more confident that their more extreme responses could accurately express their affirmation or negation, whereas the more subtle choices might convey ambiguity. Confusion about the commonly used Likert scale items resulted in an inaccurate assessment of their HIV/AIDS knowledge and awareness of risk factors.

Variations in acculturation or cultural assimilation among racial and ethnic minority men can affect their risk factors for developing disease conditions. Mortality due to cancer disproportionately affects minority men. Although cancer is the second cause of death for both men and women of each racial and ethnic group, it accounts for 16% excess mortality for Black men younger than 70 years of age (Gargiullo, Wingo, Coates, & Thompson, 2002). African American, Hispanic, Asian American/Pacific Islander, and American Indian men all have higher rates of stomach cancer than their White counterparts (Rich & Ro, 2002). Koreans generally have lower rates of stomach cancer than other persons in the United States because they traditionally consume diets lower in beef, chicken, breads, soda, and dairy products than U.S. citizens (Kim et al., 2000). However, Koreans who immigrate to the U.S. may raise their risk of stomach cancer as they become more assimilated. Notably, marital status and higher educational level acted as risk factors rather than protective factors for 41 male and 62 female Korean immigrants who, on average, had lived in the United States for eight years. Married men with at least 12 years of education reported the highest levels of dietary change. Thus risk factors for racial and ethnic minority men may require more careful assessment and may also change over time as the men acquire Western behaviors.

Disease Screening

Nurse researchers often fail to consider the effect of structural and environmental influences on the health of minority populations (Jackson, 1993).

Researchers who provide adequate descriptions of the structural and environmental characteristics of their samples rarely provide comparison data on members from the same racial and ethnic subgroup; instead, findings from minority samples are compared to either Whites or the general U.S. population. Consequently, determining which risk factors may be related to structural and environmental influences and which may be associated with behavioral factors unique to the study sample becomes difficult. For reasons that are not well understood, the mix of structural, environmental, and behavioral influences is unknown.

Approximately 30% of deaths due to heart disease occur to White men, who make up 75% of the U.S. population (CDC, 2002). Comparatively, 12.5% of the U.S. population is Latino, but approximately 24% of heart disease mortality occurs to Latino men. The cardiovascular-related mortality in African American men is largely due to uncontrolled hypertension and diabetes. Despite the increasing prevalence of heart disease, diabetes, and HIV/AIDS among minority populations, some researchers suggest that these conditions may actually be underdiagnosed in these populations because of minorities' inadequate awareness or knowledge of risk factors, their limited access to appropriate services, differences in how the disease is manifested within these populations, or even social and environmental issues, such as culture.

Researchers examined the awareness of risk factors for incidence of hypertension among a convenience sample of 448 men and 677 women, 81% of whom were Mexican American and 58% of whom had incomes below the poverty level (Jones, Ricard, Sefcik, & Miller, 2001). Investigators reported that only 53% of the sample with elevated blood pressure were aware of their potential for developing hypertension, which the investigators attributed to this population's lack of access to and contact with health care providers.

Intravenous drug users, many of whom are Latino or African American, face special risks for developing HIV/AIDS. However, HIV/AIDS may be underdiagnosed or undiagnosed among IV drug users seeking substance abuse treatment because of a failure to adequately screen this population (Williams, D'Aquila, & Williams, 1987). In one study, 181 Latino, African American, and White men and women IV drug users presenting at an urban substance abuse center for treatment were tested for HIV/AIDS status and coded to facilitate anonymous testing. Participants were asked to predict their HIV/AIDS status prior to having blood drawn. Almost 25% of the sample that had identified their status as negative tested positive for HIV/AIDS.

There are racial, ethnic, and regional differences in risk factors for HIV/AIDS that have important implications for planning prevention programs (Mukhopadhyay, 1996). Regional differences that have been documented by an analysis of the 1994 CDC AIDS Public Information Data Set revealed that the highest proportion of African Americans with HIV/AIDS is in the northeast and mid-Atlantic regions, while HIV/AIDS-infected Latino cases predominate in the northeast and southern regions. There are also regional differences in the method of transmitting HIV/AIDS. Homosexual transmission surpasses heterosexual transmission of HIV/AIDS except in the Northeast, where IV drug use predominates, and in small metropolitan and nonmetropolitan areas.

Racial and ethnic differences are supported by mortality data. African American men die from prostate, lung, colorectal, esophageal, and stomach cancer more frequently than men in any other racial and ethnic group (Rich & Ro, 2002). These disproportionate mortality rates can be attributed to both high-risk behaviors as well as to inadequate health care.

The numbers of African Americans who participate in cancer clinical trials are quite low. Misperceptions about the purpose of clinical trials and other research designs may contribute to their low participation. When queried about the low participation of African Americans, a sample of 123 male and 97 female African Americans with an average household income of $30,000 stated their belief that only persons diagnosed with cancer were eligible to participate in cancer research (Millon-Underwood, Sanders, & Davis, 1992). They also expressed confusion about eligibility criteria, although 61% knew someone with cancer and 45% viewed themselves as being at risk to develop cancer. Fifty-seven percent of the group believed either that cancer research was nonefficacious or that the consequences of participating in such research were unknown. They suggested that cancer patients might participate in cancer clinical trials because these patients might be seeking hope of a cure, be willing to sacrifice themselves for a cure, or be willing to help future generations fight cancer.

Using a social marketing model, Zimmerman (1997) conducted a study with 51 Latino men, predominantly Mexican American, who had recently undergone a prostate screening exam to identify factors that influenced their participation in prostate screening exams. They cited sources of information such as newspapers, friends, family, and church. These men cited low-cost health services and conveniently located screening sites with evening and weekend hours of operation that permitted walk-in visits as a motive for participation, and only 4% cited the actual digital rectal exam (DRE) as a barrier.

Health care providers may fail to screen at-risk minority men for diabetes because the disease process may manifest differently among some racial and ethnic groups in comparison to Whites. CDC data do not distinguish between diabetes type 1 and type 2 as causes of the disproportionate mortality due to diabetes mellitus among minority men. American Indians, Alaska Natives, African Americans, and Latinos are about twice as likely as Whites to have a diagnosis of diabetes (CDC, 2002). Approximately 10% of all Hispanic/Latino populations have diabetes, and almost one fourth of Mexican Americans and Puerto Ricans and 32% of African Americans are estimated to have diabetes due to genetic and behavioral risk factors. The incidence of diabetes within the American Indian/Alaskan Native populations varies considerably by tribe, but the highest incidence of diabetes in the United States is believed to occur within the Pima Tribe in Arizona, with a prevalence rate of approximately 50% in adults 30–64 years of age. American Indians and Alaskan Native populations are almost three times as likely to have diabetes as non-Hispanic Whites of the same age. The incidence of diabetes among Asian/Pacific Islanders has not been determined, but some researchers believe that some ethnic subgroups, such as Hawaiians, are at increased risk for development of type 2 diabetes.

Researchers hypothesize that many African Americans with type 2 diabetes are undiagnosed because of differences in the presenting signs and symptoms (Chasens, Umlauf, Pillion, & Singh, 2000). In one study, the investigators examined links among symptoms of nocturia, excessive daytime sleepiness (EDS), and obstructive sleep apnea (OSA) in a sample of 87 African American men and women using a conceptual model specially developed for EDS and OSA. This model had not been tested with African American populations. They proposed that rather than being a manifestation of glycosuria or prostatism, nocturia may actually be a secondary symptom of undiagnosed OSA and may contribute to the obesity risk factor for type 2 diabetes among African Americans. Study participants with either diabetes or EDS reported a fourfold risk of OSA in comparison to those without either diabetes or EDS.

Researchers proposed that the incidence of depression may also be underdiagnosed in African Americans with HIV/AIDS because of cultural differences in how the disease manifests (Lyon & Munro, 2001). An increase in viral load was associated with increases in symptoms of depression for 79 African Americans with HIV/AIDS, although none had a previous diagnosis of depression. The investigators did not speculate about how cultural factors might influence how depression is manifested. However, future qualitative research studies with ethnic minority men on this topic could illuminate the influence of gender, race, and ethnicity.

In combination, these findings suggest that life for racial and ethnic minority men may simply be more complex than for White men and that therefore health-promoting behaviors are important but have lower priority than other, more immediate concerns. Social, environmental, and cultural factors may affect the willingness and ability of racial and ethic minority men to participate in health-promoting behaviors. None of the researchers deconstructed or defined the concepts of race, ethnicity, or culture, although these factors were consistently cited as predictors for lower levels of health-promoting knowledge and behaviors. It may be that the concepts of race, ethnicity, and culture may sometimes be used as proxies for social and environmental influences on health-promoting behaviors for minority men, such as participation in screening and in behaviors such as changing exercise or diet habits.

An investigation of structural and environmental influences involved a telephone intervention to reduce salt intake among a small convenience sample of very-low-income, African American elderly men ($n = 5$) and women ($n = 21$) that was effective for a 3-week study period (Freeman-McGuire, 1997). Unfortunately, the lifestyle complexity that accompanies poverty, including limited access to supportive health services, undoubtedly impaired these seniors' ability to maintain their behavioral changes for a prolonged time period.

Another example of the complexity of life for African American men revolves around cancer screening. African Americans' lower level of participation in cancer screening in comparison to the general population has been attributed to cultural values of fatalism or learned helplessness, which suggests that some African Americans may feel incapable of exerting influence over their health status, do not value health, or lack cancer prevention knowledge (Underwood, 1992). However, 62% of 189 African American men, mean age 53.8 years, who declined to participate in a free prostate cancer screening program scored similar to 60 White men of the same age on measures of perceived benefits of prostate cancer screening (Tingen, Weinrich, Boyd, & Weinrich, 1997). This sample included low- to middle-income men, 46% of whom had some high school or college.

Davis (2000) identified stages of change for low-income elderly African American men (11) and women (26) diagnosed with hypertension who were living in a public housing complex to determine their responsiveness to an intervention to improve cardiovascular status. The study demonstrated that despite poverty and advanced age, not all elderly African Americans are resistant to incorporating health-promoting behaviors, such as changes in diet or exercise.

In a randomized clinical trial a subsample of 19 urban African American men, 18 to 49 years of age who were diagnosed with hypertension demonstrated adequate knowledge of cardiac disease risk factors but cited multiple social, cultural, and personal barriers that interfered with their ability to institute change (Rose, Kim, Dennison, & Hill, 2000). Their ability to comply with the health-related demands of planning for regular appointments, medications, and lifestyle changes in diet and exercise to prevent hypertension-related complications fit poorly with the complexity of meeting their daily life concerns. Other investigators used the Health Belief Model to explain reasons why a subsample of 988 African American and 444 White men refused to participate in a free prostate cancer screening program after receiving an educational intervention (Weinrich, Reynolds, Tingen, & Starr, 2000). These men were participants in a larger study described later in this chapter (Weinrich, Greiner, Reis-Starr, Yoon, & Weinrich, 1998) whose purpose was to identify factors that influence participation in a free prostate cancer screening program. The men reported putting off the screening, inability to identify an appropriate health care provider, and inconvenience as reasons for nonparticipation. Another subgroup of this same study sampled 377 African American and 172 White men 40–70 years of age. These men identified additional barriers to receiving either a DRE or a prostate specific antigen (PSA) blood test (Boyd, Weinrich, Weinrich, & Norton, 2001); these included sociocultural barriers such as difficulty using the health care system, difficulty finding time for appointments, the tendency to ignore program reminders, and no access to telephones.

Learning about cancer risk factors and warning signs may not be a priority in the lives of African American men who do not perceive themselves as being susceptible to developing cancer. Two studies of African American men and women reported that most either did not perceive themselves as being susceptible or underestimated their risk of developing cancer (Millon-Underwood et al., 1992; Underwood, 1991). Ninety-nine percent of a group of 123 men and 97 women viewed themselves as having low susceptibility to cancer (Millon-Underwood et al., 1992). The fact that only 12% of this group had received a physical exam in the past 3 years and that most had a little knowledge of both risk factors and warning signs is noteworthy. Another group of 354 African American men, mean age of 43.9 years with an average of 15 years of education, also underestimated the incidence of cancer among African Americans (Underwood, 1991). Still another study assessed the knowledge and perceptions of 211 African American men, mean age of 23 years with some college education. Approximately 75% of these men underestimated their own susceptibility to testicular cancer (Millon-Underwood & Sanders, 1991).

Social and environmental influences may contribute to differences in the level of knowledge and awareness of and attitude toward cancer and cancer screening among African American men. Most (87%) of 320 African American men living in the southern United States were interested in receiving genetic testing for susceptibility to prostate cancer. However, some confused genetic testing for susceptibility with screening to detect prostate cancer (Weinrich, Royal, et al., 2002). Those who reported not being interested were typically unmarried and expressed concern about possible future discrimination for themselves and their families if their test results were unfavorable.

In another study, 108 African American men also demonstrated low levels of knowledge (Agho & Lewis, 2001). Yet those who were younger and had lower educational and income levels scored higher on levels of prostate cancer knowledge. The findings may be misleading without additional socioeconomic characteristics of the sample. In general, the sample was well educated and included 60.8% with health insurance, 86.2% below 50 years of age, almost 40% with more than a high school education, and over 40% with a yearly income of over $40,000. Another study of 613 African American men who routinely participated in church-based PSA screening exams also demonstrated greater knowledge, but younger age and low education and income levels were associated with more negative attitudes toward a DRE (Gelfand, Parzuchowski, Cort, & Powell, 1995). The median income for this sample was $35,000, most had insurance, and only four men had ever refused to undergo a DRE.

Notably, age, education, and marital status did not predict participation in free prostate screening that included both DRE and PSA for 115 African American and 179 White men after a work site educational intervention in the southern United States (Weinrich, Greiner, et al., 1998). Instead, participation was associated with White race, proximity to work site, and ability to participate during working hours. Because of frequent underemployment, minority men are more likely to be employed in jobs that require late hours, mandatory overtime, and shift changes.

Several researchers used small samples of African American men to identify beliefs, attitudes, and practices regarding prostate cancer screening. Regardless of whether they regularly received prostate screening exam-inations, African American men expressed doubts about the efficacy of prostate cancer screening and treatment procedures, were concerned about the discomfort of the digital rectal exam (DRE), and worried about the potential impact of treatment for prostate cancer on their sexual function and their self-images (Clarke-Tasker & Wade, 2002; Fearing, Bell, New-ton, & Lambert, 2000; Watts, 1994).

Social connections are a major influential environmental factor in men's participation in screening. Minority men's connections to their families and communities or lack thereof seem to exert strong influence on their health behaviors. White married men with at least a high school education were most likely to participate in prostate cancer screening (Tingen, Weinrich, Boyd, & Weinrich, 1998). Marital status may indicate men's connectedness to their families and to their communities. If so, the poverty and social isolation that affect all too many African American men may have significant adverse consequences for their health, as researchers consistently identified marital status as a predictor for participation in prostate cancer screening programs (Weinrich, Faison-Smith, Hudson-Priest, Royal, & Powell, 2002; Weinrich, Reynolds, et al., 2000; Weinrich, Royal, et al., 2002; Weinrich, Weinrich, et al., 2001).

Unmarried, older African American men in poverty who had less than a high school education and who lived alone were more likely than either young African American men or White men of any age to report their health status as being either fair or poor (Weinrich, Weinrich, et al., 2001). Being unmarried was correlated with not participating in prostate cancer screening programs for both White and African American men. But for African American men, being unmarried was also associated with having less knowledge of their families' health history and reporting poorer health status.

African American men who are isolated or separated from their fami-lies may lack knowledge of their own health risk factors because they lack information of their families' health histories. Researchers speculated that the opportunity to participate in a free prostate cancer screening program heightened awareness of the disease and led minority men to engage in conversations with family members about this topic (Weinrich, Faison-Smith, et al., 2002), conversations that may have led to changes in family history reports 1 year later. The African American men in the sample of 96 men who were most likely to make changes in family history after one year were unmarried, had low income, and did not participate in the free prostate cancer screening program.

African American ethnicity was a strong predictor of not participating in free prostate screening, even when urinary symptoms suggested prostate enlargement (Weinrich, Weinrich, et al., 1998). Perhaps some African American men pay less attention to specific symptoms indicative of prostate cancer because they are used to general poor health. As unmarried men who live alone in poverty, their poor health status may reflect their overall social isolation and their limited ability to gain access to health care services.

Regular attendance at church may also indicate minority men's connectedness to their families or communities. African American men who participated in face-to-face educational programs, particularly church-based educational programs in churches whose members shared their personal experiences with prostate cancer, were more likely than those who received educational video interventions to undergo free prostate screening exams (Tingen et al., 1998; Weinrich, Holdford, et al., 1998). Having a congregation member diagnosed with cancer in the last year increased participation in church-based prostate cancer screening education for 393 African American men (Weinrich, Holdford, et al., 1998). There were, however, no significant differences in participation in the free prostate cancer screening program among men who regularly attended church and had been previously exposed to information about prostate cancer or had previously undergone prostate cancer screening.

In terms of another screening focus, regular church attendance may also have confounded results in a study conducted to determine differences in levels of adherence to prescribed regimens for hypertension among African Americans who attended a church with a blood pressure screening program in comparison to those who attended a church without that program (Smith, 1989). The investigator found no significant differences in adherence between the two church congregations.

Social, environmental, and cultural factors may also affect the willingness and ability of racial and ethic minority men to participate in health-promoting behaviors. Elderly African American men (400) and women (565) demonstrated greater knowledge of hypertension and greater adherence to medication use than younger men and women, all of whom had been diagnosed with hypertension (Wieck, 1997). Barriers to adherence included long lines in clinics and losing wages when appointments conflicted with working hours. Nevertheless, 64% of both young and elderly persons reported their health as good to excellent, regardless of their adherence with their prescribed regimen.

Cultural factors may affect risk factors as well as the ability of health care providers to assess risk factors. Instruments that are valid cross-culturally do not necessarily mean that the concept under study is also valid cross-culturally (Porter & Villarruel, 1993). Several researchers identified culturally specific concepts for African American and Latino samples. The following studies used small samples, but in combination they provide support for the idea that concepts differ across cultures. Thirty low-income African American men and women defined the concept of stress as a consequence of their inability to manage the multiple obligations of their complex lives because of inadequate resources for themselves and their families. In comparison, the concept of worry was defined as involving social concerns about themselves, their children, kin, and communities (Boutain, 2001).

In another study, a group of 10 Latino immigrants and their families identified culturally specific concepts such as *animo*, the need to have a positive mental disposition, drive, or energy to be able to handle adversity, and *comodo*, the state of being or achieving comfort, along with less culturally specific comfort needs such as pain relief (Arruda, Larson, & Meleis, 1992). Still another study of 12 Latino, 42 African American, and 44 White men and women identified racial and ethnic differences in spirituality and mastery over stress for HIV/AIDS infected persons. African Americans scored higher on using spirituality as a strategy to combat stress, whereas mastery over stress was a more important value for Latino persons (Gray, 2002). A very cautious interpretation of these findings might suggest that since stress for African Americans involves having inadequate resources to meet family needs, spirituality, or turning to an external higher power, may be an appropriate coping response. In comparison, Latino persons value mastery over stress, which is consistent with the concept of *animo*, an internal drive or energy, cited previously.

Family and community relations seem to be an equally important influence on the health-promoting behaviors of Latino men. A predominantly Puerto Rican sample of college men reported lower intentions to use condoms and also reported using condoms less frequently in comparison to the women in the sample (Jemmott et al., 2002). Their beliefs about partner and peer approval and about impulse control predicted their intent to use condoms to prevent HIV/AIDS. Similarly, Mexican American men reported needing to feel trust in their relationships before introducing the topic of condoms (McQuiston & Gordon, 2000).

These studies illustrate that some racial and ethnic minority men may not participate in cancer screening procedures or other health protection behaviors for other reasons besides lack of awareness or inadequate knowledge of risk factors and screening procedures. Social and environmental factors, particularly marital status, seem to influence the willingness of minority men to participate in health promotion behaviors.

Disease Management

Researchers identified racial and ethnic disparities in the health care management of persons already diagnosed with the targeted disease conditions, although the mechanisms remain unknown. A chart audit of 19 Latino men and women, 43 African American men and women, and 75 White men and women demonstrated that regular access to health care services was not associated with better management of hypertension and diabetes for Latino and African American men and women even when access to health care services was controlled (Baumann, Chang, & Hoebeke, 2002). Using national guidelines for treatment and information from patient charts for the past three visits, researchers found that, in comparison with White patients, Latinos and African Americans received fewer influenza vaccinations, had less than optimal glycemic control, and had additional risk factors for cardiac disease and diabetes, such as smoking and obesity, that were not documented as diagnosed risk factors.

Researchers also audited the charts of 44 African American and 598 White patients hospitalized after an acute myocardial infarction to explore racial differences in treatment. African American patients were 32% less likely to receive a coronary artery bypass graft (CABG) and one fifth less likely to undergo revascularization procedures, even after diagnostic angiography and controlling for severity of myocardial infarction, preexisting comorbidity, clinical history, and presence of anginal symptoms (Funk, Ostfeld, Chang, & Lee, 2002). The differences could reflect either overuse of the procedure with White patients or underuse of the procedure with African American patients, who often have lower levels of insurance coverage.

Despite providing detailed descriptions of the race and ethnicity of samples, some researchers did not discuss any of their findings in relation to race and/or ethnicity. This flaw negates the heterogeneity among and within groups and the specificity of factors for one subgroup versus another. The following three studies illustrate these points. Nurse practitioners managed 22 Latino, 20 African American, and 59 White men and women with HIV/AIDS on AZT in an outpatient primary care setting (Cox, Martin, Styer, & Beall, 1990). Longevity improved, but there was no attempt to correlate findings with race, ethnicity, range of lifestyle patterns, behaviors, or environmental conditions.

In another study, an examination of the Minimum Data Set files for all New York nursing home residents for 1997 determined that nursing home patients with HIV/AIDS are increasingly more likely to be younger, male, and to be either Latino or African American in comparison to traditional nursing home patients (Shin, Newman, Gebbie, & Fillmore, 2002). Nursing home patients with HIV/AIDS also tend to have more symptoms of depression, use more psychiatric medications, and have greater incidences of bowel and bladder incontinence, all of which require greater amounts of nursing care than that given traditional nursing home patients. Despite identifying the increasing prevalence of minority men requiring nursing home care, the investigators neglected to identify culture- or gender-specific implications for care.

Finally, a randomized clinical trial was designed to test the effect of adding aloe vera lotion to treatment regimens to reduce adverse skin reactions or radiation dermatitis related to high-dose chemotherapy among 73 Latino (35%), African American (26%), and White (39%) men and women with cancer (Olsen et al., 2001). Results indicated that adding aloe vera was only protective for those patients who demonstrated some resistance to radiation dermatitis. None of these studies identified differences associated with the race or ethnicity of the subjects.

Racial and ethnic disparities in health care management for minority populations have also been attributed to differences between the primarily White, middle-class culture of health care providers and the cultures of racial and ethnic minorities. Thus, the remaining articles in this section examined possible racial and ethnic differences in response to the experience of having a disease condition and differences in responses to disease management. The Visual Analog Scale (VAS), Memorial Pain Scale (MPS), and Face Scale were equally useful in assessing differences in response to cancer pain in Latino (23.5%), African American (11.8), Asian/ Pacific Islander (7.9%), or White patients (56.9%) (Ramer et al., 1999). However, since the total sample size was 51 men and women, the small numbers of racial and ethnic minorities may have affected the findings. Still, Asian patients not only reported the highest levels of pain but also reported being least satisfied with pain relief measures.

There may be some limits to the influences of racial and ethnic differences. Neither language acculturation nor socioeconomic status predicted health-related quality of life for monolingual and bilingual Spanish-speaking Latino HIV/AIDS patients (van Servellen, Chang, & Lombardi, 2002). Researchers examined language acculturation and socioeconomic status to determine if these specific factors caused differences in health-related quality-of-life ratings for 89 monolingual and bilingual Spanish-speaking men and women. They found instead that health-related quality of life was negatively correlated with increased HIV/AIDS symptoms. It may be that language acculturation and socioeconomic status are more important to general quality of life, but the pain and discomfort of HIV/AIDS-related symptoms may take precedence over any other life concerns.

Overall quality of life was rated as being high for both dyad members of 61 African American and 62 White cancer survivors and family member dyads (Mellon, 2002). These dyads were interviewed to identify the meaning of breast, colon, prostate, and uterine cancer illness for the survivor and its effect on the family. The investigator attributed the high-level ratings to the similarity in themes for both dyad members.

Although social support has previously been identified as a mediator of self-efficacy, neither the size of their social support network nor satisfaction with social support was correlated with glucose control or self-efficacy for a sample of 30 male and 65 female insulin-dependent Latino diabetics, 95% of whom were Puerto Rican (Gleeson-Kreig, Bernal, & Woolley, 2002). Levels of social support were more predictive for African Americans. Lower levels of social support were associated with higher serum glucose levels, manifested by glycosylated hemoglobin (GHb) levels and higher basal metabolic index (BMIs), for 104 African Americans with type 2 diabetes, seven of whom were men, but not for a matched White sample (Bailey & Lherisson-Cedeno, 1997). In general, diabetic functional status was best predicted by educational level for a sample of 133 African American men and women with diabetes, but there were also gender differences (Montague, 2002). Men reported greater self-efficacy in monitoring glucose levels, adhering to prescribed regimens, and controlling their diabetes than women.

DISCUSSION

The findings in this review have implications for nursing research, education, and practice. The special health risks faced by all men in the United States are aggravated by social and environmental influences when those men are members of racial or ethnic minorities, particularly for heart disease, cancer, diabetes, and HIV/AIDS. The limitations of this review include possibly missing important studies that were published in non-nursing journals. Nevertheless, this review does demonstrate that some work has been done in nursing research to address the four adult health disparities targeted by DHHS—heart disease, cancer, diabetes, and HIV/AIDS—although much more is certainly needed.

The findings from this review suggest that when considering the health of minority men it is essential to consider social and environmental factors such as regional differences, language, acculturation, and changes in cultural habits caused by assimilation. Failure to consider these factors may result in underdiagnosis of DHHS-targeted illnesses: appropriate racial and ethnic subgroups may not be targeted and inappropriate assessment and screening procedures may be used. Nurse researchers should consider a new approach to preventive health care and disease management for minority men that can take place within the context of their families, work, churches, and communities. Consequently, the family rather than the individual should become the unit of analysis in research studies of minority men. Interdisciplinary research with sociologists and medical anthropologists will facilitate this transition and will help us examine the structural and environmental nuances that influence the health behaviors of minority populations.

Future research should be based upon literature reviews that have identified gaps in what is known and that have established theoretical or conceptual frameworks that have been tested with or adapted to specific racial and ethnic populations and subgroups. Conceptual or theoretical literature generates appropriate research questions and hypotheses that can contribute to our understanding of discipline-related concepts (LoBiondo-Wood & Haber, 1998). A review of the scholarly literature can ascertain what is known or yet to be determined about a concept or a problem, thereby establishing priority areas for future research. Meta-analysis, an increasingly accepted research technique in behavioral sciences, can be used to combine study results in order to draw conclusions from a large number of research studies (Baumgartner, Strong, & Hensley, 2002). Only then can empirical studies uncover new knowledge that can lead to the development, validation, or refinement of theories that can then promote changes in clinical practice (LoBiondo-Wood & Haber, 1998). Future research based on gaps identified in existing literature and theoretically guided research can contribute to a national strategy to guide efforts in investigating structural social, cultural, environmental influences on the health and health behaviors of racial and ethnic minority men.

Gender differences in causes of mortality research and clinical activities to promote health and prevent diseases among men have not received the same attention recently devoted to women's health. Low levels of known risk factors for major chronic diseases identified during routine health maintenance visits (blood pressure, serum glucose, smoking, and obesity) are strong predictors for continued good health in old age (Reed et al., 1998). Women use more primary care services and diagnostic services then men by incorporating health maintenance issues with their visits for family planning, pregnancy, and childbirth (Bertakis, Azari, Helms, Callahan, & Robbins, 2000; Dean & Downey, 1998). Men utilize fewer primary care health services and receive less health maintenance. Instead, men's use of more acute and expensive health services, such as emergency care, hospitalizations, and home health care visits, increases as they age, while their visits to primary care providers continue to decrease (Murphy & Hepworth, 1995).

Nurses and physicians rarely provide men with the skills to promote and maintain health through either verbal instruction or educational brochures (Dean & Downey, 1998). This review provides an important contribution to knowledge about the DHHS-targeted areas of health disparities, but there are still many important gaps to be addressed. In addition to learning about the mechanisms of health disparities, we need to know more about preventing, assessing, and managing the leading causes of morbidity and mortality for minority men.

REFERENCES

Agho, A., & Lewis, M. A. (2001). Correlates of actual and perceived knowledge of prostate cancer among African Americans. *Cancer Nursing, 24*, 165–171.

American Cancer Society. Retrieved March 01, 2003, from www.cancer.org/downloads/STT/CancerFacts&Figures2002TM.pdf

Arruda, E. N., Larson, P. J., & Meleis, A. F. (1992). Comfort: Immigrant Hispanic cancer patients' views. *Cancer Nursing, 16*, 387–394.

Bailey, B. J., & Lherisson-Cedeno, D. (1997). Diabetes outcomes and practices: Comparison of African Americans and Caucasians. *Journal of the National Black Nurses Association, 9*, 66–75.

Baumann, L. C., Chang, M., & Hoebeke, R. (2002). Clinical outcomes for low-income adults with hypertension and diabetes. *Nursing Research, 51*, 191–198.

Baumgartner, T. A., Strong, C. H., & Hensley, L. D. (2002). *Conducting and reading research in health and human services* (3rd ed.). Boston: McGraw-Hill.

Bertakis, K. D., Azari, R., Helms, L. J., Callahan, E. J., & Robbins, J. (2000). Gender differences in the utilization of health care services. *Journal of Family Practice, 49,* 147–152.

Boutain, D. M. (2001). Discourses of worry, stress, and high blood pressure in rural south Louisiana. *Journal of Nursing Scholarship, 33,* 225–230.

Boyd, M. D., Weinrich, S. P., Weinrich, M., & Norton, A. (2001). Obstacles to prostate cancer screening in African-American men. *Journal of the National Black Nurses Association, 12,* 1–5.

Centers for Disease Control (CDC). (1986, February 28). Perspectives in disease prevention and health promotion report of the Secretary's Task Force on Black and Minority Health. *Morbidity and Mortality Weekly Report, 35,* 109–112.

Centers for Disease Control (CDC). (2001, September 21). Deaths: Final data for 1999. *National Center for Health Statistics Report, 49*(12).

Centers for Disease Control (CDC). (2002, September 16). Deaths: Final data for 2000. *National Vital Statistics Report, 50*(15), Retrieved January 25, 2003, from http://www.cdc.gov/nchs/data/dvs/nvsr50_15_p9.pdf

Chasens, E. R., Umlauf, M. G., Pillion, D. J., & Singh, K. P. (2000). Sleep apnea symptoms, nocturia, and diabetes in African-American community dwelling older adults. *Journal of the National Black Nurses Association, 11,* 25–33.

Clarke-Tasker, V. A., & Wade, R. (2002). What we thought we knew: African American males' perceptions of prostate cancer and screening methods. *ABNF Journal, 13,* 56–59.

Cox, P. H., Martin, M. A., Styer, C. M., & Beall, G. N. (1990). Outcomes of treatment with AZT of patients with AIDS and symptomatic HIV infection. *Nurse Practitioner, 15,* 36, 39–40, 42–44.

Davis, L. (2000). Exercise and dietary behaviors in African American elders: Stages of change in efficacy expectancies. *ABNF Journal, 11,* 56–58.

Dean, M., & Downey, P. (1998). Preventive healthcare: Are men offered enough? *Journal of Clinical Nursing, 7,* 564–565.

Doyal, L. (2001). Sex, gender, and health: The need for a new approach. *BMJ, 323,* 1061–1063.

Fearing, A., Bell, D., Newton, M., & Lambert, S. (2000). Prostate screening health beliefs and practices of African American men. *ABNF Journal, 11,* 141–143.

Freeman-McGuire, M. (1997). Community-based hypertensive education for African American seniors: A replication study. *Journal of the National Black Nurses Association, 9,* 57–68.

Funk, M., Ostfeld, A. M., Chang, V. M., & Lee, F. A. (2002). Racial differences in the use of cardiac procedures in patents with acute myocardial infarction. *Nursing Research, 51,* 148–157.

Gargiullo, P., Wingo, P. A., Coates, R. J., & Thompson, T. D. (2002). Recent trends in mortality rates for four major cancers, by sex and race/ethnicity—United States, 1990–1998. *MMWR, 51*(3), 49–53. Retrieved February 19, 2003, from http://www.cdc.gov/mmwr/preview/mmwrhtml/mm5103a1.htm

Gelfand, D. E., Parzuchowski, J., Cort, M., & Powell, I. (1995). Digital rectal examinations and prostate cancer screening: Attitudes of African American men. *Oncology Nursing Forum, 22,* 1253–1255.

Gleeson-Kreig, J., Bernal, H., & Woolley, S. (2002). The role of social support in the self-management of Diabetes Mellitus among a Hispanic population. *Public Health Nursing, 19,* 215–222.

Gray, J. (2002). Racial/ethnic differences in psychosocial factors among persons living with HIV/AIDS. *Journal of Multicultural Nursing and Health, 8,* 50–60.

Hoyert, D. L., Arias, E., Smith, B. L., Murphy, S. L., & Kochanek, K. D. (2001). *Deaths: Final data for 1999.* Atlanta, GA: Centers for Disease Control and Prevention.

Jackson, E. M. (1993). Whiting-out the difference: Why U.S. nursing research fails black families. *Medical Anthropology Quarterly, 7,* 363–385.

Jemmott, L. S., Jemmott, J. B., & Villarruel, A. M. (2002). Predicting intentions and condom use among Latino college students. *Journal of the Association of Nurses in AIDS Care, 13,* 59–69.

Jones, R. A. P., Ricard, R., Sefcik, E., & Miller, M. E. (2001). The health risk of hypertension in south Texas: A demographic profile. *Holistic Nurse Practitioner, 15,* 35–44.

Kim, K. K., Yu, E. S. H., Chen, E. H., Cross, N., Kim, J., & Brintnall, R. A. (2000). Nutritional status of Korean Americans: Implications for cancer risk. *Oncology Nursing Forum, 27,* 1573–1583.

Lillie-Blanton, M., Brodie, M., Rowland, D., Altman, D., & McIntosh, M. (2000). Race, ethnicity, and the health care system: Public perceptions and experiences. *Medical Care Research and Review, 57*(Suppl.), 218–235.

LoBiondo-Wood, G., & Haber, J. (1998). *Nursing research: Methods, critical appraisal, and utilization* (4th ed.). St. Louis: Mosby.

Lyon, D. E., & Munro, C. (2001). Disease severity and symptoms of depression in Black Americans infected with HIV. *Applied Nursing Research, 14,* 3–10.

McQuiston, C., & Gordon, A. (2000). The timing is never right: Mexican views of condom use. *Health Care for Women International, 21,* 277–290.

McQuiston, C., Larson, K., Parrado, E. A., & Flaskerud, J. H. (2002). AIDS knowledge and measurement considerations with unacculturated Latinos. *Western Journal of Nursing Research, 24,* 354–372.

Mellon, S. (2002). Comparisons between cancer survivors and family members on meaning of the illness and family quality of life. *Oncology Nursing Forum, 29,* 1117–1125.

Millon-Underwood, S., & Sanders, E. (1990). Factors contributing to health promotion behaviors among African-American men. *Oncology Nursing Forum, 17,* 707–712.

Millon-Underwood, S., & Sanders, E. (1991). Testicular self-examination among African-American men. *Journal of the National Black Nurses Association, 5,* 18–28.

Millon-Underwood, S., Sanders, E., & Davis, M. (1992). Determinants of participation in state-of-the-art cancer prevention, early detection/screening, and treatment trials among African Americans. *Cancer Nursing, 16,* 25–33.

Montague, M. C. (2002). Psychosocial and functional outcomes in African Americans with Diabetes Mellitus. *ABNF Journal, 13,* 103–109.

Mukhopadhyay, A. (1996). HIV/AIDS: An overview of national demographics. *ABNF Journal, 7*(2), 37–41.

Murphy, J. F., & Hepworth, J. T. (1996). Age and gender differences in health services utilization. *Research in Nursing and Health, 19,* 323–329.

National Center for Health Statistics. (2002). HHS report finds health improves for most racial, ethnic groups but disparities remain in some areas. Retrieved January 23, 2003, from http://www.cdc.gov/nchs/releases/02news/healthimpr.htm

Olsen, D. L., Raub, W., Bradley, C., Johnson, M., Macias, J. L., Love, V., et al. (2001). The effect of aloe vera gel/mild soap versus mild soap alone in preventing skin reactions in patients undergoing radiation therapy. *Oncology Nursing Forum, 28,* 543–547.

Porter, C. P., & Villarruel, A. M. (1993). Nursing research with African American and Hispanic people: Guidelines for action. *Nursing Outlook, 41,* 59–67.

Ramer, L., Richardson, J. L., Cohen, M. Z., Bedney, C., Danley, K. L., & Judge, E. A. (1999). Multimeasure pain assessment in an ethnically diverse group of patients with cancer. *Journal of Transcultural Nursing, 10,* 94–101.

Reed, D. M., Foley, D. J., White, L. R., Heimovitz, H., Burchfiel, C. M., & Kamal, M. (1998). Predictors of healthy aging in men with high life expectancies. *American Journal of Public Health, 88,* 1463–1468.

Rich, J. A., & Ro, M. (2002). *A poor man's plight: Uncovering the disparity in men's health.* Battle Creek, MI: W. K. Kellogg Foundation.

Rose, L. E., Kim, M. T., Dennison, C. R., & Hill, M. N. (2000). The contexts of adherence for African Americans with high blood pressure. *Journal of Advanced Nursing, 32,* 587–594.

Schulman, K. A., Berlin, J. A., Harless, W., Kerner, J. F., Sistrunk, S., Gersh, B. J., et al. (1999). The effect of race and sex on physicians' recommendations for cardiac catheterization. *New England Journal of Medicine, 340,* 618–626.

Shin, J. K., Newman, L. S., Gebbie, K. M., & Fillmore, H. H. (2002). Quality of care measurement in nursing home AIDS care: A pilot study. *Journal of the Association of Nurses in AIDS Care, 13,* 70–76.

Smedley, B. D., Stith, A. Y., & Nelson, A. R. (Eds.). (2002). *Unequal treatment: Confronting racial and ethnic disparities in health care.* Washington, DC: National Academies Press.

Smith, E. D. (1989). The role of Black churches in supporting compliance with antihypertension regimens. *Public Health Nursing, 6,* 212–217.

Tingen, M. S., Weinrich, S. P., Boyd, M. D., & Weinrich, M. C. (1997). Search and research. Prostate cancer screening: Predictors of participation. *Journal of the American Academy of Nurse Practitioners, 9,* 557–567.

Tingen, M. S., Weinrich, S. P., Boyd, M. D., & Weinrich, M. C. (1998). Perceived benefits: A predictor of participation in prostate cancer screening. *Cancer Nursing, 21,* 349–357.

Underwood, S. (1991). African American men: Perceptual determinants of early cancer detection and risk reduction. *Cancer Nursing, 14*(6), 281–288.

Underwood, S. (1992). Cancer risk reduction and early detection behaviors among Black men: Focus on learned helplessness. *Journal of Community Health Nursing, 9,* 21–31.

van Servellen, G., Chang, B., & Lombardi, E. (2002). Acculturation, socioeconomic vulnerability, and quality of life in Spanish-speaking and bilingual Latino HIV-infected men and women. *Western Journal of Nursing Research, 24*, 246–263.

Weinrich, S., Holdford, D., Boyd, M., Creanga, D., Cover, K., Johnson, A., Frank-Stromborg, M., & Weinrich, M. (1998). Prostate cancer education in African American churches. *Public Health Nursing, 15*, 188–195.

Weinrich, S., Royal, C., Pettaway, C. A., Dunston, G., Faison-Smith, L., Hudson-Priest, J., et al. (2002). Interest in genetic prostate cancer susceptibility testing among African American men. *Cancer Nursing, 25*, 28–34.

Weinrich, S. P., Faison-Smith, L., Hudson-Priest, J., Royal, C., & Powell, I. (2002). Stability of self-reported family history of prostate cancer among African American men. *Journal of Nursing Measurement, 10*, 39–46.

Weinrich, S. P., Greiner, E., Reis-Starr, C., Yoon, S., & Weinrich, M. (1998). Predictors of participation in prostate cancer screening at worksites. *Journal of Community Health Nursing, 15*, 113–129.

Weinrich, S. P., Reynolds, W. A., Tingen, M. S., & Starr, C. R. (2000). Barriers to prostate screening. *Cancer Nursing, 23*, 117–121.

Weinrich, S. P., Weinrich, M., Boyd, M., & Atkinson, C. (1998). The impact of prostate cancer knowledge on cancer screening. *Oncology Nursing Forum, 25*, 527–534.

Weinrich, S. P., Weinrich, M. C., Priest, J., Fodi, C., & Talley, C. B. (2001). Perceived health status in African American and Caucasian men 40 to 70 years old. *Holistic Nursing Practice, 16*, 65–72.

Wieck, K. L. (1997). Hypertension in an inner-city minority population. *Journal of Cardiovascular Nursing, 11*, 41–49.

Williams, A. B., D'Aquila, R. T., & Williams, A. E. (1987). HIV infection in intravenous drug abusers. *Image: Journal of Nursing Scholarship, 19*, 179–183.

Zimmerman, S. M. (1997). Factors influencing Hispanic participation in prostate cancer screening. *Oncology Nursing Forum, 24*, 499–504.

Chapter 6

Immigration and Health

DeAnne K. Hilfinger Messias and Mercedes Rubio

ABSTRACT

The purpose of this integrated review was to examine research on the relationships between immigration and health. The review was limited to studies of immigration into North America published since 1994. The results suggested that, although recent research has furthered the understanding of immigration and health, the multiple health effects of the various social and cultural processes immigrants undergo are still not clearly understood. In addition, research on acculturation has not clarified the positive or negative effects of acculturation on health. The incorporation of transnational perspectives and contemporary concepts and frameworks such as biculturalism, undocumentedness, and transitions was noted as a significant contribution from recent research. The results of this integrative review indicate that interdisciplinary research on immigration and health is moving in new directions. The reviewers provide suggestions for future research on health disparities as well as on possible health protective factors among diverse immigrant populations.

Keywords: acculturation, immigrants, immigration

The effects of immigration on health and the potential for health disparities among immigrant groups and between native-born and immigrant populations are areas of increasing interest to nurses, nurse researchers, and other health professionals. The historical implications of health and human migration have long been recognized. In the United States today, the well-

101

being of immigrants is not only a public health concern but also a complex social, cultural, economic, and political issue. Immigration scholars come from diverse disciplines and backgrounds, including nursing, public health, epidemiology, psychology, sociology, anthropology, demography, economics, political science, history, and women's studies. Immigration and health researchers attempt to describe, explain, and predict situations, contexts, and factors that link human migration, health, and illness.

Research, practice, and anecdotal experience suggest that in terms of physical, psychological, and social health, migration may be successful, unsuccessful, or relatively uneventful (Hull, 1979). A wide range of factors have been identified as possible contributors to the prevalence of physical and mental illness among immigrants and refugees (Flaskerud & Kim, 1999; Palinkas, Pierce, Rosbrook, Pickwell, & Ball, 2003). Premigration and home country factors include unsanitary living conditions and endemic diseases (e.g., tuberculosis, malaria, hepatitis) and the social, political, and environmental conditions surrounding the decision to immigrate. Social isolation, cultural conflicts, poor social integration and assimilation, role changes and identity crises, low socioeconomic status, racial discrimination, and acquired risks for chronic diseases such as cancer, diabetes, hypertension and coronary heart disease, and mental illness are examples of host country factors that may contribute to health disparities among immigrants. Although much of the prior medical literature on immigrants has focused on the prevalence of particular diseases or health-related conditions immigrants bring with them, more recently researchers have begun to focus on how immigrants maintain, improve, or regain their health throughout the immigration process (Choudhry, 1998; Miller & Chandler, 2002; Misra, Patel, Davies, & Russo, 2000; Song, Sohng, & Yeom, 2002).

A set of traditional assumptions about the relationships of immigration and health has influenced both research and practice. Foremost among these are the selective nature of migration as a predictor of immigrant health, the negative effects of immigration on health, and positive health-related outcomes of immigration. Reflecting on the diversity of human migration experiences, it is not surprising that there has been research-based evidence to both support and refute assumptions about the relationships between immigration and health, as well as considerable theoretical critiques of these traditional assumptions. Acculturation has been an important concept in the immigration literature, yet there is little consensus among researchers and theorists about the complex relationships among

immigration, acculturation, and health or how to best measure acculturation. Unfortunately, many studies of immigrants and ethnic groups (e.g.,
Hispanics/Latinos, Asian Americans) lack any specific immigration indicators or variables, such as immigration status, country of birth, generational
history, or length of time in the United States. Such studies undoubtedly
contribute to knowledge development on health disparities, but by not
including immigration variables or indicators, they do little to further
understanding of the relationships between immigration processes and
immigrant health status, outcomes, and practices. Comparison of immigration studies is often problematic because of the multiplicity of variables
that could potentially influence immigrant health outcomes, behaviors,
and practices (Kasl & Berkman, 1983). However, the opportunity to explore this diversity is one of the most stimulating challenges for nursing
and health researchers.

The purpose of this integrative review was to examine the current
body of literature that does address relationships between immigration and
health. Although migration is a global phenomenon, the primary focus of
this review was research related to immigration into North America (United
States and Canada). Other recent integrative reviews have examined the
research related to immigrant women's health (Aroian, 2001), language
(Peragallo, Fox, & Alba, 2000), and the birth-weight paradox among
Mexican immigrant childbearing women (Callister & Birkhead, 2002).
Therefore, this review is more conceptual and methodological, examining
research that has supported, challenged, and expanded assumptions about
the relationships between immigration and health and the methods and
instruments used to explore these relationships.

We initiated the review with broad searches of electronic databases
from the social science, public health, and nursing literature using keywords
such as *immigrant, migration, acculturation,* and *health.* We also conducted manual searches of specialized journals (e.g., *Journal of Immigrant
Health; Transcultural Nursing*) and identified other potential sources
through journal article reference lists, professional publications, and dissertation abstracts. We limited the review to studies published since 1994,
although in our discussion of conceptual frameworks we have sited classic
works from as far back as 1926.

Based on the U.S. Census demographic categories, the most frequently
studied immigrant groups were Hispanics ($n = 19$) and Asian/Pacific
Islanders ($n = 13$). In terms of specific country of origin, Mexican immigrants were included in 13 of the 16 studies of Hispanic immigrants.

Countries of origin in the studies of Asian/Pacific Islander immigrant populations included Korea, Japan, the Philippines, India, Vietnam, and China. Of the studies reviewed, the only specific Arab country of origin studied was Jordan; European populations included immigrants (primarily refugees) from the former Soviet Union ($n = 2$). Only two studies included in this review were of African-born immigrants. Rather than studying a broad demographic group or country of origin, several researchers restricted their studies to more specific immigrant subgroups, such as Gujurati Asian Indians; indigenous Mixtec, Zapotec, and Triquis immigrants from the state of Oaxaca, Mexico; Chaldean Americans; and Soviet Jews. Other investigators conducted broader epidemiological studies ($n = 12$) of foreign-born immigrants or conducted studies that included both foreign-born and U.S.-born populations.

This review is organized into four major sections: selective migration and health; positive and negative effects of immigration on health; acculturation as an independent variable affecting immigrant health; and research using contemporary frameworks and concepts.

SELECTIVE MIGRATION AND HEALTH

The concept of selective migration, also known as the healthy migrant effect, reflects the assumption of a process of natural selection of healthy individuals as immigrants. Thus immigrants are viewed as a healthy and resilient group of people, willing and able to respond to the myriad possible health hazards of migration, such as increased risk of communicable disease, increased mental and emotional stress, and reduced access to medical care (Evans, 1987). As a result of the healthy migrant effect, newcomers have better health status or outcomes than the native-born person.

Support for the healthy migrant effect has come from several recent studies that examined the hypothesis that migration selectivity would account for differences in birth weights (Kelaher & Jessop, 2002; Weeks, Rumbaut, & Ojeda, 1999). Kelaher and Jessop used prenatal care service data, which included self-reports of previous low-birth-weight births (less than 2,500 grams at birth). The results indicated that Latina women born in the United States (USB) were significantly more likely to have low-birth-weight infants than both documented and undocumented foreign-born Latinas. Because no significant differences were found between documented and undocumented foreign-born Latinas, the researchers suggested that both official screening and selective migration might play a role in the lower rates of low birth weights among foreign-born Latinas compared to USB Latinas. Of note in this study is the fact that the researchers included Puerto Rican women in the USB group, a methodological decision that highlights a potential conceptual conundrum. Although Puerto Rican women who move to the mainland United States are migrants in geographic and cultural contexts, technically they are not transnational immigrants, because they are U.S. citizens and therefore not subject to U.S. government immigration restrictions. However, by including these women in the USB group, the researchers may have masked the effects of migration among this group.

Evidence from recent qualitative research suggests that prior to migration some individuals actively seek to ensure that they are healthy. Messias (2002) identified premigration health practices, such as going for gynecological checkups, taking care of dental needs, and stocking up on medications, as measures to ensure health among Brazilian immigrant women who had come to the United States with the express intention of settling, at least temporarily. One of the study participants described her premigration health concerns as follows: "I wanted to be well to come here, so I went to several doctors before coming. . . . I was concerned about not bringing any disease with me, in coming here" (Messias, 2002, p. 85).

The results of other recent studies highlight the mixed support and implications of the notion of selective migration. Siegel, Horan, and Teferra (2001) conducted a survey of health status, health behaviors, and health care access and utilization among African-born residents in Washington, DC, and compared the results to data from the Behavioral Risk Factor Surveillance Survey, the National Health Interview Survey for Virginia residents, and other demographic data for the Washington metropolitan area. Compared to the local and regional population, the African immigrants were less likely to report being told they had high cholesterol or to use tobacco or alcohol. However, they were much more likely to be uninsured or report not being able to see a physician because of cost. The African women in the sample were also less likely to ever have had a mammogram or Pap smear. These results suggest that these immigrants may have been relatively healthier upon arrival, but the barriers to health care they face in the United States may result in increased future health risks. Using death data from the 1997 Multiple Cause of Death data file and population data from the 1997 Current Population Survey, Rubia, Marcos, and Muennig (2002) found all-cause, age-adjusted mortality rates for foreign-born individuals to be significantly lower than the rates among native-born individuals. However, deaths due to ischemic heart disease and stroke were significantly higher among foreign-born females than among native-born females. A similar Canadian study involving a random sample (N = 180,350) of female immigrants supported the notion that immigrants, upon arrival, tend to have lower mortality risk when compared to Canadian-born residents (Payne et al., 2002). However, as might be expected, increased vulnerability was found among certain immigrant subgroups, particularly refugee women and immigrants with lower educational levels.

A study of blood lead (BPb) levels among a cohort of refugee children less than 7 years of age in Massachusetts by Geltman, Brown, and Cochran (2001) challenged the assumption of the healthy migrant effect, particularly among refugee populations. The researchers found elevated BPb levels in 11.3% of the sample (N = 693), a prevalence 2.7 times that of comparably aged U.S.-born children. Country of birth was the strongest predictor of elevated BPb levels, with prevalence ranging from 0% among Bosnian refugee children born in Germany to 27% among Vietnamese and African children and 40% among children born in Cuba and Haiti. This type of research supports the need to tailor clinical screening guidelines to specific immigrant and refugee populations.

Although some existing research does support the concept of selective migration as a predictor of immigrant health, determining when and if it will occur remains a challenge to both researchers and practitioners (Hull, 1979). There is a definite need for further research on identifying and predicting the mechanisms related to selective migration and the healthy migrant effect. For example, although intentional migrants who enter the country on immigrant visas must submit to premigration health screenings in their home country, immigrants who arrive via irregular channels or who enter on other types of visas (e.g., tourist visas) evade the highly selective pressures of an immigrant screening process. Some of these immigrants may be more likely to have characteristics associated with the risk factors for greater disease potential (Gushulak & MacPherson, 2000). Because health status at the time of migration does not necessarily predict future health outcomes, there is also an urgent need for more transnational and longitudinal studies. Such research could examine the relationship of preexisting health and social factors to the decision to migrate; the effect of immigration health screening on migration and subsequent health status; and changes in health status and health practices before and after migration.

Further research is needed to explain existing disparities in the level of immigrant health and to determine whether certain immigrants were healthier to start with (selective migration) or whether their health status improved (positive effect) or declined (negative effect) over time as a result of migration.

OPPOSING ASSUMPTIONS: POSITIVE OR NEGATIVE EFFECTS OF IMMIGRATION ON HEALTH

There are two contrasting assumptions regarding the effect of immigration on health. One premise is that many migrants undertake the move with the express desire to better their living conditions, economic status, lifestyle, or personal development and that these expectations are often at least partially realized, with positive effects in terms of individual and collective health (Evans, 1987). The assumption of positive effects of immigration on health is based on Gordon's (1964) classic conceptualization of acculturation and assimilation as vehicles for upward mobility and improved quality of life and the impetus for achieving the "American dream." Among many researchers and practitioners, acculturation has been assumed to be a desired social outcome as well as a beneficial health-related outcome of immigration. Gordon's critics have argued that while the classic model of structural and cultural assimilation may have validity as a framework for explaining the experiences of European immigrants, these assumptions do not apply to the current wave of non-European immigrants (Almaguer, 1994; Portes & Rumbaut, 2001; Rumbaut, 1994). The changing demographics of the latest wave of immigration to the United States call into question the classic assumption of the positive effect of acculturation on immigrant health.

Anticipation of a "better life" certainly plays a critical role in current migratory trends; it is also true that many new immigrants arrive with university degrees and previous professional experience. The results of several recent studies of immigrants from Brazil (Margolis, 1994; Messias, 2001, 2002), the former Soviet Union (Miller & Chandler, 2002), and Korea (Shin & Shin, 1999) suggest that rather than experiencing upward social mobility, highly educated professionals often experience the opposite. Shin and Shin's phenomenological study of the lived experiences of Korean immigrant women supported the notion that these highly educated women had subscribed to the vague dream of a better life through immigration. However, they experienced ongoing conflicts as they dealt with changing expectations and difficulties in fulfilling immigrant women's roles within the contexts of two different cultures. Some found their former education or careers irrelevant to their current situations and employment. Others, who had previously been full-time homemakers, were forced to enter the workforce because of economic pressures, which resulted in an increased workload, role conflict, and loss of personal time. Such research highlights the need to consider premigration contexts as well as postmigration social and environmental contexts and individual and collective processes of adaptation and acculturation in relation to health.

The opposing view is that the immigration process itself is inherently difficult, stressful, and often even hazardous, and the lifestyle changes and adjustments that accompany immigration bring with them a new set of health risks. Support for the negative effect of immigration is rooted in the early 20th-century sociological research of the Chicago School (Burgess, 1926; Park, Burgess, & McKenzie, 1925; Thrasher, 1927; Wirth, 1928) and others (Cowan, 1982; Galarza, 1964; Handlin, 1973; Poyo, 1989; Samora, 1971), which focused on the hardships and sacrifices of immigrants and described direct and indirect effects on their health. More recently, researchers have challenged the assumption of immigration as inherently stressful by attempting to identify specific relationships among immigrant characteristics and experiences in terms of both positive and negative health outcomes (Berry, 1994, 1997).

There is evidence from recent research that, for many immigrants, the migratory passage itself is dangerous and stressful and that certain health risks are associated with environmental factors and modes of travel and entry (Gushulak & MacPherson, 2000; McGuire, 2001; McGuire & Georges, 2003). McGuire conducted a binational grounded theory study exploring the transnational migration and health experiences in indigenous Oaxacan women. Data collection included participant observation and interviews in Oaxaca, Mexico, along the U.S.-Mexico border and in the interior of California. The research clearly identified multiple risks, dangers, and stresses these women confronted in the process of crossing the border. The decision to leave home, family, and community in remote rural mountainous regions of Oaxaca was in and of itself frightening and risky. Fear of the inherent dangers of the migratory journey often prompted the women to leave their children behind in the care of relatives rather than risk bringing them to the United States, although this meant carrying an added emotional burden of suffering and pain. However, fears about the journey were not unfounded, as evidenced by their reports of numerous physical health risks. These included injuries (e.g., fractures, snake bites, scorpion stings, punctures or impalement by cactus needles or nettles), heat, cold, hunger, thirst, and bodily weakness from the rigorous physical work involved in the migratory travel. Along the way, they were subject to violence and extortion by the coyotes paid to smuggle them across the most patrolled border in the world, and they risked capture and deportation by the border patrol. For women who were successful in crossing the border, this extraordinary feat became a pivotal event in their personal histories as well as part of the collective narratives of their communities in Oaxaca, Texas, and California.

Other researchers have highlighted the social and emotional costs of immigration on health and well-being. The results of a qualitative study of Jordanian immigrant women (Hattar-Pollara & Meleis, 1995) delineated the postmigration stressors of daily family life. The participants identified various sources of stress related to the initial difficulties of settling into an unfamiliar culture. These immigrant women needed to master new skills to deal with ordinary daily tasks such as shopping, using public transportation, writing checks, and paying bills. Interfacing with the U.S. educational system in which their children studied was another significant source of stress. A more persistent, long-term stressor was the emotional toll of loneliness, nostalgia, being a foreigner, and diminished social networks. The researchers noted that for all of these immigrant women, the fundamental differences between Arab and American cultures created significant pressure from within their families and the Jordanian immigrant community to maintain ethnic continuity. As a result, these immigrant women felt a strong need to maintain their identities as Jordanian women, wives, and mothers.

The results of Miller and Chandler's (2002) study of recent immigrants from the former Soviet Union (FSU) provided further evidence of the negative health impact of immigration-related stress. The investigators used the Demands of Immigration Scale (Aroian & Schappler-Morris, 1996) to measure acculturative stress and a modified Russian-language version of the Resilience Scale (Aroain, Schappler-Morris, Neary, Spitzer, & Tran, 1997) to assess a personality style that facilitates adaptation among immigrants. Symptoms of depression were measured by a Russian version of the Center for Epidemiological Studies–Depression (CES-D) Scale. The results indicated high levels of depressive symptoms, with close to 84% reporting a score above 16 on the CES-D, the cutoff indicating possible clinical depression in the U.S. population. Depressive symptoms were significantly positively correlated with Demands of Immigration scores (-0.396; $p = 0.01$) and age (0.154; $p = 0.05$) and significantly negatively correlated with English proficiency (-0.252; $p = 0.05$), English usage (-0.344; $p = 0.01$), and resilience (-0.336; $p = 0.05$). The only significant correlation with the Resilience Scale was English usage (0.190; $p = 0.01$). An interesting finding from the regression analysis was that English usage (e.g., working and living in proximity with English speakers and being exposed to English in the context of daily life), but not proficiency (self-reported language ability), contributed significantly to the CES-D. The authors identified several important areas for further research. These include studies of the psychological benefits and risks of residing and socializing in coethnic communities as compared with more mainstream cultural groups and further investigations of the strengths and resources that may protect immigrant women from the effects of acculturative stress and enhance their immigration transitions. In a study of substance use and other maladaptive behaviors among Latino youth, Cabrera Strait (2001) found that youths who had problems learning English experienced more acculturative stress than those who did not report English-language difficulties. After controlling for gender, age, and socioeconomic status, the study found that Latino youths who experienced more acculturative stress consumed more alcohol than those who experienced less acculturative stress. The results of these studies also suggest the need for further research on the role of language and, more specifically, clarification of the interactions of English-language usage, contexts, and abilities on the social, psychological, and physical health of immigrants across the lifespan.

Negative health outcomes may also be the result of immigrant relocation to destinations where they are exposed to diseases that are less prevalent in their population of origin. Higher behavioral risk practices, ranging from dietary changes to tobacco and alcohol use, commercial sex work, and violent behavior, as well as environmental health risks associated with crowded housing, unregulated work environments, and lack of access to health care services, have all been identified as factors contributing to the deterioration of health status following migration (Cabrera Strait, 2001; Gushulak & MacPherson, 2000; Hummer, Rogers, Nam, & LeClere, 1999; Singh & Yu, 1996). Descriptive, cross-sectional studies have documented changing behavioral and social patterns among immigrants. For example, Yang and Read (1996) conducted a mail survey among Asian-born residents ($N = 124$) in Nevada. The study was designed to compare the fat, cholesterol, and fiber content between pre- and postmigration dietary intake. The results indicated postmigration increases in fat and cholesterol intake and decreased carbohydrate and fiber intake. However, compared with current U.S. dietary patterns, these Asian immigrants' current diets were relatively low-fat, high-carbohydrate, and high-fiber diets. In order to understand the mechanisms involved and the long-term health effects of dietary changes on immigrant health status, more longitudinal studies are needed. As this review has indicated, a variety of factors, ranging from premigration health status and health risks related to the migratory passage to the social, cultural, environmental, and health sector contexts of settling into the host country may contribute either positively or negatively to the health status of immigrants. Researchers continue to search for explanations as to the specific mechanisms that may contribute to positive or negative health outcomes among different immigrant groups. One of those explanations is acculturation, addressed in the following section.

ACCULTURATION AS AN INDEPENDENT VARIABLE AFFECTING HEALTH

Acculturation is one of the most frequently used variables in studies of immigration and health. Researchers have examined acculturation as an independent variable in relationship to a wide variety of health-related outcomes. Among the research we reviewed, acculturation was studied in relation to specific health behaviors or risks such as diet and physical exercise (Huang et al., 1996; Misra et al., 2000; Song et al., 2002), breast self-examination (Peragallo et al., 2000), alcohol or drug use or dependence (Cabrera Strait, 2001; Khoury, Warheit, Vega, Zimmerman, & Gil, 1996), and sexual behaviors (Villarruel, Langfeld, & Porter, 2003). Others examined the association between acculturation and health service utilization (Amaro & de la Torre, 2002; Lee, 2000; Vega, Kolody, Aguilar-Gaxiola, & Catalana, 1999) and medical procedures such as hysterectomy (Brett & Higgins, 2003). Specific health outcomes studied in relation to acculturation include birth weight (Ventura, Martin, Curtin, Mathews, & Park, 2000; Weigers & Sherraden, 2001), immunization status (Prislin, Suarez, Simspon, & Dyer, 1998), hypertension (Dallo & James, 2000; Juarabe, 1998; Luepker, 2001; Wei et al., 1996), and depressive symptoms (González, Haan, & Hinton, 2001; Miller & Chandler, 2002; Shen & Tekeuchi, 2001). However, the considerable variation found in the operationalization of acculturation across these studies constitutes a major critique of the current research on immigration, acculturation, and health.

Single-Item Proxy Measures

The intent of acculturation measures is to determine the degree to which immigrants have integrated and incorporated values, beliefs, attitudes, and practices of the host society into their lives (Peragallo et al., 2000). Existing scales of acculturation fall within three broad types: single-item proxy measures, multidimensional scales, and a combination of these two. Single-item proxy measures of acculturation, such as generational distance, place of birth, language of interview, or length of time spent in the host country, have been used in studies of a wide range of immigrant groups and health indicators (Brett & Higgins, 2003, Ebin et al., 2001; van Servellen, Chang, & Lombardi, 2002) and have had variable results. Using data from the 1998–1999 National Health Interview Survey, Brett and Higgins used three single-item proxies (country of origin, time in the United States, and language of interview) in their study of hysterectomy prevalence among Hispanic ($n = 4,684$) and non-Hispanic White ($n = 20604$) women. After adjusting for educational attainment, no differences in hysterectomy rates were found between the Hispanic and non-Hispanic White women. Among the Hispanic women, risk of hysterectomy was not associated with acculturation as measured by either place of birth or length of time in the United States.

However, women who had higher levels of acculturation as measured by choice of language of interview (those who chose English) were more likely to have a hysterectomy than those with lower levels of acculturation (those who chose to be interviewed in Spanish). This finding poses some unanswered questions as to why women who were more comfortable speaking English had higher rates of hysterectomies. For example, were they more likely to seek health care services for identified health problems, or were they more likely to have employer-provided or government insurance than other Hispanic women with more limited English skills? Comparing the results of this investigation with the findings of Miller and Chandler's (2002) research suggests the need for further clarification of the role of English-language acquisition, ability, comfort in relation to immigrant health status, and its relation to health outcomes and health care utilization.

Huang et al. (1996) used two single-item proxies of acculturation (place of birth and generational distance) in their study of diet, physical activity, and risk of diabetes in a sample of 8,006 Japanese American men in Hawaii. The investigators found better health habits (i.e., a lower-fat diet and more physical activity) among Japanese-born men in comparison to their Hawaii-born counterparts, providing support for the notion of acculturation as a health risk among this particular population. A study of health promotion behaviors of Gujurati Asian Indian immigrants (Misra et al., 2000) found that respondents who had lived in the United States for more than 20 years were more physically active, were more responsible for their health, and practiced better stress management skills than immigrants who were in the country less than 20 years. In a study of elderly Korean immigrants, Song et al. (2002) found no association between length of residence in the United States and health-promoting behaviors, as measured by the Health Promoting Lifestyle Profile (HPLP). However, significant correlations were found between total HPLP scores and self-efficacy, level of education, and economic status. Immigrants who engaged in more exercise had a higher economic status than those who did not engage in regular exercise. The results of these studies suggest that multiple social, economic, and cultural factors are part of a complex equation between acculturation and health, which single-item proxies of acculturation are unable to capture.

Multiitem Acculturation Scales and Combined Measures

Despite the widespread use of single-item proxy measures of acculturation, these measures have been criticized as lacking depth and content. As a result, various multivariate acculturation scales have been developed. Language use, preference, and proficiency have been the focus of multivariate scales such as the Bicultural Involvement Questionnaire (Szapocznik, Kurtines, & Fernandez, 1980) and the Bidimensional Acculturation Scale (Marin & Gamba, 1996). Ethnic identification, values, and structural location have also been incorporated into several multivariate acculturation scales (Cuellar, Harris, & Jasso; 1980; Marin, Sabogal, Marin, Ortero-Sabogal, & Perez-Stable, 1987; Mendoza, 1989).

Much like single-item proxy scales, multivariate acculturation scales have been used to explore a variety of health behaviors, risks, and outcomes. For example, Prislin and colleagues (1998) used a multidimensional scale to examine the relationship between acculturation of Mexican American mothers in Texas and the immunization status of their children, ages 3 to 24 months. The investigators used a revised version (Dawson, Crano, & Borgoon, 1996) of the Acculturation Rating Scale for Mexican Americans (ARSMA; Cuellar et al., 1980), a 10-item scale that takes into account language preferences, ethnic identity, music and television viewing preferences, place where reared, and contacts with Mexico. The results indicated that incomplete immunization was more likely among more acculturated Mexican American women. Specifically, mothers with low levels of acculturation were 2.6 times more likely to have their children properly immunized than women with high levels of acculturation. The relationship remained significant even after adjusting for other covariates of immunization (e.g., education, income, and health coverage). González et al. (2001) employed the same instrument in their study of immigration, acculturation, and prevalence of depression in older Mexican Americans. The higher prevalence and risk of depression among immigrants than among U.S.-born Mexican Americans was contradictory to findings of previous research on the same population.

One methodological strategy researchers have adopted is to tailor multivariate acculturation measures to specific populations. A case in point is A Short Acculturation Scale for Hispanics (ASASH; Marin et al., 1987), a 12-item, 5-point Likert scale measure that evaluates the extent to which respondents engage in behaviors related to culture of origin or the host culture. Peragallo et al. (2000) used ASASH in their study of breast self-examination (BSE) among immigrant Latina women ($N = 111$) in an urban Midwest area. The majority of the immigrant women (84.7%) scored low on the ASASH acculturation measure, and 85% reported they did not practice BSE. In contrast to other studies of acculturation and positive health behaviors, this study showed that Latina women with high levels of acculturation were twice as likely to practice correct BSE as women with low acculturation (OR odds ratio 2.1).

Interestingly, De la Cruz, Padilla, and Agustin (2000) opted to adapt the ASASH for use with Filipino Americans, producing A Short Acculturation Scale for Filipino Americans (ASASFA) in English and Tagalog. The authors cited both measurement and cultural factors that contributed to their decision. Measurement factors included the psychometric soundness, practical length, and lack of sociodemographics (generation, length of residence, age at immigration, etc.) of the ASASH, which allowed for these to be used as correlates of acculturation. The common culture and history of Spanish colonization between Filipinos and Mexican Americans also contributed to the decision to adopt the ASASH rather than create another instrument for use with Filipino immigrants.

Other researchers have responded to the challenges presented by both single-item proxy measures and multivariate acculturation scales by combining both types of measures. A case in point is the study of acculturation and generational distance on sexual behaviors of Latino preadolescents and adolescents (Villarruel et al., 2003). In addition to using ASASH (Marin et al., 1987), the investigators determined generational distance by several questions related to place of birth of the respondent and the respondent's parents. The acculturation measure that was significantly related to differences in intimate behaviors and intercourse was generational difference. That is, third-generation adolescents engaged in more intimate sexual behaviors and sexual intercourse than their first-generation counterparts.

In a study of the relationship of acculturation to a network of psychosocial correlates relevant to mental health among Chinese Americans (N = 983), Shen and Takeuchi (2001) also combined multiple acculturation measures. The 14-item acculturation scale, modified from the work of Burnam, Hough, Karno, Escobar, and Telles (1987), included daily language use and preference in a variety of situations, patterns of social contact, and participation in cultural events. The researchers measured generational status from the nativity status of the respondent and the respondent's parents and also used length of time in the United States as an indicator of acculturation. Findings included an association of higher levels of acculturation with higher stress, which in turn contributed to elevated depressive symptoms. In addition, higher stress was related to lower perceived levels of health, which also contributes to depressive symptoms. However, neither generational status nor length of time in the United States was related to the mental health outcome variables in this study. A covariate of mental health, immigrant socioeconomic status, was measured in terms of education and income levels and found to be directly and indirectly related to mental health outcomes.

This review of recent research on acculturation and health confirms previous critiques that the association between acculturation and health depends in large part on how acculturation is conceptualized and measured. The most widely used acculturation scales have high reliability scores (i.e., alpha coefficients above 0.80) and account for differences across and within groups (Ebin et al., 2001; Marin & Marin, 1991). However, inconsistent and inconclusive research findings have been attributed to the lack of standardization, reliability, and validity of acculturation measures as well as to the diversity of measurement scales (Marin & Gamba, 1996; Marin & Marin, 1991; Peragallo et al., 2000). In spite of efforts over several decades to develop and refine acculturation scales, this review of recent research demonstrates little progress toward increasing substantive knowledge about the complex relationships between acculturation and immigrant health. As the mixed results of these various studies suggest, further research is needed to identify the social, cultural, and environmental mechanisms contributing to these changes in health behaviors among individual immigrants and specific immigrant groups. Few researchers have conducted comparative studies, another promising area for future research. Suggestions for comparative studies include the interactions of acculturation and health between different immigrant groups and contexts, across the lifespan, and transgenerationally.

CONTEMPORARY CONCEPTS AND FRAMEWORKS FOR RESEARCH ON IMMIGRATION AND HEALTH

Traditional models of immigration and health have been critiqued for ethnocentric bias, lack of empirical support, and lack of applicability to very diverse, heterogeneous populations of immigrants. In response to these methodological and conceptual challenges, and in the context of an increasingly global and interconnected world, immigration scholars have begun to rethink and reconceptualize immigration experiences, moving away from linear, ethnocentric models of acculturation to more fluid, dynamic explanations of immigration experiences (Portes & Zhou, 1993). This section contains a review of research based on more contemporary concepts and frameworks such as biculturalism, transnationalism, undocumentedness, and transitions.

Biculturalism

In contrast to the traditional linear conceptualization of acculturation, biculturalism reflects the position that acculturation to the new culture and adherence to values and behaviors of the culture of origin are independent (Birman, 1998; Phinney, 2003). Biculturalism assumes that it is possible for an individual to have a sense of belonging in two cultures without compromising his or her sense of cultural identity (LaFromboise, Coleman, & Gerton, 1993). Researchers using bicultural models reflect the notion that since immigrants may identify with more than one culture, cultural identification can be assessed on several independent dimensions and change can be measured along each dimension (Bourhis, Moise, Perreault, & Senecal, 1997). One of the better known and widely used bicultural models was developed within cross-cultural psychology (Berry, 1994, 1997; Berry, Kim, Minde, & Mok, 1987; Berry, Kim, Power, Young, & Bujaki, 1989; Bourhis et al., 1997; Sayegh & Lasry, 1993). The model consists of four identifiable immigrant acculturation patterns—assimilation, integration, separation, and marginalization—which reflect how immigrants engage with and make sense of the social contexts of both their home and host society.

Applying a bicultural matrix model in relation to health, Lee, Sobal, and Frongillo (2000) explored the relationships of traditional, bicultural, and acculturated perspectives on health behaviors using a random sample of individuals with Korean surnames. The analysis included five health dimensions—smoking, physical activity, fat intake, body weight, and overall health. The results indicated that bicultural men are less likely to smoke than men with lower or higher levels of acculturation. Further, acculturated men had higher mean Body Mass Index than traditional Koreans. This linear relationship persisted after other variables associated with body weight were accounted for (i.e., age, socioeconomic status, and health behaviors). In terms of self-rated health, men in the acculturated and bicultural groups reported more positive health than those with a traditional Korean cultural orientation. However, physical activity and fat intake were unrelated to acculturation patterns. Although this study highlighted interesting similarities and differences in health and acculturation patterns, the results did little to clarify the multiple mechanisms that may factor into health outcomes among individuals with varying cultural orientations. In a study of diet and acculturation in Chinese American and Chinese Canadian women (Satia-Abouta, Patterson, Kristal, The, & Tu, 2002), researchers found stronger preferences for the traditional Chinese diet among older adults, who often had younger, highly educated family members living in the household. Although these women were categorized as more "Western" on the dietary acculturation scale, the researchers suggested that their dietary patterns might actually be more bicultural, in that they eat more Western foods outside the home but follow the Chinese dietary practices of elder family members at home.

The meaning of biculturalism, as perceived and experienced by second-generation Chinese American women, was explored in a recent qualitative study (Willgerodt, Miller, & McElmurry, 2002). The initial step was the convening of a focus group of Asian American women identified as community experts. These women were asked to define biculturalism and describe how they arrived at their self-identification. Then they were asked to provide feedback on a proposed interview guide for the study of biculturalism. The second phase of the study involved individual, semi-structured interviews with a purposive sample ($N = 15$) of second-generation Chinese American women. Based on the focus group feedback and the definitional inconsistencies in the use and meaning of *bicultural, Chinese American,* and *second generation,* the investigators did not use any of these terms in the final interview guide. Rather, they asked the participants to relate their parents' immigration history and asked them to describe their experiences growing up as an American with parents who came from China and to identify any situations where they expressed more characteristics from one culture than the other. An important result of this study, in terms of conceptualizing ethnic identity development (Phinney, Horenczyk, Liebkind, & Vedder, 2001), was that although ethnic identity formation among these second-generation Chinese immigrants clearly began in childhood, it was a dynamic, continuous process that continued throughout adolescence, with significant associations to the developmental transitions of adulthood. The results of this research not only expanded the concept of biculturalism but also lent support for the applicability of another contemporary immigration and health framework, that of transitions, addressed in the next section.

IMMIGRATION, TRANSITIONS, AND HEALTH

Particularly within nursing, a transition framework is one of the more recent conceptual approaches to understanding and explaining the relationships of migration and health (Meleis, Sawyer, Im, Messias, & Schumacher, 2000). Transition has been broadly conceptualized as the passage between one life phase, condition, or status to another, associated with some degree of self-redefinition within the individual experiencing the transition (Chick & Meleis, 1986). Immigration, like other life transitions, is not a linear process, nor does it occur in isolation. The migration transition in itself is multiple in nature, possibly involving transitions in employment, social networks, and socioeconomic status. Immigration transitions may well coincide with occupational, educational, or professional transitions; birth, marriage, divorce, death of loved ones, or other family role transitions; developmental transitions such as adolescence or menopause; or health-illness transitions (Birman & Trickett, 2001; Im & Meleis, 2000; Meleis et al., 2000; Messias, 2001, 2002).

McGuire (2002) described the migration experiences of indigenous Mexican women as "crossing myriad borders," a metaphor to express the multiple transitions that these women must negotiate when relocating north of the border. The results of a qualitative study of Brazilian women indicated their immigration transition experiences to be *multiple and complex* in nature, involving situational, developmental, and health-illness transitions (Messias, 2001, 2002). What characterized these Brazilians' immigration experiences as transitions was not so much the movement across national borders but the resulting passages between different life phases, conditions, and statuses, accompanied by some degree of self-redefinition. All of the women ($N = 26$) experienced some form of work or occupational transition in conjunction with their transnational migration. These migratory occupational transitions were embedded in social transitions, which in many cases translated into downward social mobility. For many, migration signified the transition from being a Brazilian professional, employee, student, or middle-class housewife to immigrant domestic worker. Domestic or food service work was a temporary steppingstone for some, a long-term career change for others. In several cases, the physical and emotional overload and stress associated with domestic work and employment were identified as factors that diminished their health and quality of life as immigrants. However, others reported a sense of satisfaction, competence, personal growth, and well-being as a result of their immigrant work experiences.

A transition framework also guided research on the meanings of menopause and symptom experiences among midlife Korean immigrant women (Im, 1997; Im & Meleis, 2000; Im, Meleis, & Lee, 1999). The research was a cross-sectional descriptive study consisting of both quantitative and qualitative methods. Data on perceived symptoms were collected using the Cornell Medical Index, supplemented by 14 questions on menopausal symptoms based on previous research of both Western and Korean women and open-ended questions about perceived causes and symptom management strategies. Although no general patterns were found, the most prevalent symptoms reported during the past 6 months were impaired vision for reading, aches in back of neck and skull, and complete exhaustion. In contrast to studies of Western women, but consistent with other studies of Asian women, these immigrant Korean women were less likely to experience vasomotor symptoms associated with the Western, medical phenomenon of menopause (e.g., hot flashes, dizziness, or night sweats). Overall, the immigrant women attributed their symptoms to aging, psychological stress, and physical overwork; none of the participants connected menopause with pathological changes. The qualitative data indicated that most of the participants were unclear about the biological processes related to menopause, but none connected menopause with any pathological changes or considered it a disease needing medical treatment. For most of the women, family health and economic and social concerns took precedence over the menopause transition, which merited little attention or energy. The authors suggested that having to deal with multiple situational transitions related to migration contributed to the fact that these Korean immigrants placed less emphasis and priority on the health and developmental transition of menopause.

In their study of Soviet Jewish refugee adolescents and parents, Birman and Trickett (2001) identified various factors that may mediate the multiple transitions within the migration experience. These include the context of the sending society, the context of the receiving society, age at migration, and gender. Possible mediating factors within the sending and receiving societies include labor and economic conditions, the political climate, immigration policies, public opinion around migration and immigrants, and access to social migration networks.

A positive trend within the immigration and health research arena, as presented in these studies, is the recognition of the ways in which developmental, situational, organizational, and health-illness transitions often overlap and interact, creating complex, multiple transitions.

Transnational Perspectives and Practices

Transnationalism refers to social processes in which migrants establish social fields that cross geographic, cultural, and political borders (Glick Schiller, Basch, & Blanc-Szanton, 1992a, 1992b; Rogler, 1994). This is another more contemporary concept incorporated into research on migration and health. Several recent studies have provided support for the notion of transnational immigrant health practices, in which immigrants move back and forth between and among different formal and informal health care systems in home and host countries. These studies have documented some of the ways in which immigrant women utilize transnational social and kinship networks as important sources of health information, transportation, employment, and social support.

Transnational health practices that Messias (2002) identified among Brazilian immigrants included maintaining a personal stock of prescription medications from Brazil for the purposes of self-medication and sharing with family and friends and continued reliance on some type of Brazilian health resources and services. For some this was accomplished during trips home; others simply put health care "on hold" until some indefinite point in the future when they planned to return to Brazil. Several women reported having used Brazilian doctors, nurses, and dentists living in the area as a source of information, advice, and formal and informal health care. Similarly, Lee (2000) reported a common practice among Korean immigrants of returning to Korea for the tests and treatment of cancer or other medical conditions. Structural barriers to health care in the United States, including the costs of health care and health insurance, as well as language barriers and lack of time, were identified as contributing to this transnational practice of seeking health care. Messias identified a variety of syncretic combinations of health care strategies, as well as examples of selective inclusion or elimination of home- or host-based approaches among the Brazilian immigrants. The investigator emphasized the point that immigrants may have different degrees of fluidity in their adoption of transnational health care frameworks, approaches, or perspectives.

Clark's (2002) longitudinal ethnographic study of Mexican immigrant women's personal expertise in recognizing and treating children's ailments is another example of research that has explored the complex dynamics of immigrants' transnational lives and health practices. The research provided examples of how immigration status, access to transportation, language ability, and intra- and extrafamiliar gender negotiations intersected with the complexities and cultural biases of the U.S. health care services as immigrant women took care of their children's health. The results demonstrated how these immigrant women's work of family health maintenance occurred within dynamic contexts created by the intersections of family, culture, class, immigration status, changing U.S. immigration and welfare legislation, and a complex, multilayered health care system.

Qualitative researchers have used innovative methodologies to document and explore the transnational social networks of pregnant Mexican immigrants. To extend the qualitative data collected through focus groups, Bender and Castro (2000) used photonarratives and documentation of local kin networks. The photonarrative method consisted of having the women take photographs of people, places, and things that were important to them and then explain the significance of the photos. The diagrams of participants' extended family networks were a way of documenting the immigrant women's social connections in both home and host societies. In her longitudinal ethnographic study of social support among Mexican-origin women in their last trimester of pregnancy through the first month postpartum, Clark (2001) also employed innovative methodological approaches. The study explored the density, distribution, and stability of social networks from the perspectives of the women (emic) and the nurse researchers (etic). Data for the etic perspective included information gathered through the interviews on social support, accumulated observational information recorded in field notes throughout the 4-month perinatal period, and the genogram of the family. The resulting comparison and juxtaposition of both emic and etic perspectives highlighted the differences of these two perspectives. For these *Mexicanas*, social support in the perinatal period encompassed daily instrumental help, emotional support, and the perception that others can be counted on to "be there" for them. In contrast, the etic typologies developed by the nurses on the research team identified "disconnections in social support for immigrant women with the lowest levels of acculturation and poorest English language skills, and failed support for women who encountered aggravation and antagonism from family and friends who they believed should have offered support instead" (p. 1315). The only consistent pattern of the etic support typology in relation to acculturation or immigration status was that women with a pattern of disconnected social support were typically new immigrants separated from key members of their traditional support network. The results of Clark's study not only highlighted differences and ambiguities in the emic and etic perceptions of social support but also provided support for the need to examine more closely ethnocentric biases of the conceptual frameworks and theories that undergird immigration and health research. Through the use of such innovative, participatory research methods and transnational perspectives, these studies have made significant contributions to the efforts to incorporate transnational perspectives and frameworks to immigration and health research.

Exploring Another Dimension of the Immigration Experience: Undocumentedness

Undocumentedness is one of the most recent concepts incorporated into the theoretical and research literature on immigration and health (Messias, 1996). In relation to international migration, *undocumentedness* technically refers to the state of lacking a written record of proof of legal immigration or citizenship status. In contrast to the concepts of assimilation and acculturation, undocumentedness reflects the marginalization and vulnerability of immigrants who are not legally incorporated into the social life of the host nation as a result of social and political power inequalities. McGuire's (2001, 2002; McGuire & Georges, 2003) research among indigenous immigrant women from Mexico who were of Mixtec, Zapotec, and Triquis origin illustrated the power differentials related to immigration status. The findings demonstrated the high degree of agency in decisions to leave home and in attending to their personal and family health care needs within culturally familiar venues. However, on arrival in the United States, undocumentedness emerged as a major barrier to seeking health care, further complicating language differences and the cultural milieu of health care agencies. The results of the study indicated that indigenous immigrant women's ability to manage the health care of their families was significantly compromised by undocumentedness, reinforcing impoverishment and its associated elevated health risks. In contrast, possession of legal documents expanded indigenous immigrant women's repertoire of possibilities for health care access along the U.S.-Mexican border.

Similar findings were reported from a study of day laborers in San Francisco (Walter, Bourgois, Loinaz, & Schillinger, 2002). These researchers found evidence of increasing health and economic risks to border passage, as undocumented immigrants cross through dangerous, remote areas to avoid increases in border security. For many of these men, this meant they had incurred significant debts to the "coyotes" who provided assistance in crossing the border. The researchers noted that the day labor was "a form of indenture that makes it difficult to leave dangerous or abusive work environments" (p. 223). Further risks to their health included homelessness or overcrowded, shared housing arrangements. On the job, lack of training and experience, inadequate safety equipment, and economic pressures increase the risk of injury and disability, ranging from dermatitis, chronic allergic conjunctivitis, musculoskeletal injuries, joint pain, overuse syndromes and more serious injuries from burns, lacerations, and crush injuries, as well as anxiety, depression, and drug or alcohol abuse.

In situations of unequal social power, such as encounters between health care providers and immigrant patients, fear and distrust related to undocumentedness and other cultural, economic, social, or political factors may be heightened. To determine the extent to which concerns about immigration status served as a deterrent to seeking care, the Project HOPE Undocumented Immigrant Health Care Access Survey was conducted in two Texas communities and two California communities (Berk & Schur, 2001). Using U.S. Census data, neighborhoods likely to have concentrations of undocumented Latinos were identified, and in-person interviews using trained Latino interviewers fluent in Spanish screened 7,342 households for study eligibility. Of 1,171 eligible respondents, 973 participated in the study. Fear about getting medical care was operationalized as a "yes" response to the question "At some time were you afraid you would not receive medical service because you did not have 'papers'?" (p. 153). The results indicated that across all four sites, 39% of undocumented Latino adults reported having feared they would not receive medical care because of their undocumented status. No associations were found between fear about immigration status and age, sex, or years in the United States. However, of particular note was the indication that undocumented immigrants who reported fear they would not receive services were substantially more likely to report actually having been unable to get the care they needed (14%) or get a prescription filled (9.6%) than those not expressing fear (3% and 2.2%, respectively).

Research with undocumented populations presents specific methodological challenges related to disclosure. Although determining nativity or length of stay may be fairly straightforward, identifying and documenting immigration status presents legal and methodological challenges (Messias, 1996). Although higher rates of undocumentedness have been identified among certain segments of the immigrant population, they often involve groups that are difficult for researchers to reach. A study of day laborers of Mexican and Central American origin in Los Angeles reported that 95% were undocumented upon entering the United States (Valenzuela, 1999). Women, estimated to make up half of the undocumented population in the country, often work in the informal sector, cleaning, cooking, and providing child and elder care in private homes, and thus limiting access by researchers (Chavez, Hubbell, Mishra, & Valdez, 1997; Walter et al., 2002).

Methodological, ethical, and political issues complicate research on undocumentedness. Recruitment of samples of immigrant populations in a manner that both protects confidentiality and is nonthreatening to the status of undocumented persons is a major ethical and methodological challenge (Kelaher & Jessop, 2002; Messias, 1996). Although it is not possible to distinguish the citizenship or immigration status of foreign-born persons in most epidemiological data sets (Korenbrot, Dudley, & Greene, 2000), health systems administrative databases "often inadvertently capture this information because immigration status may affect program eligibility and billing" (Kelaher & Jessop, 2002, p. 2172). In their study of immigration status and birth weights, Kelaher and Jessop developed a method to classify immigration status. Foreign-born Latinas who presented a resident status card or reported a Social Security number at intake were classified as *documented*; those who did not present a resident status card or had missing data recorded for the resident status variable and no Social Security number recorded in the administrative database were classified as *undocumented*.

Determining immigration status is often difficult or impossible, particularly for researchers using large national data sets (Rubia et al., 2002). For example, there is no way to separate foreign-born populations by country or region of birth within the National Health and Nutrition Examination Survey. Similarly, the annual morbidity and mortality rate summaries published by the Centers for Disease Control and Prevention, which track mortality by age, gender, income, and race, to date have not included foreign birth or immigration status as a variable. Despite these limitations, as this review has indicated, a growing number of researchers have responded creatively to the need to include immigration status, particularly undocumentedness, in research on immigrant health behaviors, outcomes, and access to care.

SUMMARY AND FUTURE DIRECTIONS

The dynamic nature of global migration and the increasingly transnational contexts of migrants' lives, social relationships, and health practices are challenging researchers to expand their frameworks, methodologies, and even the geographic boundaries of their research. The results of this integrative review provide some indications that interdisciplinary research on immigration and health is moving in new directions. However, in order to advance knowledge and provide direction for interventions aimed at reducing health disparities among immigrant populations, certain areas warrant further attention. Particularly among intentional migrants, there is a definite need for binational and multinational research on premigration health status and practices, in order to identify possible mechanisms involved in selective migration and the healthy migrant effect. Transnational research focusing on both premigration as well as return migration health issues is needed. Health researchers have not yet begun to explore the roles and relationships of health and illness to return migration (either permanent or temporary), a neglected phenomenon among immigration scholars in general (Gmelch, 1980). Transnational, fluid migrant families dealing with temporary, intermittent, or lengthy separations provide a promising area of study for family health researchers.

The results of recent qualitative studies and studies employing multivariate instruments have furthered the understanding of acculturation and immigrant health. However, the multiple health effects of the various social and cultural processes immigrants undergo are still not clearly understood, nor has the acculturation research clarified the opposing assumptions of positive or negative effects of acculturation on health. To date, researchers employing multivariate models have not adequately explored the extent to which acculturation and socioeconomic status operate independently and jointly in the distribution of health and health disparities. Within the current context of the U.S. health care system, characterized by both increasing costs and rapidly rising uninsurance rates, the relationship of immigrants' financial resources (or lack thereof) and health cannot be ignored.

There are several other methodological and conceptualization issues that need to be addressed. In many of the studies reviewed, the variance explained by acculturation in the regression models was not stated. Typically, the correlation among acculturation and health measures and the reliability of the acculturation scales were indicated, but not the R^2 of the regression models. The explanatory power or robustness of acculturation and its relationship to health remains unclear. Moreover, often researchers do not justify their choice of one particular acculturation measure over another, making it difficult to ascertain if the acculturation measure was used out of convenience, for its high correlation with the outcome variable, or for its high alpha reliability score.

The dynamic interactions of acculturation, language, social context, and psychological well-being and the need to develop and test more complex models to explain these relationships were noted by the authors of several of the studies in this review (González et al., 2001; Miller & Chandler, 2002). In addition to language, nativity, immigration status, and length of time in the host country, health researchers need to pay more attention to immigrants' host and home country community associations and contacts. Among different immigrant groups, settlement patterns vary among different immigrant groups, depending on factors such as geography, U.S. immigration and resettlement policies, and changing economic opportunities.

The existing research does not do justice to the wide diversity of immigrants currently living in the United States and to their varying immigration contexts. Retrospective studies would be useful in elucidating possible relationships between settlement patterns and immigrant health. As part of the settlement process, contextual information such as neighborhood characteristics, racial/ethnic segregation, and racial discrimination are needed. These contextual factors may shape the acculturation process, relate to access to health services, and relate to health prevention and promotion mechanisms, in addition to independently influencing health disparities (Pickett & Pearl, 2001; Raudenbush & Sampson, 1999).

To better understand the health implications of widely disparate immigration contexts and populations, more research is needed on understudied populations, such as immigrants and refugees from Africa and Arab countries. Another virtually unstudied phenomenon is the health of American emigrants and ex-patriots. In addition to studies of health risks, a stronger focus on the health resources of individual immigrants and immigrant groups is needed. Intervention research is needed to determine the effectiveness of programs designed to promote health, improve health status, and reverse preexisting as well as acquired health risks among immigrants. In addition, such studies could further knowledge about immigration and health transitions by identifying the most propitious points in time for health interventions in relation to immigration and other lifespan transitions.

To further understanding of documented health disparities as well as possible health protective factors among diverse immigrant populations, researchers must design both cross-sectional and longitudinal studies to examine more closely possible interactions between migration, demographic variables, and social and environmental contexts as well as the intersections of gender, class, ethnicity, nativity, and immigration status on health risks, practices, and outcomes. The health impact of immigration policy is of increasing importance and an area that few researchers have addressed to date. In light of recent federal welfare and immigration policy reforms after September 11, 2001, citizenship and immigration status will be a variable of increasing interest to researchers studying health and health care disparities.

REFERENCES

Almaguer, T. (1994). *Racial fault lines: The historical origins of White supremacy in California.* Berkeley: University of California Press.

Amaro, H., & de la Torre, A. (2002). Public health needs and scientific opportunities in research for Latinas. *American Journal of Public Health, 92,* 525–529.

Aroian, K. J. (2001). Immigrant women and their health. In J. J. Fitzpatrick (Ed.), *Annual review of nursing research* (Vol. 19, pp. 179–226). New York: Springer Publishing Co.

Aroian, K. J., & Schappler-Morris, N. (1996). Using qualitative data for estimating construct validity of standardized measures. *Journal of Nursing Measurement, 4,* 59–74.

Aroian, K. J., Schappler-Morris, N., Neary, S., Spitzer, A., & Tran, T. V. (1997). Psychometric evaluation of the Russian language version of the Resilience Scale. *Journal of Nursing Measurement, 5,* 151–164.

Bender, D. E., & Castro, D. (2000). Explaining the birth weight paradox: Latina immigrants' perceptions of resilience and risk. *Journal of Immigrant Health, 2,* 155–173.

Berk, M. L., & Schur, C. L. (2001). The effect of fear on access to care among undocumented Latino immigrants. *Journal of Immigrant Health, 3,* 151–156.

Berry, J. W. (1994). Acculturation and adaptation: An overview. In A. M. Bouvy, F. J. R. van de Vijve, P. Boski, & P. Schmitz (Eds.), *Journeys into cross-cultural psychology* (pp. 129–141). Amsterdam: Swets & Zeitlinger.

Berry, J. W. (1997). Immigration, acculturation, and adaptation. *Applied Psychology, 46,* 5–68.

Berry, J. W., Kim, U., Minde, T., & Mok, D. (1987). Comparative studies of acculturative stress. *International Migration Review, 21,* 491–511.

Berry, J. W., Kim, U., Power, S., Young, M., & Bujaki, M. (1989). Acculturation attitudes in plural societies. *Applied Psychology, 38,* 185–206.

Birman, D. (1998). Biculturalism and perceived competence of Latino immigrant adolescents. *American Journal of Community Psychology, 263,* 335–354.

Birman, D., & Trickett, E. J. (2001). Cultural transitions in first-generation immigrants: Acculturation of Soviet Jewish refugee adolescents and parents. *Journal of Cross-Cultural Psychology, 32,* 456–477.

Bourhis, R., Moise, C., Perreault, S., & Senecal, S. (1997). Towards an interactive acculturation model: A social psychological approach. *International Journal of Psychology, 32,* 369–386.

Brett, K. M., & Higgins, J. A. (2003). Hysterectomy prevalence by Hispanic ethnicity: Evidence from a national survey. *American Journal of Public Health, 93*, 307–312.

Burgess, E. W. (Ed.). (1926). *The urban community.* Chicago: University of Chicago Press.

Burnam, M. A., Hough, R. L., Karno, M., Escobar, J. I., & Telles, C. A. (1987). Acculturation and lifetime prevalence of psychiatric disorders among Mexican Americans in Los Angels. *Journal of Health and Social Behavior, 28*, 89–102.

Cabrera Strait, S. (2001). *Examining the influence of acculturative stress on substance use and related maladaptive behavior among* Latino *youth.* Unpublished doctoral dissertation, Claremont Graduate University, Claremont: California.

Callister, L. C., & Birkhead, A. (2002). Acculturation and perinatal outcomes in Mexican immigrant childbearing women: An integrative review. *Journal of Perinatal and Neonatal Nursing, 16*, 22–38.

Chavez, L. R., Hubbell, F. A., Mishra, S. I., & Valdez, R. B. (1997). Undocumented Latina immigrants in Orange County, California: A comparative analysis. *International Migration Review, 31*, 88–108.

Chick, N., & Meleis, A.I. (1986). Transitions: A nursing concern. In P. L. Chinn (Ed.), *Nursing research methodology* (pp. 237–257). Boulder, CO: Aspen.

Choudhry, U. K. (1998). Health promotion among immigrant women from India living in Canada. *Image: Journal of Nursing Scholarship, 30*, 269–274.

Clark, L. (2001). *La familia:* Methodological issues in the assessment of perinatal social support for Mexicanas living in the United States. *Social Science and Medicine, 53*, 1303–1320.

Clark, L. (2002). Mexican-origin mothers' experiences using children's health care services. *Western Journal of Nursing Research, 24*, 159–179.

Cowan, P. (1982). *An orphan in history: Retrieving a Jewish legacy.* New York: Doubleday.

Cuellar, I., Harris, L. C., & Jasso, R. (1980). An acculturation scale for Mexican American normal and clinical populations. *Hispanic Journal of Behavioral Science, 2*, 199–217.

Dallo, F. J., & James, S. A. (2000). Acculturation and blood pressure in a community-based sample of Chaldean-American women. *Journal of Immigrant Health, 2*, 145–153.

Dawson, E. J., Crano, W. D., & Borgoon, M. (1996). Refining the meaning and measurement of acculturation: Revisiting a novel methodological approach. *International Journal of Intercultural Relations, 20*, 97–114.

De la Cruz, F. A., Padilla, G. V., & Agustin, E. O. (2000). Adapting a measure of acculturation for cross-cultural research. *Journal of Transcultural Nursing, 11*, 191–198.

Ebin, V. J., Sneed, C. D., Morisky, D. E., Rotheram-Borus, M. J., Magnusson, A. M., & Malotte, C. K. (2001). Acculturation and interrelationship between problem and health-promoting behaviors among Latino adolescents. *Journal of Adolescent Health, 28*, 62–72.

Evans, J. (1987). Introduction: Migration and health. *International Migration Review, 21*, v–xiv.

Flaskerud, J. H., & Kim, S. (1999). Health problems of Asian and Latino immigrants. *Nursing Clinics of North America, 34,* 359–380.

Galarza, E. (1964). *Merchants of labor: The Mexican bracero story.* Santa Barbara, CA: NcNally & Loftin.

Geltman, P. L., Brown, M. J., & Cochran, J. (2001). Lead poisoning among refugee children resettled in Massachusetts, 1995–1999. *Pediatrics, 108,* 158–162.

Glick Schiller, N., Basch, L., & Blanc-Szanton, C. (1992a). Towards a definition of transnationalism: Introductory remarks and research questions. In N. Glick Schiller, L. Basch, & C. Blanc-Szanton (Eds.), *Towards a transnational perspective on migration: Race, class, ethnicity, and nationalism reconsidered* (Vol. 645, pp. ix–xv). New York: New York Academy of Sciences.

Glick Schiller, N., Basch, L., & Blanc-Szanton, C. (1992b). Transnationalism: A new analytic framework for understanding migration. In N. Glick Schiller, L. Basch, & C. Blanc-Szanton (Eds.), *Towards a transnational perspective on migration: Race, class, ethnicity, and nationalism reconsidered* (Vol. 645, pp. 1–24). New York: New York Academy of Sciences.

Gmelch, G. (1980). Return migration. *Annual Review of Anthropology, 9,* 135–159.

González, H. M., Haan, M. N, & Hinton, L. (2001). Acculturation and the prevalence of depression in older Mexican Americans: Baseline results of the Sacramento Area Latino Study on Aging. *American Geriatrics Society, 49,* 948–953.

Gordon, M. M. (1964). *Assimilation in American life.* New York: Oxford University Press.

Gushulak, B. D., & MacPherson, D. W. (2000). Health issues associated with the smuggling and trafficking of migrants. *Journal of Immigrant Health, 2,* 67–78.

Handlin, O. (1973). *The uprooted: The epic story of the great migration that made the American people.* Boston: Little, Brown. (Original work published 1951)

Hattar-Pollara, M., & Meleis, A. I. (1995). The stress of immigration and the daily lived experiences of Jordanian immigrant women in the United States. *Western Journal of Nursing Research, 17,* 521–539.

Huang, B., Rodriguez, B., Burchfiel, C. M., Chyou, P., Curb, J. D., & Yano, K. (1996). Acculturation and prevalence of diabetes among Japanese-American men in Hawaii. *American Journal of Epidemiology, 144,* 674–681.

Hull, D. (1979). Migration, adaptation and illness: A review. *Social Science and Medicine, 13A,* 25–36.

Hummer, R. A., Rogers, R. G., Nam, C. B., & LeClere, F. B. (1999). Race/ethnicity, nativity, and U.S. adult mortality. *Social Science Quarterly, 80,* 136–153.

Im, E. O. (1997). *Neglecting and ignoring menopause within a gendered multiple transitional context: Low income Korean immigrant women.* Unpublished doctoral dissertation, University of California, San Francisco.

Im, E. O., & Meleis, A. I. (2000). Meanings of menopause to Korean immigrant women. *Western Journal of Nursing Research, 22,* 84–102.

Im, E. O., Meleis, A. I., & Lee, K. A. (1999). Symptom experience during menopausal transition: Low income Korean immigrant women. *Women and Health, 29,* 53–67.

Juarabe, T. E. (1998). Risk factors for cardiovascular disease in Latina women. *Progress in Cardiovascular Nursing, 13,* 17–27.

Kasl, S. V., & Berkman, L. (1983). Health consequences of the experience of migration. *Annual Review of Public Health, 4,* 69–90.

Kelaher, M., & Jessop, D. J. (2002). Differences in low-birthweight among documented and undocumented foreign-born and US-born Latinas. *Social Science and Medicine, 55,* 2171–2175.

Khoury, E. L., Warheit, G. J., Vega, W. A., Zimmerman, R. S., & Gil, A. G. (1996). Gender and ethnic differences in prevalence of alcohol, cigarette and illicit drug use among an ethnically diverse sample of Hispanic, African American, and non-Hispanic White adolescents. *Women & Health, 24,* 21–40.

Korenbrot, C. C., Dudley, R. A., & Greene, J. D. (2000). Changes in births to foreign-born women after welfare and immigration policy reforms in California. *Maternal and Child Health Journal, 4,* 241–250.

LaFromboise, T., Coleman, H., & Gerton, J. (1993). Psychological impact of biculturalism: Evidence and theory. *Psychological Bulletin, 114,* 395–412.

Lee, M. C. (2000). Knowledge, barriers, and motivators related to cervical cancer screening among Korean-American women: A focus group approach. *Cancer Nursing, 23,* 168–175.

Lee, S. K., Sobal, J., & Frongillo Jr., E. A. (2000). Acculturation and health in Korean Americans. *Social Science and Medicine, 51,* 159–173.

Luepker, R. (2001). Cardiovascular disease among Mexican Americans. *American Journal of Medicine, 110,* 147–148.

Margolis, M. S. (1994). *Little Brazil: An ethnography of Brazilian immigrants in New York City.* Princeton, NJ: Princeton University Press.

Marin, G., & Gamba, R. J. (1996). A new measurement of acculturation for Hispanics: The bidimensional acculturation scale for Hispanics (BAS). *Hispanic Journal of Behavioral Science, 18,* 297–318.

Marin, G., & Marin, B. V. (1991). *Research with Hispanic populations* (Applied Social Research Method Series, Vol. 23). New Park, CA: Sage Publication.

Marin, G., Sabogal, F., Marin, B., Ortero-Sabogal, R., & Perez-Stable, E. (1987). Development of a short acculturation scale for Hispanics. *Hispanic Journal of Behavioral Science, 9,* 183–205.

McGuire, S. (2001). *Crossing myriad borders: A dimensional analysis of the migration and health experiences of indigenous Oaxacan women.* Unpublished doctoral dissertation, University of San Diego, California.

McGuire, S. (2002). Agency, initiative, and obstacles to health among indigenous immigrant women. *Proceedings of the 35th Annual Communicating Nursing Research Conference/16th Annual WIN Assembly* (p. 229), Palm Springs, California.

McGuire, S., & Georges, J. (2003). Undocumentedness and liminality as health variables. *Advances in Nursing Science, 16,* 185–195.

Meleis, A. I., Sawyer, L. M., Im, E., Messias, D. K. H., & Schumacher, K. (2000). Experiencing transitions: An emerging middle-range theory. *Advances in Nursing Science, 23,* 12–28.

Mendoza, R. H. (1989). An empirical scale to measure type and degree of acculturation in Mexican-American adolescents and adults. *Journal of Cross-Cultural Psychology, 20,* 372–385.

Messias, D. K. H. (1996). Concept development: Exploring undocumentedness. *Scholarly Inquiry for Nursing Practice: An International Journal, 10,* 235–252.

Messias, D. K. H. (2001). Transnational perspectives on women's domestic work: Experiences of Brazilian immigrants in the United States. *Women & Health, 33,* 1–20.

Messias, D. K. H. (2002). Transnational health resources, practices, and perspectives: Brazilian immigrant women's narratives. *Journal of Immigrant Health, 4,* 183–200.

Miller, A. M., & Chandler, P. J. (2002). Acculturation, resilience, and depression in midlife women from the former Soviet Union. *Nursing Research, 51,* 26–32.

Misra, R., Patel, T., Davies, D., & Russo, T. (2000). Health promotion behaviors of Gujurati Asian Indian immigrants in the United States. *Journal of Immigrant Health, 2*(4), 223–230.

Palinkas, L., Pierce, J., Rosbrook, B., Pickwell, S., & Ball, D. (2003). Cigarette smoking behavior and beliefs of Hispanics in California. *American Journal of Preventive Medicine, 9,* 331–337.

Park, R. E., Burgess, E. W., & McKenzie, R. D. (1925). *The city.* Chicago: University of Chicago Press.

Payne, J., Desmeules, M., Gold, J., Cao, Z., Vissandjee, B., Lafrance, B., Fair, M., & Mao, Y. (2002). Gender relevant determinants of mortality in female immigrants. *Annals of Epidemiology, 12,* 533–534.

Peragallo, N. P., Fox, P. G., & Alba, M. L. (2000). Acculturation and breast self-examination among immigrant Latina women in the USA. *International Nursing Review, 47,* 38–45.

Phinney, J. S. (2003). Ethnic identity and acculturation. In K. M. Chun, P. B. Organista, & G. Marin (Eds.), *Acculturation: Advances in theory, measurement and applied research* (pp. 63–81). Washington, DC: American Psychological Association.

Phinney, J. S., Horenczyk, G., Liebkind, K., & Vedder, P. (2001). Ethnic identity, immigration, and well-being: An international perspective. *Journal of Social Issues, 57,* 493–510.

Pickett, K. E., & Pearl, M. (2001). Multilevel analyses of neighbourhood socioeconomic context and health outcomes: A critical review. *Journal of Epidemiology Community Health, 55,* 111–122.

Portes, A., & Rumbaut, R. G. (2001). *Legacies: The story of the immigrant second generation.* Berkeley: University of California Press.

Portes, A., & Zhou, M. (1993). The New School Generation: Segmented assimilation and its variants. *Annals, American Academy of Political and Social Science, 530,* 4–96.

Poyo, G. E. (1989). *With all and for the good of all: The emergence of popular nationalism in the Cuban communities of the United States, 1848–1898.* Durham, NC: Duke University Press.

Prislin, R., Suarez, L., Simspon, D. M., & Dyer, J. A. (1998). When acculturation hurts: The case of immunization. *Social Science and Medicine, 47,* 1947–1956.

Raudenbush, S. W., & Sampson, R. J. (1999). Ecometrics: Towards a science of assessing ecological settings, with application to the systematic social observation of neighborhoods. *Sociological Methodology, 29,* 1–41.

Rogler, L. (1994). International migrations: A framework for directing research. *American Psychologist, 49*, 701–708.

Rubia, M., Marcos, I., & Muennig, P. A. (2002). Increased risk of heart disease and stroke among foreign-born females residing in the United States. *American Journal of Preventive Medicine, 22*, 30–35.

Rumbaut, R. G. (1994). The crucible within: Ethnic identity, self-esteem, and segmented assimilation among children of immigrants. *International Migration Review, 28*, 748–794.

Samora, J. (1971). *Los mojados: The wetback story.* Notre Dame, IN: University of Notre Dame Press.

Satia-Abouta, J., Patterson, R. E., Kristal, A. R., The, C., & Tu, S. (2002). Psychosocial predictors of diet and acculturation in Chinese American and Chinese Canadian women. *Ethnicity and Health, 7*(1), 21–39.

Sayegh, L., & Lasry, J.-C. (1993). Acculturation, stress et santé mentale chez des immigrants libanais à Montréal. *Santé mentale au Québec, 18*(1), 23–52.

Shen, B. J., & Takeuchi, D. T. (2001). A structural model of acculturation and mental health status among Chinese Americans. *American Journal of Community Psychology, 29*, 387–417.

Shin, R. K. R., & Shin, C. (1999). The lived experience of Korean immigrant women acculturating into the United States. *Health Care for Women International, 20*, 603–617.

Siegel, J. E., Horan, S. A., & Teferra, T. (2001). Health and health care status of African-born residents of metropolitan Washington, DC. *Journal of Immigrant Health, 3*(4), 213–224.

Singh, G. K., & Yu, S. M. (1996). Adverse pregnancy outcomes: Differences between U.S. and foreign-born women in major U.S. racial and ethnic groups. *American Journal of Public Health, 86*, 837–843.

Song, K-Y., Sohng, S., & Yeom, H-A. (2002). Health-promoting behaviors of elderly Korean immigrants in the United States. *Public Health Nursing, 19*(4), 294–300.

Szapocznik, J., Kurtines, W. M., & Fernandez, T. (1980). Bicultural involvement and adjustment in Hispanic-American youth. *International Journal of Intercultural Relations, 4*, 353–365.

Thrasher, M. (1927). *The gang: A study of 1,313 gangs in Chicago.* Chicago: University of Chicago Press.

Valenzuela, V. (1999). *Day laborers in Southern California: Preliminary findings from the day labor survey.* University of California Los Angeles Center for the Study of Urban Poverty Working Paper Series, May, 1999, 1–19.

van Servellen, G., Chang, B., & Lombardi, E. (2002). Acculturation, socioeconomic vulnerability, and quality of life in Spanish-speaking and bilingual Latino HIV-infected men and women. *Western Journal of Nursing Research, 24*, 246–263.

Vega, W. A., Kolody, B., Aguilar-Gaxiola, S., & Catalana, R. (1999). Gaps in service utilization by Mexican-Americans with mental health problems. *American Journal of Psychiatry, 156*, 928–934.

Ventura, S. J., Martin, J. A., Curtin, S. C., Mathews, T. J., & Park, M. M. (2000). Births: Final data for 1998. *National Vital Statistics Report, 48*, 3.

Villarruel, A. M., Langfeld, C., & Porter, C. (2003). Sexual behavior of Latino pre-adolescents and adolescents: The relationship of acculturation and generational history. *Hispanic Health Care International, 1,* 24–30.

Walter, N., Bourgois, P., Loinaz, M., & Schillinger, D. (2002). Social context of work injury among undocumented day laborers in San Francisco. *Journal of General Internal Medicine, 17,* 221–229.

Weeks, J. R., Rumbaut, R. G., & Ojeda, N. (1999). Reproductive outcomes among Mexico-born women in San Diego and Tijuana: Testing the migration selectivity hypothesis. *Journal of Immigrant Health, 1,* 77–83.

Wei, M., Valdez, R. A., Mitchell, B. D., Haffner, S. M., Stern, M. P., & Hazuda, H. P. (1996). Migration status, socioeconomic status, and mortality rates in Mexican Americans and non-Hispanic Whites: The San Antonio heart study. *Annuals of Epidemiology, 6,* 307–313.

Weigers, M. E., & Sherraden, M. S. (2001). A critical examination of acculturation: The impact of health behaviors, social support, and economic resources on birthweight among women of Mexican descent. *International Migration Review, 35,* 804–839.

Willgerodt, M. A., Miller, A. M., & McElmurry, B. J. (2002). Becoming bicultural: Chinese American women and their development. *Health Care for Women International, 23,* 467–480.

Wirth, L. (1928). *The ghetto.* Chicago: University of Chicago Press.

Yang, W., & Read, M. (1996). Dietary pattern changes of Asian immigrants. *Nutrition Research, 16,* 1277–1293.

Chapter 7

Health Disparities Among Asian Americans and Pacific Islanders

M. Christina Esperat, Jillian Inouye, Elizabeth W. Gonzalez, Donna C. Owen, and Du Feng

ABSTRACT

The Asian American and Pacific Islander (AAPI) group is the fastest-growing minority group in the United States. AAPIs have been touted in the literature as the "model minority" because of their achievements in the socioeconomic and educational spheres, which in certain categories are beyond the average levels of the dominant majority. However, generalizations such as these are very misleading, because they mask the glaring health disparities that are experienced by subgroups within the AAPI population. The purpose of this chapter is to explore the literature dealing with health disparities among AAPIs. Twenty-eight usable research reports were reviewed after a thorough review of the literature that spanned the years between 1990 and 2003. The review has revealed that the predominant psychosocial and cultural variables studied in research dealing with AAPI are acculturation, family and social networks, help-seeking behaviors, and cultural brokering. In general, research conducted on this group tended to be at the descriptive and comparative-correlational levels; more studies that investigate the effects of interventions to reduce or eliminate health disparities on this group are needed. The challenge is to build a body of knowledge on which to base future action.

Keywords: Asian-Pacific Islanders, health disparities

THE MYTH OF THE "MODEL MINORITY"

The Asian American and Pacific Islander (AAPI) group is the fastest-growing minority group in the United States. As a collective group, AAPIs are extremely diverse, representing more than 60 different ethnic groups that speak more than 100 different languages (Institute of Medicine, 2002; Office of Minority and Multicultural Health, 2000). The Asians within this group originate from Asia and Southeast Asia, with the largest subgroups consisting of Chinese, Filipinos, Japanese, and Koreans. Pacific Islanders, on the other hand, are not all immigrants; many of them reside in the Pacific Rim, where they are native to the islands of Polynesia (Hawaii, Samoa and Tonga), Micronesia (Marianas, Marshalls, Gilbert, to name a few), and Melanesia (Fiji).

AAPIs now constitute over 12 million people, about 5% of the total U.S. population. The diversity of this group has not been elucidated fully in national surveys (National Heart, Lung and Blood Institute, 2000). This group is very poorly understood in many majority reports detailing the needs of ethnic minority groups (Lin-Fu, 1993). AAPIs have been touted in the literature as the "model minority" because of their achievements in the socioeconomic and educational spheres, which in certain categories are beyond the average levels of the dominant majority. This label can only be characterized as a fallacy, and it is misleading and dangerous for several reasons. It does not recognize the huge diversity within the AAPI group in most parameters for measuring social, economic, and educational status, particularly when these are quantified and presented statistically as means for the group as a whole. The label also tends to blind people to the real needs and problems of AAPI subgroups, or it provides an excuse, whether intentionally or unintentionally, to not address those needs and problems aggressively. When specific issues relative to subgroups of AAPI are disaggregated from the whole, it is very evident that these subgroups suffer significant disparities in health and health care.

HEALTH DISPARITIES IN ASIAN AMERICANS AND PACIFIC ISLANDERS

When the leading causes of death in the United States are broken down, the conditions that are identified cluster around chronic health problems. Cardiovascular disease continues to rank as the leading cause of death, followed closely by cancer. The literature shows that the overall death rate due to coronary heart disease in AAPIs is lower than that of the general population. It is, however, the leading cause of death within this population for both males and females. The age-adjusted stroke death rates declined 8.1% from 1990 to 1998 (American Heart Association, 2003).

These statistics are an example of isolated facts on which the "model minority" stereotype is based. It masks the significant differences within the subgroups, which show alarming trends, and further underscores the need to highlight knowledge needs in specific areas regarding health disparities among specific subgroups. For example, Native Hawaiians have double the rate of coronary artery disease (CAD) than Caucasians and other AAPIs; Asian Indians have 2 to 4 times higher rates of CAD at all ages, and 5 to 10 times higher in younger age groups—in spite of the fact that they have no additional risk factors and nearly half are vegetarians (Office of Minority and Multicultural Health, 2000). Filipino Americans exhibit higher levels of high blood pressure than other AAPIs, and in one study (Stavig, Igra, & Leonard, 1988), Filipinos ages 50 years and older had a hypertension prevalence rate of 60–65%, compared to the overall U.S. prevalence rate of 47% in that age group. Within AAPI subgroups, smoking rates are highest among Laotians (92%), followed by Vietnamese (65%) and Cambodians (71%). Yet when the data on rates of smoking are aggregated, AAPIs as a group show only an 18% rate (Office of Minority and Multicultural Health, 2000), illustrating how disaggregating data can more accurately reflect the real problems in these health disparities within a heterogeneous group. These are but a few examples of the health disparities that become apparent once the data are disaggregated.

The purpose of this chapter is to review research dealing with health disparities among Asian American and Pacific Islander (AAPI) people within American society. Being an AAPI in American society is defined by challenges of unique experiences shaped by both internal and external realities. At the same time, it also means living through a collective experience common to the group. To begin to understand how health disparities are engendered in AAPIs, it is necessary to determine what factors shape their overall experiences within the health care system and how they respond within those experiences. Psychosocial and cultural factors were a major focus in this exploration of the literature. Thus this integrative literature review is directed by the following research questions: What are the psychosocial and cultural factors that influence health disparities among AAPIs? Among those, are there specific factors that predominate in influencing the outcomes of their health experiences?

METHODS

An initial search cast a narrow net to determine the most effective methodology. The initial search was limited to the traditional electronic search engines used in nursing research—CINAHL, PubMED, and MEDLINE—using various permutations of the following keywords: *health behaviors, help seeking, self efficacy, social support, health disparities, minority,* and *Asian Americans, Pacific Islanders,* inclusive of the years 1995–2003. As the initial search results were evaluated, a decision was made to also include the PYCHLIT, PSYCHINFO, ERIC, HealthSTAR, ACP Journal Club, and National Library of Medicine databases. Because the initial search yielded few relevant results, it was decided to expand the time frame for the search to include studies from 1960. Keywords relative to the most common chronic diseases were added to the search terms: *cardiovascular disease, cancer, diabetes,* and *mental health illness.* The authors were assigned specific keywords to use in the searches and specific databases to search. At the conclusion of the searches, the authors reviewed the abstracts and made decisions on which articles to retrieve.

Direct retrieval from library resources as well as through interlibrary loan produced over 150 articles. The majority of the articles were research reports, but some were conceptual or theoretical articles. Only research reports are included in this review. After the initial review, 33 research reports were fully reviewed, and out of those, 28 were finally included in the review covering those published between 1990 and 2003. Studies were categorized by comparing the predominant issues raised across all the studies reviewed. They were placed in one category that was most representative of the main focus of the study. If a study also contributed information about other categories, then it was also discussed in those categories.

THE IMPACT OF SPECIFIC PSYCHOSOCIAL AND CULTURAL VARIABLES

Acculturation

The sociocultural context of people's experiences when they migrate to a new culture is expressed in part by their degree of adaptation to the challenges of a whole new way of life. Across a significant number of the articles reviewed (see Table 7.1), acculturation was identified and tested as a predictor of health attitudes, behaviors, and outcomes (Jones, Jaceldo, Lee, Zhang, & Meleis, 2001; Kagawa-Singer, Wellisch, & Durvasula, 1997; Maxwell, Bastani, & Warda, 1998; Mehta, 1998; Shen &

TABLE 7.1 Studies in Asian American and Pacific Islander Groups, 1990–2003

Author(s)	Design	Sample	Concepts	Measures
Abe-Kim, Takeuchi, & Hwang (2002)	Descriptive	N = 1,503 Chinese Americans	Help-seeking behavior Emotional stress Physical health Mood Access to care Social network	Frequency of medical and informal services sought Occurrence of 10 negative events during preceding 12 months Self-rating physical health Symptom Checklist-90-Revised 3 items that represent beliefs and attitudes affecting access to care Positive and Negative Social Interactions Scale
Akutsu, Snowden, & Organista (1996)	Descriptive	N = 1,095 African A., 2,168 Asian A., 1,385 Hispanic, 2,273 Caucasian	Social network Access to mental health care	Interviews about specific mental health needs and social network
Arnault (2002)	Grounded theory	N = 25 Japanese wives in USA	Help-seeking behavior	Participants asked to give examples of situations in which they needed help or provided help to others in a support group
Barnes et al. (1998)	Descriptive	N = 31 terminally ill cancer patients (9 Chinese, 12 Latino, 10 Caucasian)		Open-ended interviews in English, Cantonese, and Spanish
Braun & Brown (1998)	Qualitative	N = not identified, Vietnamese, Chinese, Japanese, and Filipino Americans	Support network in caregiving	In-depth interview

(continued)

TABLE 7.1 *(continued)*

Author(s)	Design	Sample	Concepts	Measures
Braun, Takamura, & Mougeot (1996)	Descriptive, qualitative	N = 39 Vietnamese immigrants	Cultural brokering	Focus group, key informant interviews
Huang et al. (1996)	Survey	N = 7,956 Japanese American men	Acculturation	Acculturation measured by place of birth (Japan vs. Hawaii), number of years lived in Japan, and self-reported current diet type (Oriental, mixed, or Western)
Jones et al. (2001)	Descriptive, comparative, correlational	N = 29 Chinese American; 21 Filipino American women	Acculturation	Adaptation of Acculturation Rating Scale for Mexican Americans
			Role integration	Structured interview to determine role occupancy and involvement; role satisfaction instrument
			Perceived health	Cantril Ladder to measure perceived health, Health Perception Questionnaire, Bradburn's Affect Balance Scale
Joun et al. (2000)	Descriptive survey	N = 428 Korean Americans	Acculturation Health behavior	Investigator-developed survey in Korean Mammography use
Kagawa-Singer & Pourat (2000)	Epidemiologic secondary analysis of NHIS population survey (1993–1994)	N = 528 with six AAPI subgroups	Health behaviors	Rates of cervical and mammogram screening

TABLE 7.1 *(continued)*

Author(s)	Design	Sample	Concepts	Measures
Kagawa-Singer & Wellisch (2003)	Descriptive survey	$N = 46$ women who completed breast cancer treatment (18 Chinese A., 15 Japanese A., 13 Caucasian)	Acculturation Experience with breast cancer	Suinn-Lew Acculturation Scale Qualitative breast cancer experience
Kagawa-Singer et al. (1997)	Descriptive, exploratory	$N = 34$ women (12 Caucasian, 11 Chinese, 11 Japanese American)	Social support Acculturation Health symptoms Depression Experience with breast cancer	Arizona Social Support Interview Schedule Suinn-Lew Acculturation Scale Weiner-Adler Health Symptoms CES-D Questionnaire of Breast Cancer Experience
Kim et al. (2000)	Descriptive survey	$N = 318$ Korean A. (159 men and 159 women)	Health behavior	National Health Interview Survey cancer control supplement—translated into Korean language
Ma et al. (2002)	Cross-sectional survey	$N = 1,374$ Chinese, Korean, Vietnamese, and Cambodians	Health behavior	Questionnaire based on standard instruments used in national health surveys
Maxwell et al. (1998)	Descriptive survey	$N = 218$ Filipino A., 229 Korean A., 50 years and older	Acculturation Health behavior	Acculturation tool developed for Southeast Asians Interviews conducted in Tagalog or English and Korean language on use of mammography

(continued)

141

TABLE 7.1 *(continued)*

Author(s)	Design	Sample	Concepts	Measures
Maxwell et al. (2002)	Randomized clinical trial	N = 483 Filipino women > 40 years old	Exercise	Exercise Assessment tool (National Health & Nutrition Examination Survey II)
			Cancer screening education	Single-session teaching intervention
Mehta (1998)	Survey	N = 195 first-generation immigrants who were born in India	Acculturation	Acculturation measured using a modified version of American International Relations Scale with 3 subscales: perceived acceptance, cultural orientation, and language usage
			Mental health	Mental health measured by the Langner Index
Narikiyo & Kameoka (1992)	Descriptive	N = 144 Japanese, 144 Caucasian	Help-seeking	Questionnaire to assess causal attribution for mental illness and attitudes toward help-seeking
Sadler et al. (2001)	Descriptive, correlational	N = 194 American Asian Indian women	Acculturation Health behavior	Investigator-developed instrument BSE adherence and mammography use
Shen & Takeuchi (2001)	Descriptive	N = 983 Chinese Americans, the majority of whom were immigrants	Acculturation Depression	Suinn-Lew Acculturation Scale Center for Epidemiologic Scale on Depression
Shin (2002)	Descriptive, qualitative	N = 70 Korean immigrants	Help-seeking behavior	In-depth interviews

TABLE 7.1 *(continued)*

Author(s)	Design	Sample	Concepts	Measures
Maxwell et al. (2002)	Randomized clinical trial	N = 483 Filipino women > 40 years old	Exercise	Exercise Assessment tool (National Health & Nutrition Examination Survey II)
			Cancer screening education	Single-session teaching intervention
Mehta (1998)	Survey	N = 195 first-generation immigrants who were born in India	Acculturation	Acculturation measured using a modified version of American International Relations Scale with 3 subscales: perceived acceptance, cultural orientation, and language usage
			Mental health	Mental health measured by the Langner Index
Narikiyo & Kameoka (1992)	Descriptive	N = 144 Japanese, 144 Caucasian	Help-seeking	Questionnaire to assess causal attribution for mental illness and attitudes toward help-seeking
Sadler et al. (2001)	Descriptive, correlational	N= 194 American Asian Indian women	Acculturation Health behavior	Investigator-developed instrument BSE adherence and mammography use
Shen & Takeuchi (2001)	Descriptive	N = 983 Chinese Americans, the majority of whom were immigrants	Acculturation Depression	Suinn-Lew Acculturation Scale Center for Epidemiologic Scale on Depression
Shin (2002)	Descriptive, qualitative	N = 70 Korean immigrants	Help-seeking behavior	In-depth interviews

Takeuchi, 2001; Tabora & Flaskerud, 1997; Tang, Solomon, & McCracken, 2001; Ying & Miller, 1992). Acculturation is a multidimensional process that results in four possible outcomes: assimilation, integration, reaffirmation of traditional culture, and marginalization (Anderson et al., 1993). Although language preference and proficiency are used extensively in the development of tools to measure acculturation, they are not the only dimensions of the concept. Acceptance, preferences for food, and friends are among the other dimensions included in the measurement of acculturation.

In general, stronger acculturation was associated with positive health factors. For instance, in the Maxwell et al. (1998) study, acculturation was positively related to the likelihood of being screened for breast cancer in Filipino and Korean women. Researchers used an acculturation measure that was developed specifically for Southeast Asians. More studies focusing on acculturation and its impact on cultural values and health-promotive and health-protective practices and behaviors need to be undertaken. For example: Does increasing acculturation among AAPIs lead to lifestyle and behavioral changes that could negate the health-protective cultural practices in these groups?

Dietary practices are an example. Generally diets in AAPI cultures are low in saturated fats, which have been identified as an important factor in cardiovascular disease. Changes in the diets of AAPIs could lead to increased risk of chronic diseases and hinder the effort to reduce or eliminate health disparities in these groups. Two studies illustrate the negative environmental effects of acculturation on health. The large Honolulu heart program that investigated 8,006 Japanese American men in Hawaii from 1965 to 1968 resulted in several studies on the effects of acculturation. One study by Huang et al. (1996) examined the change from the typical Japanese diet to a more Western diet. It found that living a typical Japanese lifestyle as compared to the more Western diet was associated with a reduced prevalence of diabetes after controlling for age, body mass index, and physical activity. The other study by Egusa and colleagues (1993) examined Westernized food and found that the intake of animal fat and simple carbohydrates was markedly greater in Japanese Americans compared to Japanese living in Japan. The authors suggest that Westernized food habits are associated with marked increases in the concentrations of serum cholesterol, triglycerides, and types IIa and IIb hyperlipidemia. These two studies suggest a risk effect of dietary acculturation on serum lipids and the incidence of diabetes in Japanese Americans.

Family and Social Networks and Support

Research on the social support structure and function for Asian Americans in general is extremely limited. Social support has been identified as a multidimensional construct involving issues such as family, tangible emotional and informational support, and network size (Marshall & Funch, 1983). Although the function and dimensions of social support may be similar for Asian Americans and Anglo-Americans, who constitute the social support network, what is considered to be appropriate social support and help, how this need is communicated, and how the needs are met appear to differ considerably. Significantly, these differences also extend to interethnic differences within the Asian American subpopulations.

For example, the use of nuclear family members as a support network was reported by Chinese Americans dealing with the experience of breast cancer (Kagawa-Singer & Wellisch, 2003; Wellisch et al., 1999) and Korean Americans who experienced emotional difficulties (Shin, 2002). Pride and fear of losing confidentiality were the main factors identified for seeking support from nuclear family members among Korean immigrants who experienced emotional difficulties. On the other hand, Vietnamese Americans and Filipino Americans reported the use of extended family members in addition to immediate family members as support networks in caring for relatives with dementia (Braun & Brown, 1998; Braun, Takamura, & Mougeot, 1996).

In traditional Chinese culture, hierarchy is important, and family members have prescribed roles according to gender, age, and birth order. Chinese Americans, Filipino Americans, and Japanese Americans report moral obligations in caring for older adults with dementia, and Chinese Americans confer decision-making authority to an eldest male family member (Barnes, Davis, Moran, Portillo, & Koenig, 1998; Levkoff, Levy, & Weitzman, 1999). Additionally, harmony and unity for the family are essential in Chinese culture. Overt displays of anger or conflict are considered shameful within many Asian cultures. The presence of conflict within the family among Chinese Americans was reported to be a powerful stressor, precipitating distress and leading to the need to seek medical and mental health services (Abe-Kim, Takeuchi, & Hwang, 2002).

Differences in perceptions and uses of social support have been reported. Wellisch and associates (1999) compared the social support of Chinese American, Japanese American, and Anglo-American women breast cancer patients. The results showed that Anglo and American women expressed greater need for supportive advice and feedback than Chinese American and Japanese American women did. This may be attributed to the fact that verbal communication is not part of traditional Asian American styles of giving or receiving support. Chinese American and Japanese American women with breast cancer did not differ in emotional or tangible social support received. However, the Japanese Americans' support networks were significantly smaller than those of the Anglo- and Chinese Americans. Chinese American women also reported that the family was most involved in their decision making regarding cancer treatment, while Japanese American women reported that female friends and coworkers were their main sources of support in making decisions.

Arnault (2002) examined how cultural factors regulate social support among Japanese American women ($N = 25$) married to Japanese American men working for a Japanese company in the United States. The findings showed that some Japanese American women were reluctant to "bother" their husbands with their problem to avoid increasing his stress and because they perceived their role as a support to the husband. However, for those who communicated their problems to their husband, support was mobilized through members of the husband's company. Specifically, the husband takes the initiative to communicate his wife's need to his superior, and the boss then communicates to his (boss's) wife, thereby mobilizing support among wives of employees. This result suggests that within this group of Japanese American women there are differences in how problems are communicated.

The family and social networks are expected to be strong influences in AAPIs, partly because many Asian and Pacific cultures have a strong sense of familial and group collectivism, where individuality is submerged in the interest of the group welfare. Several of the studies previously discussed included family and social networks as variables in the investigations (Abe-Kim et al., 2002; Arnault, 2002; Braun et al., 1996; Kagawa-Singer & Wellisch, 2003; Kagawa-Singer et al., 1997; Levkoff et al., 1999; Shin, 2002; Wellisch et al., 1999; Ying, 1990). However, only one study had a direct focus on the family in determining the effect of multiple roles of AAPI women as caregivers (Jones et al., 2001). In this study, the sample consisted of two groups of foreign-born Asian American women—Chinese ($n = 29$) and Filipino ($n = 21$). The women were caring for elderly parents. Only those women who assumed multiple roles as wife, mother, employee, and caregiver were included. The mean age was 47.8 years ($SD = 2$). All instruments were translated into Chinese and Tagalog, back-translated, and validated. There were no significant differences between groups in age, number of years living in the United States, number of years providing care, highest level of education completed, income, and the type of relationship between caregiver and care recipient. However, Filipino American caregivers were more acculturated and spent more work hours per week than the Chinese American caregivers. The results also showed that total role integration across multiple roles was positively associated with the overall health of the subjects, and total role satisfaction was positively associated with current health and psychological well-being. Role satisfaction was stronger in the Filipino subjects than in the Chinese subjects. Many of the adult roles that people occupy are defined by the family structure, and in this sense, the family is a strong influence on the total health and well-being of the individual. Still, it is rather surprising that not more studies were conducted that examine the direct role of the family in these family-oriented cultures, particularly in promoting more positive health-related perceptions, attitudes, and behaviors.

Lockery (1991) asserts that the family is the primary informal support system of racial and ethnic minorities and that it serves as the fulcrum of their social integration. More research needs to be conducted to investigate the potential strength of the family as a variable in health disparities among AAPIs. In particular, the assumption that racial and ethnic minorities have extensive social resources as a result of strong family ties needs to be tested. A large family kinship structure or a dense social network does not necessarily mean a strong and effective social support system. In fact, family support systems that may be assumed to provide relief from emotional and psychological distress may in fact be the source of such distress (Lockery, 1991).

Health Behaviors and Cancer

Several studies focused on health behaviors and cancer screening (Kagawa-Singer & Pourat, 2000; Kim et al., 2000; Ma, Tan, Freeley, & Thomas, 2002; Maxwell, Bastani, Vida, & Warda, 2002; Tanjasari et al., 2001). Cancer screening, unlike health promotion activities such as moderate exercise or healthy eating behavior, requires that AAPIs enter into the Western health care system and interact with Western health care providers in order to use health care services that detect cancer at its earliest stages. These studies demonstrated that AAPIs who engaged in risky health behaviors such as smoking or who did not adhere to regular cancer screening were significantly less knowledgeable about these health risks. Kim and associates in a study of 263 Korean American men and women reported that while 90% of the men in the study were aware of the relationship between smoking and lung cancer, less than 30% were aware of the relationship of smoking with other diseases, such as heart disease. Tanjasari and associates (2001) reported that low literacy in their native language and language barriers with health care providers had a negative impact for Hmong women ($N = 201$) in obtaining breast cancer screening. Another important finding in this study was that a significantly greater number of women (30%, $p = 0.017$) who had never had a mammogram were in poor general health. These study findings suggest that although some groups of AAPIs are acquiring knowledge about cancer screening, factors other than knowledge are determining whether screening is used.

Knowledge acquisition is an important precursor to seeking help; however, culturally based barriers to learning have been identified. In a study of 194 Asian Indian women, study subjects expressed interest in knowing more about breast cancer, but they did not believe that friends or family members would be receptive to information provided by study subjects (Sadler et al., 2001). In contrast, the importance of providing health information—specifically, giving simple information about positive aspects of exercise—was shown to improve exercise use among Korean women (Maxwell et al., 2002). These findings suggest that Asian Americans from several subgroups have not been successful in seeking out and using the resources to detect or prevent cancer in the early stages of the disease.

In summary, these studies focused primarily on identifying factors that were barriers to knowledge or to engaging in health-promoting behavior. The studies recruited only small samples of mostly women and did not include examination of help-seeking strategies that would be useful for Asian Americans.

Help-Seeking Behaviors

Gourash (1978) defined help-seeking as the process by which people use or seek to use resources they themselves cannot provide. Help-seeking also includes actions taken by an individual or family when they recognize that a health problem exists and seek advice or service from other people or organizations (Dixon, 1986). Although help-seeking has been explored in various applied contexts, such as medical and mental health settings (Fischer, Winer, & Abramowitz, 1983) and with other ethnic and racial minorities (Rew, 1997), few studies focused on this concept with Asian Americans.

In one such study, Levkoff and associates (1999) conducted a retrospective qualitative study of 40 family caregivers of elders diagnosed with Alzheimer's disease and related disorders—10 African Americans, 10 Chinese Americans, 10 Irish Americans, and 10 Puerto Ricans—to understand the help-seeking of minority family caregivers and the role of religious and ethnic factors. The Chinese American narratives contained themes of having to do with traditional Confucian ethical rules related to the decision-making authority of an eldest male family member and whether or not the rules should be followed. Although none of the Chinese Americans discussed use of prayer, beliefs about a deity, or other religious imagery related to help-seeking, there was a clear theme of moral imperative to care for the elder that was rooted in Confucianism.

A cluster of studies were reviewed that demonstrated a stronger influence of the family as opposed to health professionals in help-seeking behaviors, particularly in the area of mental health. Shin (2002) used focus groups and in-depth interviews to investigate the help-seeking behaviors of 70 Korean immigrants. Help-seeking behaviors were grouped into three categories: help-seeking from informal sources, help-seeking from formal sources, and behaviors that did not include help-seeking. Informal sources consisted of immediate family members and neighbors. Despite the high level of distress reported by Korean immigrants, they and their families did not view the symptoms as severe enough to get help from outside the family. Help-seeking from informal sources is driven by a different set of factors than help-seeking from formal services. However, studies such as those by Abe-Kim et al. (2002) have documented the importance of informal services as a critical resource for individuals in distress.

To determine the reasons for underuse of mental health services by Japanese Americans, Narikiyo and Kameoka (1992) compared perceived causes of mental illness and help-seeking preferences. Because many Asian Americans regard the use of mental health services as shameful, professionals are consulted as a last resort. The authors tested the hypothesis that illness attribution and help-seeking responses differ between Japanese and White Americans. Using several questionnaires in a descriptive study with 72 men and 72 women in each ethnic group, they found that Japanese American students were more likely than White American students to attribute mental illness to social causes, to resolve problems on their own, and to seek help from family members or friends or both. This reliance on informal supports rather than formal sources of support was consistent with findings from Shin (2002) with Korean immigrants.

In another study, Abe-Kim and associates (2002) examined predictors of help-seeking for emotional distress among 1,503 Chinese immigrants and U.S.-born Chinese Americans 18–65 years of age living in Los Angeles County. They found that Chinese immigrants and U.S.-born Chinese who experienced high levels of family conflict had a higher probability of seeking formal services, both medical and mental health care. Family conflict was the strongest predictor of help-seeking for medical care. The authors suggest that the presence of conflictual family ties precipitated help-seeking more than the absence of supportive linkages between family members. High levels of distress and lack of knowledge about services were predictors of informal help-seeking. These findings are consistent with the results of studies by Shin (2002) and Narikiyo and Kameoka (1992) on the use of informal help-seeking in different Asian American subgroups.

Finally, Pablo and Braun (1997) studied how Asian American groups in Honolulu perceived abuse or neglect and sought help. The sample consisted of 20 older women: 10 Korean and 10 Filipinos who were asked to respond to scenarios depicting abuse and help-seeking situations. Their perceptions of abuse and help-seeking were then measured. The authors compared their findings to a previous study conducted in Minnesota using the same methodology. Unexpectedly, they found that the Filipino and Korean responses were more like those of Caucasians in Minnesota than like those of the Korean group in Minnesota. That is, the Korean Americans in Minnesota were the group least likely to seek help as compared to other groups. The possible explanation offered by the investigators was that the minorities in Honolulu had better access to culturally appropriate services than in the midwestern United States. In addition, they posited that differences in acculturation and the availability of family networks may have accounted for the differences.

Experiences and perceptions of formal sources of support were explored in several studies. For example, Braun and associates (1996) explored perceptions of Vietnamese refugees' help-seeking, caregiving, and dementia perceptions within a cultural context and immigration history. Key informant interviews were conducted with four different groups of men only, women only, mixed adults, and young adults. Findings from participants suggest that help-seeking from formal sources would be considered only when dementia symptoms were severe. These formal sources consisted mainly of private physicians who spoke their language or had a bilingual staff member who could provide translation.

Kagawa-Singer and colleagues (1997), using a descriptive, exploratory study, examined differences in help-seeking behavior among Chinese American ($n = 11$), Japanese American ($n = 11$), and Anglo-American ($n = 12$) women 30 years of age and older with all stages of cancer. They completed intensive interviews at 6 months to 3 years posttreatment. One hypothesis was that Asian American women would seek assistance for psychosocial problems at a significantly lower rate than Anglo women would. This hypothesis was partially supported. Although the percentage of Asian women who requested help was lower than that of the Anglos, it was not statistically significant. There were different reactions to interactions with physicians. Acculturated Japanese Americans expressed great satisfaction, while Chinese women with low acculturation reported lower satisfaction with physician interactions.

SUMMARY

The studies reviewed above used four different AAPI subgroups: Chinese Americans, Japanese Americans, Korean Americans, and Filipino Americans. Of these, four studies included mixed samples. All of the studies addressed a mental health component, help-seeking either for mental health or for emotional problems or distress. One study focused on the perception of abuse, and others evaluated caregivers with Alzheimer's or dementia.

Primary care and general practitioners, as well as Chinese herbalists and acupuncturists, are the principal targets of formal help-seeking for mental illness by AAPIs (Narikiyo & Kameoka, 1992; Shin, 2002). These studies also reported that access to specialty health services requires multiple steps and is affected by such factors as stigma, cultural and linguistic appropriateness of services, lack of information, and geographic proximity. Thus, it seems that the difficulty in stimulating help-seeking behaviors in some groups of AAPIs becomes progressively greater as the sources of services become more structured and specialized as opposed to informal sources. In addition, there are other factors that shape perceptions and attitudes about the help-seeking process. Levkoff et al. (1999) suggest that such factors as religious and ethnic affiliations should be considered in seeking support and assistance for family caregivers of ethnic minority clients with Alzheimer's disease.

Results from the study with Korean immigrants (Shin, 2002) and the study with Japanese Americans (Narikiyo & Kameoka, 1992) suggest that non-help-seeking behaviors are influenced by established ways of coping with emotional difficulties. Subjects in these two studies reported that they had to overcome their mental distress by using willpower and solitary coping responses, such as suppressing feelings and ignoring experiences. They attributed mental illnesses to social causes and attempted to resolve problems on their own. These attitudes and beliefs are consistent with the values of self discipline, emotional restraint, and reliance on oneself that appear to be consistent with Korean and Japanese Americans' cultural values.

Studies on help-seeking behaviors in relation to mental health, emotional issues, or psychosocial variables revealed that Asian Americans sought professional assistance for psychosocial problems at a significantly lower rate than Whites, had difficulty communicating with physicians, used lay referral networks and community-based programs rather than the formal health care providers, found language to be a barrier to help-seeking, and attempted to resolve problems on their own or sought help from family, friends, or even neighbors before utilizing formal services. Furthermore, while family conflict predicted service use, family support did not predict help-seeking behaviors.

These results are consistent with the cultural and spiritual beliefs and values of the AAPIs (Inouye, 2001) regarding collectivism, family, harmony, self-help, and informal help-seeking behaviors (Shin, 2002). Pescosolido and Boyer (1999) suggest that the network-episode model of help-seeking, which uses relationship-oriented variables, provides a more useful conceptualization of help-seeking. This model contextualizes individual help-seeking behavior within an interpersonal network and may be more applicable for development of interventions and programs because of Asian Americans' use of informal support systems (Abe-Kim et al., 2002).

A phenomenon described in the studies of help-seeking in AAPIs, particularly for mental health problems, such as major depression, is that the psychological conceptualization of a disorder leads to avoidance of professional or formal services. It also results in turning more toward informal sources of support such as family and friends, or themselves (Ying, 1990). In contrast, those who hold a physical conceptualization of their discomforts were more likely to seek professional medical services.

This supports the results of Lin and Cheung's investigation (1999), which showed that AAPI patients tend to focus more on physical rather than emotional discomforts, which results in somatization of psychological complaints.

Cultural Brokering

Cultural brokering and cultural liaisons can be a potentially effective approach in improving the ability to deliver mental health services to AAPI populations (Braun et al., 1996; Shin, 2002). In determining the underutilization of mental health services among Korean immigrants ($N = 70$) and formal health services among Vietnamese immigrants, barriers such as stigma, the cultural appropriateness of the intervention, lack of available services with bilingual and bicultural staff, finances, lack of information, and geographic proximity were identified as problems. The use of a lay referral network system was reported as an effective pathway for accessing mental health services (Shin, 2002). Braun et al. (1996) discussed young adults having to almost manipulate the elder into seeing a doctor by using sweet talk.

Akutsu, Snowden, and Organista (1996) discussed referrals by other ethnic minorities from natural help-giving and lay referral sources. Kagawa-Singer et al. (1997) found greater participation in the decision-making process if the husband, adult children, and/or friends were included in discussions when treatment options were presented. Narikiyo and Kameoka (1992) reported that Japanese American subjects rated family, friends, and self-help and support groups as significantly more helpful than White American subjects. Finally, Shin (2002) discussed cultural brokering by mental health providers between populations and other providers to negotiate a meaningful system for successful treatment.

The influence of informal sources of support, lay workers, culturally based interventions, and barriers to care suggests that bicultural and bilingual brokers are more sensitive to cultural issues and can communicate with racial and ethnic minorities in their native language. These cultural brokers can facilitate understanding and use of services by members of racial and ethnic minority populations within the contexts of their belief systems. Culturally and linguistically appropriate services are increasingly becoming a standard of care, particularly in service delivery to racial and ethnic minority populations. Interventions aimed at changing perceptions, attitudes, behaviors, and practices need to investigate the efficacy of cultural brokers and liaisons in promoting such changes in special populations. Some of the relevant issues are the familiarity with the culture and proficiency in the native languages of the cultural brokers; the use of family members as cultural liaisons also needs to be studied: How acceptable are younger family members as communication links where sensitive information from elders is the subject of the communication?

GENERAL OBSERVATIONS ON THE STATE OF THE LITERATURE ON AAPIS

In general, the literature on the factors or variables that influence health disparities among AAPIs is relatively sparse. The review process revealed the following findings about the state of the research literature on AAPIs. First, the observation reported in the Institute of Medicine report (2002) that there is a paucity in the literature on health disparities in AAPIs was resoundingly supported. Compared to the substantial body of literature on the health of African Americans and the growing literature focusing on Hispanics, the research on AAPIs is woefully scarce. The implications of this insufficiency are significant, given the fact that this group is the fastest-growing U.S. subpopulation.

There is also a predominance of studies focusing on particular groups with the AAPI population. Eleven of the 28 studies were about Chinese Americans; in contrast, there were only 2 studies focusing on Filipinos, even though this group constitutes the second-largest group of AAPIs. And there was only 1 research study that investigated the Asian Indian group. It is also apparent that within the body of literature, descriptive studies predominate, with limited comparative and correlational designs used to discover meaningful relationships among important variables. In addition, several of the studies were qualitative in nature. This is understandable, given the state of the science in this area; however, it is imperative that investigations must move beyond description if the literature is to have significance in the effort to address AAPI health disparities.

The research uncovered by the review also shows significant design and methodological limitations that must be addressed if the results are to be used for programmatic and policy decisions to address the problem. In general, although the range was wide—from a relatively small number of 25 subjects (Arnault, 2002) to a high of 7,956 subjects in a population-based study (Huang et al., 1996), the sample sizes in these studies tended to be small; even the epidemiological surveys yielded relatively smaller sample sizes than those used in national surveys. Studies that compared groups and correlated variables of interest used sample sizes that would have serious problems in deriving meaningful or generalizable results. Few of the studies reported using power analysis to determine sample sizes. A significant proportion reported the use of convenience samples. Several of the studies used instruments that were developed and tested using normative populations but were adapted and translated into the native languages of the population samples of interest. Still, there were some that reported using only English versions of the instruments. There are specific biases in these limitations; these issues seriously limit the generalizability of the results of these studies.

CONCLUSIONS AND RECOMMENDATIONS

This review has shed some light on the psychosocial and cultural factors in health disparities experienced by AAPIs. Several studies investigated the influence of acculturation on behaviors inherent in cultural practices (e.g., dietary practices) that are assumed to have health promotive and protective benefits in the larger ethnic groups within the AAPIs. Although acculturation was found to be positively related to health-promoting behaviors such as participation in screening programs, a greater level of acculturation was linked to increased risk of chronic disease such as diabetes and hyperlipidemia when dietary practices changed and Japanese men assimilated the Western diet into their eating practices. Not enough is known about the influence of acculturation on the changing health practices among the smaller subgroups. More studies to investigate the influence of acculturation on health behaviors in other AAPI subgroups are necessary.

The influence of family and social networks on the help-seeking behaviors of AAPIs was elucidated by several studies that show different patterns of help-seeking behaviors directed at specific sources. Most of the studies of help-seeking were found in the mental health literature. Research needs to be expanded to explore help-seeking behaviors in health promotion and disease prevention programs, not only in the area of mental health, but also in other aspects of the health and well-being of these groups.

The review also showed the obvious lack of studies on the influence of family and social networks on the health of AAPIs. Because family and kinship structures are so important in the cultures of AAPIs in American society, we should investigate the determinants and predictors of health-promoting behaviors emanating from these structures, as well as processes within them that could be formulated and directed toward more positive health outcomes. In addition, investigations need to be carried out that determine what health promotive and protective cultural practices could be supported and maintained by family relationships.

At the level of description, there needs to be more research that looks at comparisons between subgroups of AAPIs on the conventional indices of health. Because AAPIs are an extremely heterogeneous group, it is an error to rely on aggregate data to determine the existence of health disparities. In looking at psychosocial and cultural factors, this becomes even more critical. With such disparate groups of immigrant and native cultures, the fallacy found in the conventional indices becomes more conspicuous. Beyond the level of description, the review revealed an almost total absence of studies using designs that reliably test interventions aimed at improving health outcomes of AAPIs. This defines the state of the science in this area, and an aggressive approach is needed to increase the knowledge base on the health of a group within American society that will only continue to grow in the coming years.

One issue that is crucial to the type of research needed is effective recruitment and retention of subjects from AAPI groups. As evidenced by the literature review, the average sample sizes were small, which limits the ability of these studies to translate into meaningful and generalizable results. There needs to be a concerted effort to develop models and designs that optimize the ability of investigators to access minority populations. For example, community-based participatory research, using gatekeepers in the community and indigenous outreach or lay workers as an integral part of the research team, should be explored. Too often, the research enterprise invokes an ivory-tower image that researchers and investigators do little to dispel. This creates a chasm between researchers and subjects that is hard to breach once the study commences. Investigating the use of cultural brokers or liaisons as an intervention may also improve our ability to recruit the needed numbers of subjects from within the community to be studied, adding power to the investigation.

Health disparities in the AAPI group will continue to be a problem in the future. Comparatively little is known about specific influencing factors, particularly those in the psychosocial and cultural realms, and the challenge to build the body of knowledge on which to base action relative to this problem is one that will face scholars and scientists in the years to come. Thus, scholars and scientists must be open to new ways of thinking about issues relative to knowledge building and generation so that innovative models for research can be nurtured, enhanced, and tested.

REFERENCES

Abe-Kim, J., Takeuchi, D., & Hwang, W. C. (2002). Predictors of help-seeking for emotional distress among Chinese Americans: Family matters. *Journal of Consulting and Clinical Psychology, 70,* 1186–1190.

Akutsu, P. D., Snowden, L. R., & Organista, K. C. (1996). Referral patterns in ethnic-specific and mainstream programs for ethnic minorities and Whites. *Journal of Counseling Psychology, 43*(1), 56–64.

American Heart Association. *Statistical Fact Sheet—Populations.* Retrieved January 25, 2003, from http://americanheart.org/downloadable/heart/StatsBook.pdf

Anderson, J., Moeschberger, M., Chen, M., Kunn, P., Wewers, M., & Guthrie, R. (1993). An acculturation scale for Southeast Asians. *Social Psychiatry and Psychiatric Epidemiology, 28,* 134–141.

Arnault, D. (2002). Help-seeking and social support in Japanese sojourners. *Western Journal of Nursing Research, 24,* 295–306.

Barnes, D. M., Davis, A. J., Moran, T., Portillo, C. J., & Koenig, B. A. (1998). Informed consent in a multicultural cancer patient population: Implications for nursing practice. *Nursing Ethics, 5,* 412–423.

Braun, K., & Brown, C. (1998). Perceptions of dementia, caregiving, and help-seeking among Asian and Pacific Islander Americans. *Health and Social Work, 23,* 262–274.

Braun, K., Takamura, J., & Mougeot, T. (1996). Perceptions of dementia, caregiving, and help seeking among recent Vietnamese immigrants. *Journal of Cross-Cultural Gerontology, 11,* 213–228.

Dixon, M. (1986). Families of adolescent clients and non-clients: Their environments and help-seeking behaviors. *Advances in Nursing Science, 8,* 75–88.

Egusa, G., Murakami, F., Ito, C., Matsumoto, Y., Kado, S., Okamura, M., et al. (1993). Westernized food habits and concentrations of serum lipids in the Japanese. *Atherosclerosis, 100,* 249–255.

Fisher, E. H., Winer, D., & Abramowitz, S. I. (1983). Seeking professional help for psychological problems. In A. Nadler, J. D. Fisher, & B. M. DePaulo (Eds.), *New directions in helping:* (Vol. 3). *Applied perspectives in help-seeking and receiving* (pp. 163–185). New York: Academic Press.

Gourash, N. (1978). Help-seeking: A review of the literature. *American Journal of Community Psychology, 6,* 412–213.

Huang, B., Rodriguez, B., Burchfiel, C., Chyou, P., Curb, J. D., & Yano, K. (1996). Acculturation and prevalence of diabetes among Japanese-American men in Hawaii. *American Journal of Epidemiology, 144,* 674–681.

Inouye, J. (2001). Bridging cultures: Asians and Pacific Islanders and nursing. In J. M. Dochterman & H. K. Graces (Eds.), *Current issues in nursing* (6th ed., pp. 520–528). St. Louis: Mosby.

Institute of Medicine. (2002). *Unequal treatment: Confronting racial and ethnic disparities in health care.* Washington, DC: National Academy Press.

Jones, P., Jaceldo, K., Lee, J., Zhang, X., & Meleis, A. (2001). Role integration and perceived health in Asian American women caregivers. *Research in Nursing and Health, 24,* 133–144.

Joun, H-S., Yoonjoung, C., & Kim, M. T. (2000). Cancer screening behavior among Korean American women. *Cancer Detection and Prevention, 24,* 589–601.

Kagawa-Singer, M., & Pourat, N. (2000). Asian American and Pacific Islander breast and cervical carcinoma screening rates and Healthy People 2000 objectives. *Cancer, 89,* 696–705.

Kagawa-Singer, M., & Wellisch, D. K. (2003). Breast cancer patients' perceptions of their husbands support in a cross-cultural context. *Psycho-Oncology, 12,* 24–37.

Kagawa-Singer, M., Wellisch, D. K., & Durvasula, R. (1997). Impact of breast cancer on Asian American and Anglo American Women. *Culture, Medicine, and Psychiatry, 21,* 449–480.

Kim, K. K., Yu, E., Chen, E. H., Kim, J., Brintnall, R., & Vance, S. (2000). Smoking behavior, knowledge, and beliefs among Korean Americans. *Cancer Practice, 8,* 223–230.

Levkoff, S., Levy, B., & Weitzman, P. F. (1999). The role of religion and ethnicity in help-seeking of family caregivers of elders with Alzheimer's disease and related disorders. *Journal of Cross-Cultural Gerontology, 14,* 335–356.

Lin, K., & Cheung, F. (1999). Mental health issues for Asian Americans. *Psychiatric Services, 50,* 774–780.

Lin-Fu, J. (1993). Asian and Pacific Islander Americans: An overview of demographic characteristics and health care issues. *Asian American and Pacific Islander Journal of Health, 1,* 20–36.

Lockery, S. A. (1991). Caregiving among racial and ethnic minority elders: Family and social supports. *American Society on Aging, 15,* 58–62.

Ma, G., Tan, Y., Freeley, R., & Thomas, P. (2002). Perceived risks of certain types of cancer and heart disease among Asian American smokers and non-smokers. *Journal of Community Health, 27,* 233–246.

Marshall, J., & Funch, D. (1983). Social environment and breast cancer: A cohort analysis of patient survival. *Cancer, 52,* 1546–1550.

Maxwell, A., Bastani, R., Vida, P., & Warda, U. (2002). Physical activity among older Filipino-American women. *Women & Health, 36,* 67–79.

Maxwell, A., Bastani, R., & Warda, U. (1998). Misconceptions and mammography use among Filipino and Korean-American women. *Ethnicity and Disease, 8,* 377–384.

Mehta, S. (1998). Relationship between acculturation and mental health for Asian Indian immigrants in the United States. *Genetic, Social, and General Psychology Monographs, 124,* 61–78.

Narikiyo, T., & Kameoka, V. (1992) Attributions of mental illness and judgments about help-seeking among Japanese-American and White American students. *Journal of Counseling-Psychology, 39,* 363–369.

National Heart, Lung and Blood Institute. (2000). *Addressing cardiovascular health in Asian Americans and Pacific Islanders* (NIH Publication No. 00-3647). Bethesda, MD: Author.

Office of Minority and Multicultural Health. (2000). *The health of minorities in New Jersey, Part III*. Trenton, NJ: Office of Minority and Multicultural Health, New Jersey Department of Health and Senior Services.

Pablo, S., & Braun, K. (1997). Perceptions of elder abuse and neglect and help-seeking patterns among Filipino and Korean elderly women in Honolulu. *Journal of Elder Abuse and Neglect, 92*, 63–76.

Pescosolido, B. A., & Boyer, C. A. (1999). How do people come to use mental health services? Current knowledge and changing perspectives. In A. Horwitz & T. Scheid (Eds.), *The sociology of mental illness* (pp. 392–411). New York: Cambridge University Press.

Rew, L. (1997). Health-related, help-seeking behaviors in female Mexican-American adolescents. *Journal of the Society of Pediatric Nurses, 2*, 156–161.

Sadler, G. B., Dhanjal, S. K., Shah, N. B., Shah, R. B., Ko, C., Anghel, M., et al. (2001). Asian Indian women: Knowledge, attitudes, and behaviors towards breast cancer early detection. *Public Health Nursing, 18*, 357–363.

Shen, B., & Takeuchi, D. (2001). A structural model of acculturation and mental health status among Chinese Americans. *American Journal of Community Psychology, 29*, 387–418.

Shin, J. (2002). Help-seeking behaviors by Korean immigrants for depression. *Issues in Mental Health, 23*(5), 461–476.

Stavig, G. R., Igra, A., & Leonard, A. R. (1988). Hypertension and related health issues among Asian and Pacific Islanders in California. *Public Health Reports, 103*, 28–37.

Tabora, B., & Flaskerud, J. (1997). Mental health beliefs, practices and knowledge of Chinese American immigrant women. *Issues in Mental Health Nursing, 18*, 173–189.

Tang, T. S., Solomon, L. J., & McCracken, L. M. (2001). Barriers to fecal occult blood testing (FOBT) and sigmoidoscopy among older Chinese-American women. *Cancer Practice, 9*, 277–282.

Tanjasiri, S. P., Kagawa-Singer, M., Foo, M. A., Chao, M., Linayao-Putman, I., Lor, Y., et al. (2001). Breast cancer screening among Hmong women in California. *Journal of Cancer Education, 16*, 50–54.

Wellisch, D., Kagawa-Singer, M., Reid, S. L., Lin, Y-J., Nishikawa-Lee, S., & Wellisch, M. (1999). An exploratory study of social support: A cross-cultural comparison of Chinese-, Japanese-, and Anglo-American breast cancer patients. *Psycho-Oncology, 8*, 207–219.

Ying, Y. (1990). Explanatory models of major depression and implications for help-seeking among immigrant Chinese-American women. *Culture, Medicine and Psychiatry, 14*, 393–408.

Ying, Y. W., & Miller, L. S. (1992). Help-seeking behavior and attitudes of Chinese Americans regarding psychological problems. *American Journal of Community Psychology, 20*, 549–556.

Chapter 8

African American and Asian American Elders: An Ethnogeriatric Perspective

MELEN R. MCBRIDE AND IRENE D. LEWIS

ABSTRACT

By 2030, ethnic minority elders are expected to increase by 12%. Research about this highly diverse population is gaining momentum. This chapter summarizes selected research articles published after 1996 on access and utilization of services and resources by African American and Asian American elders. Computerized searches were made using PubMed and CINAHL (Cumulative Index of Nursing and Allied Health Literature) with the following terms used individually or combined: *health care, aging, older adults, ethnicity, access, disparities, chronic illness, community health care, health beliefs, health practices,* and *ethnogeriatrics.* Citations for 456 articles on two ethnic groups were retrieved; 155 were reviewed, and 84 citations were used for this chapter. The publications focus on African Americans (45%), Asian Americans (41%), and both groups (14%). Descriptive, exploratory, cross-sectional studies dominate the research effort, identifying unmet needs, and a limited number are on culturally appropriate and acceptable interventions. Results are discussed in the context of ethnogeriatrics, and recommendations for future studies are proposed.

Keywords: African American, Asian American, elderly, ethnogeriatrics

Ethnogeriatrics, an evolving subspecialty of geriatrics, is the synthesis of aging, health, and cultural concerns about health care and social services for older people from diverse ethnic groups, many of whom continue to experience problems in accessing health care and enjoying quality of life (Harper, 1990; Yeo, David, & Llorens, 1996; see Figure 8.1). Knowledge in the field is developing from multidisciplinary research filtered through concepts such as heterogeneity (inter- and intragroup differences); access; interaction of cultural beliefs, practices, and formal systems; and outcomes of policy and services. Conceptual frameworks have been adapted in a few studies, such as the explanatory model of health and illness (Kleinman, Eisenberg, & Good, 1978), double/triple jeopardy hypothesis of the combined effects of race/ethnicity, the aging process, and health status on quality of life (Markides & Black, 1996), the health belief model (Plowden & Miller, 2000), and the ecological approach to explain the interaction

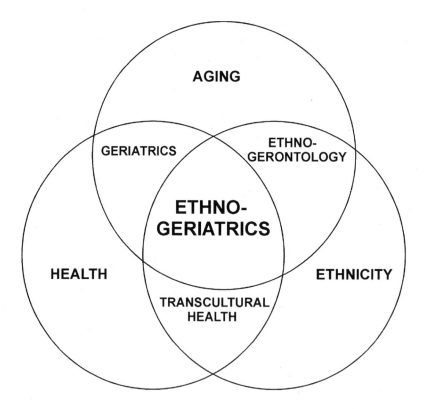

FIGURE 8.1   Domain of ethnogeriatrics.

between cultural beliefs, health behavior, and aging (Collaborative on Ethnogeriatric Education, 2000, 2001).

PURPOSE

This chapter reviews and summarizes selected research reports about health care disparities and access and utilization of resources for African American and Asian American older adults. There are five federally designated racial and ethnic minority groups—American Indian/Alaska Native, Asian American, African American, Native Hawaiian/Pacific Islander, and Hispanic/Latino American. The first four classifications are categories for race, and the fifth is a category for ethnicity (Office of Management and Budget, 2001). The terms *minority elders* or *racial and ethnic minority older adults* will be used to refer to older people of color with specific ethnic identities. We use the following definition of health disparities proposed by the National Institute of Health, Working Group on Health Disparities (2003): "Health disparities are differences in the incidence, prevalence, mortality, and burden of diseases and other adverse health conditions that exist among specific population groups in the United States."

METHOD

Ethnogeriatrics has a strong multidisciplinary focus, and research studies are reported in a variety of professional journals in the social, behavioral, medical, nursing, and public health sciences and the humanities. Computerized searches were made using PubMed, Medline, and CINAHL (Cumulative Index of Nursing and Allied Health Literature). The terms *health care, aging, ethnicity, access, disparities, ethnic minority older adults, chronic diseases* (i.e., those targeted by Healthy People 2010), *community-based health care, cultural beliefs, health practices,* and *ethnogeriatrics* were used individually or in combination. Specific populations (e.g., African American, Asian American, Filipino American, Vietnamese American) were also added to the terms. Other sources of information include the Stanford Geriatric Education Center, the Ethnogeriatric Bibliographic Database, and Dissertation Index. The review was guided by questions on (1) what is known about access to community-based health care and disparities identified or suggested by these studies, (2) issues raised by current research findings, and (3) existing and important gaps in research.

Prior to 1997, a review of the available research reports had been summarized in four health and aging monographs (McBride, Morioka-Douglas, & Yeo, 1996; McCabe & Cuellar, 1994; Richardson, 1996; Villa, Cuellar, Gamel, & Yeo, 1993) and are part of an ethnogeriatric bibliographic database at the Stanford Geriatric Education Center. The literature search for the five racial and ethnic categories resulted in 908 citations of which 456 (50.2%) titles and abstracts were considered based on selection criteria. The review was then reduced to 155 articles after limiting the review to research on African Americans ($N = 72$) and Asian Americans ($N = 83$), and 54% ($N = 84$) were used for the analysis.

The selection criteria included (1) application of the three guide questions related to health disparities and gaps in research; (2) chronic illnesses targeted in Healthy People 2010, specifically, cardiovascular disease, diabetes, and reproductive cancer (U.S. Department of Health and Human Services, 2000); (3) publication period from 1997 to present, and (4) studies conducted in the United States. The total volume of publication was too large to allow for a comprehensive review and critique on the five groups of minority elders. Therefore, we focused on the research reports on African Americans (45%), Asian Americans (41%), and on reports with both groups (14%) in the sample population (see Tables 8.1 and 8.2). A separate article is planned for the other groups.

The reports are briefly summarized and evaluated in terms of research about health disparities and ethnogeriatrics. Health status and access to health care and resources are the topics used to organize the discussion. The discussion about access to health care and resources consists of subtopics on utilization patterns, characteristics of provider and health care setting, health screening and intervention, treatment outcomes, and alternate health care options. These constructs serve as elements of an organizing framework for ethnogeriatric research. The last section of the chapter is a discussion of recommendations for infusing an ethnogeriatric context into research design, methods, sampling, measurements, and analysis.

OVERVIEW OF RESEARCH ON RACIAL AND ETHNIC MINORITY OLDER ADULTS

The Census reports that 15% of the total population in the United States are racial and ethnic minorities age 65 and older (U.S. Census Bureau,

TABLE 8.1 Selected Research Articles Reviewed on Health Status and Access to Health Care for African American and Asian American Older Adults

Study	Method	Selected findings
Abe-Kim, J., Takeuchi, D., & Hwang, W. (2002)	*Design:* Secondary analysis *Measure:* Chinese American psychiatric epidemiological data *Sample:* 1,503 Chinese Americans	Family conflict predicted use of mental health and medical services; negative life event, emotional distress, and health insurance predicted use of mental health services.
Anderson-Loftin, W., & Moneyham, J. (2000)	*Design:* Descriptive study *Measure:* Clinical outcomes, HgbA1C, lipids, BP, provider performance *Sample:* 2,000 urban African Americans with type II diabetes, randomized	First comprehensive study, in progress.

ADL = Activities of Daily living
BP = Blood pressure
CES-D = Center for Epidemiologic Studies Depression Scale
CVD = Cardiovascular disease
HCFA = Health Care Finance Administration
HgbA1C = Hemoglobin A1C
HR = Heart rate
HTN = Hypertension
NCI = National Cancer Institute
NHANES = National Health and Nutrition Examination Study
NHIS = National Health Interview Survey
OR = Odds ratio
SEER = Surveillance, Epidemiology, and End Results
SES = socioeconomic status
VA = Veterans Administration
WHO = World Health Organization

(continued)

TABLE 8.1 *(continued)*

Study	Method	Selected findings
Backus, L., Osmond, D., Grumbach, K., Vranizan, K., Phuong, L., & Bindman, A. (2001)	*Design:* Cross-sectional survey *Measure:* Questionnaire (acceptance of patients), demography, type of practice (primary care, specialist) *Sample:* 713 primary care physicians; 962 specialists	Specialists are more likely to accept new Medicaid fee-for-service patients.
Barber, K., Shaw, R., Folts, M., Taylor, D., Ryan, A., Hughes, M., Scott, V., & Abbott, R. (1998)	*Design:* Quasi-experimental study, educational and screening intervention *Measure:* Knowledge and attitude questionnaire, demography *Sample:* 944 African American and Caucasian men	African Americans have less knowledge on the basics of prostate checkup; prefer private appointment; can be reached by radio.
Baumann, L. C., Chang, M., & Hoebeke, R. (2002)	*Design:* Chart audit *Measure:* HTN and diabetes control *Sample:* 280 Blacks, Hispanics, Whites	Significant differences in blood pressure between 3 groups.
Becker, G. (2001)	*Design:* Descriptive, cross-sectional *Measure:* Semistructured interview (3 × 12 months) *Sample:* 297 mixed ethnic groups, African American, Hispanic/Latino Americans, Filipino Americans, age 23–97 years	Uninsured had poorer control of illness and lacked information about illness management.

TABLE 8.1 *(continued)*

Study	Method	Selected findings
Becker, G., Beyene, Y., Newsom, E., & Rodgers, D. (1998)	*Design:* Descriptive, cross-sectional *Measure:* Interview (structured; semistructured, in-depth) *Sample:* 35 African Americans, 55 Filipino Americans, 61 Hispanic/Latino Americans, age 50 + years	Group differences: Social, cultural, and knowledge of illness differences.
Bibb, S. C. (2001)	*Design:* Descriptive, comparative study *Measure:* Tumor registry database, secondary analysis *Sample:* 67 African Americans, 573 Whites, age 25–97 years	African American women had late-stage diagnosis, younger, lower SES. Economic access did not always result in early diagnosis; consider other factors.
Carlisle, D., Leake, B., & Shapiro, M. (1997)	*Design:* Descriptive study *Measure:* Use of cardiovascular procedures *Sample:* 104,952 hospital discharge records, African Americans, Asian Americans, Hispanic/Latino Americans, Los Angeles	Low use of procedures: African Americans, Hispanic/Latino Americans. Comparable rates to Whites: Asian Americans.
Carter, A., Borchardt, N., Cooney, M., & Greene, D. (2000)	*Design:* Descriptive, cross-sectional study *Measure:* Fasting plasma glucose, fructosamine, demographic data *Sample:* 277 patients, African Americans, Asian Americans, Hispanic/Latino Americans, mixed, Whites	Screening for diabetes: Improved detection with fructosamine levels. This test improves screening accuracy, retains ease of use, and is affordable.

(continued)

TABLE 8.1 *(continued)*

Study	Method	Selected findings
Chen, Y. (1996)	*Design:* Qualitative study *Measure:* Interview, beliefs and behaviors *Sample:* 21 Chinese American elders	Emerging theory: Conformity with nature. Interrelated constructs: Harmonizing with the environment, following bliss, listening to heaven.
Chin, M., Zhang, J., & Merrell, K. (1998)	*Design:* Retrospective, secondary analysis *Measure:* SES, clinical measures *Sample:* 1,400 Medicare beneficiaries	African Americans receive less care than Whites.
Cooley, M., & Jennings-Dozier, K. (1998)	*Design:* Descriptive, qualitative study *Measure:* Case study, explanatory model *Sample:* 2 males, African Americans	Cultural values and beliefs impact care.
Cooper-Patrick, L., Gallo, J., Gonzales, J., Powe, N., Nelson, C., & Ford, D. (1999)	*Design:* Telephone survey, November 1996 and June 1998 *Measure:* Physician's participatory decision making (PDM), SES, health status, length of patient–physician relationship *Sample:* 1,816 adults, age 18–65 years	African Americans rated physician visit as less participatory than Whites.
Corbie-Smith, G., Thomas S., & George, D. (2002)	*Design:* Survey (telephone) *Measure:* Index of trust/ regressive model *Sample:* 909 African Americans and Whites	Race strongly associated with higher distrust score.

TABLE 8.1   *(continued)*

Study	Method	Selected findings
Cotter, M., Gern, R., Ho, G., & Chang R. (2002)	*Design:* Descriptive, retrospective study *Measure:* Questionnaire, self-administered *Sample:* 953 males, mixed group (African Americans, Hispanic/Latino Americans, Whites, others)	Early onset of prostate cancer for males whose fathers had cancer; African Americans reported more family history than Whites.
Doescher, M., Saver, B., Franks, P., & Fiscella, K. (2000)	*Design:* Secondary analysis *Measure:* Scales on Satisfaction with Physician Style and Trust in Physician *Sample:* 1991–1997 Community Tracking Survey; 32,929 adult patients in primary care, White and mixed race/ethnicity	Less positive perception of physician on both scales among minority groups than among Whites.
Dunlop, D., Manheim, L., Song, J., & Chang, R. (2002)	*Design:* Secondary analysis *Measure:* SES, health needs, economic access *Sample:* 1993–1995 Asset of Health Dynamics (AHEAD) data; 1,430 African Americans, Hispanics, Whites, > 80 years	Effect of economic access on gender/ethnic disparities: Minimal effect for services covered by Medicare; significant effect on dental care—not covered by Medicare.
El-kebbi, I., Cook, C., & Ziemer, D. (2003)	*Design:* Retrospective chart analysis *Measure:* Age to A1C or HgbA1C *Sample:* 2,539 cases, mostly African Americans with type II diabetes	No significant change in BMI; nor between age groups for glucose control; baseline HgbA1C increased with decreasing age.

(continued)

TABLE 8.1   *(continued)*

Study	Method	Selected findings
Gaskin, D. J., & Hoffman, C. (2000)	*Design:* Retrospective, secondary analysis *Measure:* Admission and discharge data, SES, race/ethnicity *Sample:* Discharge data for 10 states	High rate of hospitalization for preventable conditions for African American and Hispanic older adults.
Guidry, J., Aday, L., Zhang, D., & Winn, R. (1997)	*Design:* Descriptive, comparative study *Measure:* Mailed questionnaire (assessment of barriers to treatment), demographic data *Sample:* 593 patients (African American, Asian American, Hispanic/Latino American, White) clinically diagnosed with cancer (breast, colon, cervix, prostate, and lymphoma)	Distance, no access to a car, and no driver were major barriers for African American and Hispanic Latino American patients; they may forego treatment.
Gurwitz, J., Goldberg, R., Malmgren, J., Barron, H., Tiefendrum, A., Frederick, P., & Gore, J. (2002)	*Design:* Prospective study *Measure:* National Registry of Myocardial Infarction (June 1994 to March 1998) *Sample:* 152,310 transfers; 1,674 hospitals	Hospital transfers of MI patients occurred more often for older (> 75 years) and African American patients.
Han, B., Wells, B., & Primas, M. (2003)	*Design:* Comparative study *Measure:* National Health Interview Survey, II, yes/no items *Sample:* 449 African Americans, 3,328 Whites, > 65 years	Race not associated with mammography. Barriers differ between groups.

TABLE 8.1 *(continued)*

Study	Method	Selected findings
Harada, N., Damron-Rodriguez, J., Villa, M., Washington, D., Dhanani, S., Shon, H., Chattopadhyay, M., Fishbein, H., Lee, M., Makinodan, T., & Andersen, R. (2002)	*Design:* Descriptive study *Measure:* Focus group, telephone survey, preferred VA health services *Sample:* veterans, 178 in focus group, 3,227 in survey	Preference for VA outpatient services: Associated with race/ethnicity (e.g., African American, Hispanic/Latino American) and strong veteran identity. Utilization of VA outpatient services: Associated with socioeconomic factors.
Haviland, M., Morales, L., Reise, S., & Hays, R. (2003)	*Design:* Retrospective study, secondary analysis (1998 National Research Corporation Healthcare Market Guide Survey) *Measure:* Global satisfaction ratings, composite care measures *Sample:* 120,855 cases, mixed ethnic groups	Asian/Pacific Islanders less satisfied with medical care.
Henderson, S., Magana, R., Korn, C., Genna, T., & Bretsky, P. (2002)	*Design:* Retrospective study, case review *Measure:* Degree of delay, mode of access *Sample:* 337 cases, African Americans, Asian Americans, Hispanic/Latino Americans, Whites	Average delay of 44.3 hours; Asian Americans with longest delay (92), followed by Hispanic/Latino Americans (41.5), Whites (31.6), African Americans (30.8). Asian Americans (83%) and Hispanic/Latino Americans (70%) used private transportation.

(continued)

TABLE 8.1   *(continued)*

Study	Method	Selected findings
Iwashyna, T., Curlin, F., & Christakis, N. (2002)	*Design:* Retrospective, secondary data analysis *Measure:* Demographic data *Sample:* 787,587 Medicare subscribers, Asian Americans, Hispanic/Latino Americans, Whites	Hispanic/Latino Americans and Asian Americans are less likely users of teaching hospitals than Whites.
Jennings-Dozier, K. (1999)	*Design:* Descriptive, correlational study *Measure:* Questionnaire on behavioral, normative, and control beliefs, demographic data including Pap test status *Sample:* 204 African American and Hispanic/Latino American women	Up-to-date women in the ethnic groups differ in physician choice and concern over screening services.
Jennings-Sanders, A., & Anderson, E. (2003)	*Design:* Prospective randomized study *Measure:* Secondary data analysis *Sample:* 106 African American (21%) and White women (72%)	Nurse case managers helped women to manage coexisting conditions and to navigate the health care system.
Kim, M., Han, H., Kim, K., & Duong, D. (2002)	*Design:* Descriptive study *Measure:* Demography, health behaviors, service utilization *Sample:* 205 older Korean immigrants	Common practice to use traditional Korean medicine, *hanbang*, Western medicine, or combination.

TABLE 8.1   *(continued)*

Study	Method	Selected findings
Lauderdale, D., & Goldberg, J. (1996)	*Design:* Evaluation study *Measure:* Race/ethnicity codes *Sample:* HCFA Medicare enrollees, age > 65 years	Identifiable by new codes: Asian Americans (56%), Hispanic/Latino Americans (24%), Native Americans (17%). Coded Hispanic/Latino: 18–29% born in Mexico, Puerto Rico, and Cuba; 14–73% born in nine Asian countries. Race/ethnicity code incomplete and biased.
Liburd, L., Anderson, L., Edgar, T., & Jack, L. (1999)	*Design:* Exploratory, qualitative study *Measure:* Focus group, perception of body size/shape *Sample:* 33 African American women	Middle to large size perceived to be healthier; pear-shaped body preferred. Include family in diabetes education.
Ma, G., Tan, Y., Feeley, R., & Thomas, P. (2002)	*Design:* Cross-sectional, self-report survey *Measure:* Knowledge about risks, tobacco use, demographic data *Sample:* Stratified-cluster sampling, 1,374 Chinese, Korean, Vietnamese, Cambodian Americans	Awareness of risk higher for women, more educated, nonsmokers, and former smokers.
Martin, J., Engle, V., & Graney, M. (1999)	*Design:* Exploratory *Measure:* Questionnaires on health-related hardiness *Sample:* 100 older community-living Blacks	Years of education explained 20% of variance in health-related hardiness.

(continued)

TABLE 8.1 *(continued)*

Study	Method	Selected findings
McCormick, W., Ohata, C., Uomoto, J., Young, H., Graves, A., Kukull, W., Teri, L., Vitaliano, P., Mortimer, J., McCurry, S., Bowen, J., & Larson, E. (2002)	*Design:* Cross-sectional, comparative study *Measure:* Demography, case scenarios, questionnaire *Sample:* 1,244 Japanese Americans; 1,354 Caucasian Americans	Japanese Americans rely on family; prefer home care; use nursing home if have permanent disability.
Minniefield, W., Yang, J., & Muti, P. (2001)	*Design:* Descriptive study *Measure:* Survey questionnaire *Sample:* 892 respondents (249 African Americans, 492 Whites, 71 Asian Americans, 23 Hispanic/ Latino Americans, 22 Native Americans, 35 unknown)	Trust for physicians: 46% African Americans lack trust compared to 23% Whites.
Moon, A., Lubben, J. E., & Villa, V. (1998)	*Design:* Survey *Measure:* Questionnaire *Sample:* 213 Korean Americans, 201 Hispanic/ Latino Americans, 201 non-Hispanic White Americans	Low rate of use of home and community long-term care.
Namekata, T., Moore, D., Knopp, R., Marcovina, S., Perrin, E., Hughes, D., Suzuki, K., Mori, M., Sempos, C., Hatano, S., Hayashi, C., & Hasegawa, M. (1996)	*Design:* Comparative study *Measure:* CVD screening data, 1989–1994; comparison data—NHANES data, 1988–1991, National CVD Examination survey, 1990 (Japan), Epidemiological Arteriosclerosis Research Institute data, 1989 (Japan) *Sample:* 1,466 Japanese Americans screened, Seattle, WA	Total cholesterol and triglyceride levels highest in Seattle residents. High-density lipoprotein cholesterol (HDL-C) level: Males—Seattle group and native Japanese similar; females—Japanese urban workers followed by Seattle group. Possible genetic and environmental effects.

TABLE 8.1 *(continued)*

Study	Method	Selected findings
Ness, J., Nassimiha, D., Ferea, M., & Aronow, W. (1999)	*Design:* Retrospective chart analysis *Measure:* Clinical data *Sample:* 2,003 persons, 72–88 years old, African Americans, Hispanics, Whites	Higher prevalence of stroke, neuropathy, CVD in African Americans with diabetes.
Northouse, L., Caffey, M., Deichelbohrer, L., Schmidt, L., Guziatek-Trojniak, L., West, S., Kershaw, T., & Mood, D. (1999)	*Design:* Descriptive, cross-sectional *Measure:* Stress and coping framework, quality of life *Sample:* 98 African American women, 4 years post breast cancer diagnosis	Positive illness appraisal; managing current concerns decreases symptoms of distress.
Okubo, M., Watanabe, H., Fujikawa, R., Kawamura, T., Egusa, G., & Yamakido, M. (1999)	*Design:* Descriptive study *Measure:* Glucose tolerance test, fasting plasma glucose, diabetes diagnosis *Sample:* 1,235 Japanese Americans, Hawaii and Los Angeles	Two criteria for diagnosis: World Health Organization and American Diabetes Association. Recommend: Fasting plasma glucose combined with glucose tolerance test.
O'Malley, A., Mandelblatt, J., Gold, K., Cagney, K., & Kerner, J. (1997)	*Design:* Structured telephone survey *Measure:* Screening outcomes, Pap test, clinical breast exam (CBE), mammogram *Sample:* 1,420 women— Blacks (U.S.-born Blacks, English-speaking Caribbean-born Blacks, Haitian Blacks) and Hispanic/Latinos (Puerto Rican, Dominican, Columbian, and Ecuadorian), population based	Service at a usual site and having a regular physician increased participation in cancer screening.

(continued)

TABLE 8.1   *(continued)*

Study	Method	Selected findings
Phillips, J., Cohen, M., & Tarzian, A. (2001)	*Design:* Phenomenological study *Measure:* Unstructured interview, repeated twice *Sample:* 22 African American women, low income	Women wanted a holistic approach; include relationship with family and friends; approach may help transcend the silence.
Phillips, L., Hertzberg, V., & Cook, C. (2003)	*Design:* Controlled clinical trial *Measure:* Clinical outcomes, HgbA1C, lipids, blood pressure, provider performance *Sample:* 2,000 African Americans with type II diabetes, randomized groups	Ongoing study, first comprehensive diabetes intervention program for urban African Americans.
Plotnikoff, G., Numrich, C., Wu, C., Yang, D., & Xiong, P. (2002)	*Design:* Exploratory, qualitative study *Measure:* Guided interview *Sample:* 11 Hmong shamans; 32 Hmong patients	Shaman's perspectives of healing described; Hmong patients' belief described. Shamanism considered effective care irrespective of age, gender, and degree of acculturation.
Plowden, K., & Miller, J. (2000)	*Design:* Exploratory, qualitative study *Measure:* Focus group, interview *Sample:* 38 African American men, age 24–94 years	Triggers and barriers identified. Health-seeking behaviors discussed.

TABLE 8.1 *(continued)*

Study	Method	Selected findings
Pourat, N., Lubben, J., Wallace, S., & Moon, A. (1999)	*Design:* Descriptive study, population-based *Measure:* Questionnaire (Korean), CES-D scale, basic, immediate, and advanced ADLs, social network, social support *Sample:* 223 Korean immigrants, age 70–79 years	Predictors on use of traditional healers: arthritis, chronic pain, social network, social support, health insurance.
Prehn, A., Topol, B., Stewart, A., Glaser, S., O'Connor, L., & West, D. (2002)	*Design:* Population-based study *Measure:* Type of cancer therapy, SES, other demographic data *Sample:* 1,772 Asian American (Chinese and Filipino), Pacific Islander, and White women	More mastectomies for Asian American and Pacific Islander women than for White women; less alternate therapy, i.e., adjuvant therapy, radiation therapy, hormone therapy. Differences in treatment pattern not explained by SES and demographic data.
Rooks, R., Simonsick, E., Miles, T., Newman, A., Kritchevsky, S., Schulz, R., & Harris, T. (2002)	*Design:* Longitudinal clinical study *Measure:* CVD indicators, SES *Sample:* 3,075 mixed racial/ethnic groups, age 70–79 years	Strong association with CVD indicators for Blacks; SES no effect on association.
Sateren, M., Trimble, E., Abrams, J., Brawley, O., Breen, N., Ford, L., McCabe, M., Kaplan, R., Smith, M., Ungerleider, R., & Christian, M. (2002)	*Design:* Retrospective, secondary analysis *Measure:* Demographic data, health insurance, availability of oncologist, cancer program, marketing data *Sample:* 24,332 NCI patients, 12-month accrual	Lower participation for African Americans, Asian Americans, and Hispanic/Latino Americans; highest participation from suburban areas.

(continued)

TABLE 8.1 *(continued)*

Study	Method	Selected findings
Schoengerg, N. E. (1998)	*Design:* Descriptive, qualitative study *Measure:* Structured/semistructured interview *Sample:* 41 African Americans, age 65 and older	Moderately high adherence to prescribed diet associated with perceived support from family and friends.
Shakoor-Abdullah, B., Kotchen, J., Walker, W., Chelius T., & Hoffman, R. (1997)	*Design:* Cross-sectional, experimental study *Measure:* Household assessment, social support, demographic data *Sample:* 975 African Americans, age 18 and older, randomized	No SES effect on gender differences in BP; low SES effect on obesity and uninsured. Intraracial diversity, education level, and SES influence access.
Shavers, V., Lynch, C., & Burmeister, L. (2002)	*Design:* Descriptive survey *Measure:* Questionnaire on research participation *Sample:* 198 residents in Primary Metropolitan Statistical Area (PMSA), Detroit, MI	African Americans less willing to participate than Whites. Correlates: High importance of physician's race for routine medical care; belief that minorities bear most of risks of medical research; knowledge of Tuskegee Study resulted in less trust for medical researchers.
Sundquist, J., Winkleby, M., & Pudaric, S. (2002)	*Design:* Epidemiologic study, secondary data analysis *Measure:* National Health and Nutrition Survey III (NHANES III) data *Sample:* 700 African Americans, 628 Mexican Americans, 2,192 Whites, age 65–84 years	Higher prevalence of type II diabetes for African American and Mexican American women compared to White women; African American women likely to have abdominal obesity and HTN; male and female African Americans and Mexican American women are at greatest risk of CVD.

TABLE 8.1 *(continued)*

Study	Method	Selected findings
Tan, E., Lui, L., Eng, C., Jha, A., & Covinsky, K. (2003)	*Design:* Longitudinal cohort study *Measure:* Cox proportional hazards model *Sample:* 2,002 Whites, 859 Blacks	1 year after PACE enrollment, Blacks had lower mortality rate (OR = 0.67; 95% CI = 0.54–0.85, $p < 0.001$). First year, Blacks more likely to improve or less likely to have a decline in ADL than Whites ($p < 0.001$).
Utsey, S., Chae, M., Brown, C., & Kelly, D. (2002)	*Design:* Descriptive, cross-sectional *Measure:* Multigroup ethnic identity measure, index of race-related stress, WHO quality of life *Sample:* 160 African Americans, Asian Americans, Hispanic/Latino Americans	Ethnic identity and cultural racism were significant predictors of quality of life.
Vaccarino, V., Gahbauer, E., Kasl, S., Charpentier, P., Acampora, D., & Krumholz, H. (2002)	*Design:* Prospective cohort study *Measure:* CVD clinical, functional outcomes *Sample:* 82 Blacks, 316 Whites	Functional decline greater for Blacks (37.6%) than for Whites (24.7%); Blacks had 50% higher risk of death from functional decline (OR = 1.45, 95%; CI = 1.06–1.81).
Weinrich, S., Faison-Smith, L., Hudson-Priest, J., Royal, C., & Powell, I. (2002)	*Design:* Correlation study *Measure:* Self-report, 2 data collection points over 12 months *Sample:* 96 African American men	48% changed responses; self-reports changed with increased awareness of prostate cancer.
Weinrich, S., Weinrich, M., Atwood, J., Cobb, M., & Anderson, R. (1999)	*Design:* Descriptive, quasi-experimental study *Measure:* Questionnaire, demographic data, type of educational program *Sample:* 953 Blacks and Whites, age 40–70 years	Cost-effective cancer education program in work sites for African Americans.

(continued)

TABLE 8.1 *(continued)*

Study	Method	Selected findings
Wojcik, B., Spinks, M., & Optenberg, S. (1998)	*Design:* Retrospective study *Measure:* Department of Defense Central Tumor Registry data; hazard ratio adjusted for covariates *Sample:* Mixed population, age 19–97 years	Better survival rate for African American women in military than for those in SEER program. Access to full complement of treatment options a standard DOD policy. Race-related survival differences still exist.
Wright, P., Fortinsky, R., Covinsky, K., Anderson, P., & Landefeld, C. (2000)	*Design:* Cross-sectional study *Measure:* Descriptive data *Sample:* 683 Black men and women, age 70 and up, from 5 neighborhood centers	More frequent office visits associated with greater delivery of preventive services.
Yu, E., Chen, E., Kim, K., & Abdurahim, S. (2002)	*Design:* Population-based survey *Measure:* Chinese questionnaire based on NHIS instrument *Sample:* 644 Chinese Americans	Prevalence rate of smoking below Healthy People 2010 goal of < 12%.
Zhu, K., Hunter, S., Bernard, L., Payne-Wilks, K., Roland, C., & Levin, R. (2000)	*Design:* Descriptive study *Measure:* Face-to-face interviews *Sample:* 325 single African American women, 65 years and older	Access to regular physician, having medical order for repeat mammogram; women who had mammogram previous year are three times more likely to have repeat procedure.

TABLE 8.2 Research Articles Reviewed on Cancer Screening in Asian Americans

Study	Method	Select findings
Klonoff-Cohen, H., Schaffroth, L., Edelstein, S., Molgaard, C., & Saltzstein, S. (1998)	*Design:* Descriptive, cross-sectional study *Measure:* Population-based data from the Northern California Tumor Registry of NCI SEER program; tumor classification (ductal, lobular, and mixed) *Sample:* 2,759 cases diagnosed in 1988	Ductal type most common (83.6%); lobular rarest (56.3%); most tumors were localized at diagnosis (56.3%). White women had highest rates for both tumor types; African Americans had twice rate for lobular tumor compared to Whites; Asian Americans and Hispanic/Latino Americans had higher rate for ductal type, though statistically not significant.
ASIAN INDIAN Sadler, G., Dhanjal, S., Shah, N., Shah, R., Ko, C., Anghel, M., & Harshburger, R. (2001)	*Design:* Descriptive, cross-sectional study *Measure:* Questionnaire, breast cancer knowledge, attitudes, screening behaviors *Sample:* 194 American Asian Indian women, age 40 and older	Seventy percent (70%) age 50 and older had mammogram the past 12 months. Rates for annual mammography higher than for other ethnic groups; breast cancer knowledge inadequate; women willing to share knowledge with others.

FOBT = Fecal Occult Blood Test
ACS = American Cancer Society
NCI = National Cancer Institute

(continued)

TABLE 8.2   *(continued)*

Study	Method	Select findings
CAMBODIAN		
Carey Jackson, J., Taylor, V. Chitnarong, K., Mahloch, J., Fischer, M., Sam, R., & Seng, P. (2000)	*Design:* Descriptive cross-sectional study *Measure:* Ethnographic interview on barriers to cervical cancer screening, demographic data *Sample:* Cambodian Americans: 42 women for ethnographic interview; 413 for community survey	Barriers to cervical cancer screening: Traditional orientation to prevention, cause, and treatment of disease; unfamiliarity with Western concepts of early detection; limited knowledge of cervical cancer; concern over Pap test procedure; health care access issues. Results used to design culturally appropriate community education and counseling program.
Kelly, A., Fores Chacori, M., Wollan, P., Trapp, M., Weaver, A., Barrier, P., Franz, W., & Kottke, T. (1996)	*Design:* Descriptive, retrospective, intervention study *Measure:* Review of medical record for cancer screening, past year; focus group on screening practices, demographic data *Sample:* 57 Cambodian Americans, 57 non-Cambodian Americans, age > 50 years	Screening rates: Lower than for non-Cambodian group. Identified barriers: Lack of knowledge, shyness at examination, transportation, fear of technical, large medical center, individual appointments. Postintervention community screening increased almost five times from baseline.
Tu, S., Yasui, Y., Kuniyuki, A., Schwartz, S., Jackson, J., & Taylor, V. (2002)	*Design:* Cross-sectional survey *Measure:* Screening stages of adoption, demographic data *Sample:* 398 clinical breast self-exam cases; 248 mammography cases; Cambodian American women, urban, Seattle, WA	Significant association between screening stage and physician characteristics. Increased screening with Asian American female physician.

TABLE 8.2 *(continued)*

Study	Method	Select findings

CHINESE AMERICAN

Study	Method	Select findings
Facione, N., Giancarlo, C., & Chan, L. (2000)	*Design:* Descriptive, qualitive study *Measure:* Focus group on breast cancer risk, evaluation of self-discovered breast symptoms (English, Mandarin, and Cantonese) demographic data *Sample:* 45 first-generation Chinese American women	Sense of invulnerability to the disease; linking cancer to tragic luck, predominant likelihood of delay. Preserving modesty and conserving wealth and time, favored use of Chinese medicine and delay of Western treatment.
Tang, T., Solomon, J., & McCracken, L. (2000)	*Design:* Descriptive, cross-sectional study *Measure:* Questionnaire on breast cancer screening, health history, health insurance, common cultural barriers to colorectal screening, acculturation *Sample:* 100 Chinese American women, urban, East Coast, age 60 and older	Significant predictors: Insurance and acculturation for at least one mammogram; recency of medical visit for mammogram and clinical breast exam for the past year; acculturation and modesty for having had clinical breast exam at least once.
Tang, T., Solomon, J., & McCracken, L. (2001)	*Design:* Descriptive, cross-sectional study *Measure:* Questionnaire (sigmoidoscopy screening, fecal occult blood test), health history, common cultural barriers to colorectal screening, acculturation, demographic data *Sample:* 100 Chinese American women, urban, East Coast, age 60 and older	Significant predictors: Acculturation and one-time FOBT; acculturation and physician recommendation for sigmoidoscopy. No significant predictors for regular adherence to ACS recommended colorectal screening guidelines.

(continued)

TABLE 8.2 *(continued)*

Study	Method	Select findings
Taylor, V., Hislop, G., Jackson, J., Tu, S., Yasui, Y., Schwartz, S., Teh, C., Kuniyuki, A., Acorda, E., Marchand, A., & Thompson, B. (2002)	*Design:* Experimental *Measure:* Pap testing *Sample:* 402 Chinese American women	Trilingual outreach workers and direct mail improved Pap testing vs. control.
Taylor, V., Jackson, J., Tu, S., Yasui, Y., Schwartz, S., Kuniyuki, A., Acorda, E., Lin, K., & Hislop, G. (2002)	*Design:* Community-based interview *Measure:* History of Pap test, 8 facilitating factors *Sample:* 432 Chinese American women, history of at least one Pap smear and testing in the last 2 years, urban, Seattle, WA	Independent association of recent screening: Thinking Pap test necessary for sexually inactive women, less concerned with embarrassment, physician recommendation, obstetrical care in U.S., having regular provider. Pap testing lower NCI Year 2000 goals; recent test facilitated by 5 facilitating factors.

FILIPINO AMERICAN

Maxwell, A., Bastani, R., & Warda, U. (2000)	*Design:* Descriptive survey *Measure:* Questionnaire on cancer screening practices, demographic data *Sample:* 218 Filipino women; 229 Korean women, immigrants, age 50 and older, Los Angeles	Screening for Filipinos in the past two years: 48% Pap smear; 41% mammogram and clinical breast exam; 25% colorectal screening (fecal occult blood test and sigmoidoscopy). Only 14% met recommended cancer screening guidelines. Most predictive of adherence: Higher percentage of lifetime spent in U.S.; asymptomatic medical checkup.

TABLE 8.2   *(continued)*

Study	Method	Select findings
McBride, M., Pasick, R., Stewart, S., Tuason, N., Sabogal, F., & Duenas, G. (1998)	*Design:* Formative and descriptive survey *Measure:* Focus group, structured telephone interview (English, Tagalog, Illocano, Cebuano), cultural dimensions (language, traditional health beliefs, modesty, traditional gender role), and demographic data *Sample:* 6 focus groups; 875 Filipino American women (immigrant + native born), age-satisfied, randomized	Screening (Pap test) rates: 12% never had one; 5% never heard of test; 7% heard but never had test; decreased with age (53% for age 65+ years; 63% for 50–64 years); no insurance. Correlates for low screening rates: Older women (> 50 years) with high traditional health belief factor and low English-language use factor; younger women (< 50 years) with high traditional gender role values and high modesty factor.

KOREAN AMERICAN

Study	Method	Select findings
Juon, H. Choi, Y., & Kim, M. (2000)	*Design:* Descriptive, cross-sectional study *Measure:* Face-to-face interview, questionnaire on breast and cervical cancer screening behaviors, demographic data *Sample:* 438 Korean American women, age 18 and older	Screening for the past two years: 50% of younger women (> 18 years) had Pap test; 46.8% of older women (> 40 years) had mammogram. Correlates of regular medical checkup: Age, acculturation, language proficiency (mammogram), and years of life in U.S., married, and employed (Pap test).

(continued)

TABLE 8.2 *(continued)*

Study	Method	Select findings
Kim, K., Yu, E., Chen, E., Kim, J., & Brintnall, R. (1998)	*Design:* Descriptive study *Measure:* National Health Interview Survey (NHIS), Korean translation, demography *Sample:* 159 Korean American women, 104 Korean men, age 40–69 years, Chicago, IL	Knowledge correlates: Length of residence in U.S. (digital rectal exam, DRE); gender and education (fetal occult blood test, FOBT). Screening rates: Women, 11.3% (DRE) and 8.8% (FOBT); men, 13.5% (DRE), 10.68 (FOBT).
Kim, K., Yu, E., Chen, E., Kim, J., Kaufman, M., & Purkiss, J. (1999)	*Design:* Descriptive study *Measure:* 1987 Cancer Control Supplement questionnaire, Korean translation, demographic data *Sample:* 159 Korean American women, immigrants, age 40–69 years, Midwest	Knowledge: 26% never heard of Pap test. Pap test: 34% had been screened. Cited reason for non-screening: Absence of symptoms.
Maxwell, A., Bastani, R., & Warda, U. (2000)	*Design:* Descriptive survey *Measure:* Questionnaire on cancer screening practices, demographic data *Sample:* 218 Filipino American women; 229 Korean American women, immigrants, age 50 and older, Los Angeles	Screening (Koreans) in the past 2 years: 41% Pap smear; 25% mammogram and clinical breast exam; 38% colorectal screening (FOBT and sigmoidoscopy); 10% met recommended cancer screening guidelines. Most predictive of adherence: Higher percentage of lifetime spent in U.S. and asymptomatic medical checkup.

TABLE 8.2 *(continued)*

Study	Method	Select findings
Wismer, B., Moskowitz, J., Chen, A., Kang, S., Novotny, T., Min, K., Lew, R., & Tager, I. (1998)	*Design:* Descriptive, population-based survey *Measure:* Telephone interview, questionnaire on cancer screening practices, demographic data *Sample:* 1,090 Korean American women, immigrants, age 18 and older, two California counties	Screening rate in past two years, women > 50 years of age: 34% (mammogram), 32% (clinical breast exam). Correlates to screening: Regular medical checkup. Rate estimate lower than Healthy People 2000 objectives and published estimates for other groups.

VIETNAMESE AMERICAN

Schulmeister, L., & Lifsey, D. (1999)	*Design:* Descriptive, exploratory study *Measure:* Questionnaire, face-to-face interview *Sample:* 96 Vietnamese women, migrant	Knowledge of Pap test: 75% unable to explain. Screening: Less than half had test barriers: belief that their risk of cancer is low, fear of procedure, no gynecologist, and cost.

ASIAN AMERICAN

Coughlin, S., & Uhler, R. (2000)	*Design:* Descriptive, secondary analysis *Measure:* Data from Behavioral Risk Factor Surveillance System (BRFSS), 1994–1997 *Sample:* 6,048 Asian American and Pacific Islander women, 49 states	Past two years for women, > 50 years: 71.7% had mammogram; 69.5% had clinical breast exam. Having health insurance and having been to see physician were predictive of screening.

2000). By 2030, members of these groups are expected to constitute 25% of all older people in the United States (Administration on Aging, 2001; U.S. Department of Health and Human Services, 2001). This projection must guide research on older people of color to avoid creating a wider gap in knowledge, which would result in ineffective programs and overextending expectations of health care providers. Research on aging and the health of racial and ethnic minority older adults is gaining momentum. However, the accumulation of knowledge is greater for some groups than for others. We know considerably more about the aging and health issues of African Americans, Chinese Americans, Japanese Americans, and to some extent Hispanic/Latino Americans compared to American Indians/Alaska Natives, Filipino Americans, Native Hawaiians/Pacific Islanders, Southeast Asians, and South Asian/Asian Indians.

Racial and ethnic minority groups may share certain beliefs, values, and norms of behavior; however, these may be expressed in various ways between and within groups that cross social, psychological, historical, and health domains (McBride et al., 1996; Richardson, 1996; Yeo et al., 1998). Beliefs about health, illness, and accessing treatment vary and are influenced by culture, English-language proficiency, cohort experiences, immigration history, and other factors. Researchers are making efforts to study these issues; however, progress is slow. Furthermore, progress is complicated by new and more complex health issues of minority elders precipitated by numerous changes in public policy, severe cost containment programs, and a serious health manpower crisis.

SUMMARY AND CRITIQUE OF RESEARCH REPORTS

Health Status of African American and Asian American Elders

Research on chronic diseases among racial and ethnic minority elders reports variations in the prevalence and types of illness observed in different groups. The 2002 "State of Aging" report prepared by the Gerontological Society of America points out that in 1995 more African Americans ages 70 and older had high blood pressure (58.7%) compared to Whites (44%) and Hispanic/Latino Americans (22%). The data obtained from the "Second Supplement on Aging" also indicate diabetes rates in this age category to be 20.4% for Blacks, 17.4% for Hispanic/Latino Americans, and 10.9% for non-Hispanic Whites. From 1982 to 1999, self-reported health status by persons age 85 and older declined from 36% to 31% (Federal Interagency Forum on Aging-Related Statistics, 2000).

In some large databases, health status is often measured by self-reports (e.g., Pastor, Makuc, Reuben, & Xia, 2002). Self-reports provide an overview of the older person's health status; however, for greater accuracy, health status for racial and ethnic minority elders must be corroborated by clinical data, particularly for those who are monolingual and low acculturated older immigrants. Inaccurate translation of questionnaires, misinterpretation of questions, or belief about authority figures such as health professionals may generate unreliable information.

In a review of medical records, African Americans had a higher prevalence of strokes compared to Hispanic/Latinos and Whites (Ness, Nassimiha, Feria, & Aronow, 1999), which is suggestive of a group difference in hypertension and diabetes (Baumann, Chang, & Hoebeke, 2002). The prevalence of type II diabetes in African American and Mexican American women is higher than for White women, and they are at greatest risk of cardiovascular disease, along with African American men (Sundquist, Winkleby, & Pudaric, 2002). Indicators for cardiovascular disease (Rooks et al., 2002; Shakoor-Abdullah, Kotchen, Walker, Chelius, & Hoffman, 1997) and outcomes of heart disease (Vaccarino et al., 2002) have been identified in longitudinal and cross-sectional studies. Obesity is a major risk factor for diabetes in African Americans, and 25% of older African Americans (age 65 to 74 years) have the disease (National Institute of Diabetes and Digestive and Kidney Diseases [NIDDK], 2003). Higher rates are also reported for Japanese Americans, Chinese Americans, and Filipino Americans (Asian American Pacific Community Health Organizations, 2003; Choi et al., 1990; NIDDK, 2003). These data indicate that the health of members of various groups is in jeopardy.

Data from another medical record review of over 2,000 patients with diabetes showed no significant age-related changes over time in body mass index (BMI). In terms of glucose control, glycosylated hemoglobin (HgbA1C) was higher from baseline for younger African Americans (< 65 years) compared to the older group (> 65 years) (El-kebbi, Cook, & Ziemer, 2003). Clinicians may point to poor adherence to explain these findings, but there is little documentation of a patient's belief system in medical records today that can be used to fully explain these clinical outcomes. Clearly other factors influence such outcomes, such as perceptions of self or social situation. Perceptions of support from family and friends generate a moderately high adherence to a prescribed diet (Schoengerg, 1998). Perception of self has consistently been predictive of health outcomes. A case in point is the response of African American women when asked about body shape. African American women with diabetes perceived an acceptable healthy body to be a middle to large, pear-shaped body (Liburd, Anderson, Edgar, & Jack, 1999). Although this is only one study, the findings have implications for the development of empirically based interventions for diabetes management. Further explorations of the construct "perceptions" using various qualitative methodologies would be valuable approaches to increasing nursing's knowledge base about the health of racial and ethnic minority elders.

The constructs that structure interventions for members of racial and ethnic groups must be conceptualized and measured consistently in order to contribute to nursing's understanding of inter- and intragroup differences. For example, the construct "quality of life," when used as a proxy for health status, may guide health care professionals' individualized care for racial and ethnic minority older adults. Racial and ethnic minority group membership was examined in regard to race-related stress and quality of life for African Americans, Asian Americans, and Hispanics (Utsey, Chae, Brown, & Kelly, 2002). Results revealed significantly higher race-related stress and psychological scores among African Americans than for Asians and Hispanics. For each of these groups, ethnic identity and cultural racism were major predictors of quality of life. In contrast, among older African Americans (> 65 years) who are living in the community with chronic illness, years of education and functional capacity are strong determinants of health-related hardiness (Martin, Engle, & Graney, 1999). Interestingly, cultural racism does not predict quality of life for this group of older African Americans. What are the ages when cultural racism no longer creates race-related stress? What is our understanding of the meaning of quality of life for members of racial and ethnic groups? These are critical questions that must be addressed consistently for each group.

Health status information obtained from interviews of racial and ethnic minorities revealed an important association between being uninsured, poor control of chronic illness, and lack of information about illness management (Becker, 2001). African Americans who are in their fourth year of diagnosis with breast cancer state that having a positive attitude about the illness and being able to manage their life are factors that help reduce distress (Northouse et al., 1999). Health-related hardiness or being healthier is an intriguing concept that can be adapted to different groups of racial and ethnic older adults as a major determinant of health status and quality of life. Instruments that have been developed from a White cultural perspective to measure this concept may not be appropriate for the African American community. Thus, developing research tools is an active partnership process between the researcher and the racial and ethnic minority community. For example, interview questions can be crafted and tested with careful attention to the cultural context of the information being collected.

Access and Utilization of Health Care Services and Resources

UTILIZATION PATTERNS

The utilization pattern of either a single or multiple system of health care is gradually being described for different groups of racial and ethnic elders. Studies involving older patients who are active in the health care system provide important insight into the quality and type of care they receive. The findings of one survey revealed that Asian American and Pacific Islander patients who received medical care from a West Coast–based physician group had worse access to health care when compared to Whites, African Americans, Hispanics, and Native Americans (Snyder, Cunningham, Nakazano, & Hays, 2000). Although cultural factors and communication problems were suggested as possible reasons for the differences in access, these variables were not measured. Having a bilingual provider in a health care setting may decrease the psychological discomfort of an Asian American elder with limited English proficiency. Promoting a nonjudgmental attitude toward preferences for indigenous healing practices may help reduce perceived barriers to care by this group of elders (Harper, 1990; McBride et al., 1996).

Another study documented that in five health centers located in low-income neighborhoods, more preventive services were received by African American elders when frequent office visits were scheduled (Wright, Fortinsky, Covinsky, Anderson, & Landefeld, 2000). These important findings suggest the importance of relationships to perceptions of access. Many cultures value relationships as a component of personal identification and others' expectations. Frequent clinical encounters provide opportunities to build relationships, which may be a key element in consistent utilization of preventive health care services. Research about health disparities has yet to consistently include patient–provider relationships as a measurable construct. The time is right to examine this element, because downsizing of health care services and increasing experience of burnout in the workplace can negatively affect how health care services are used. How much these system-based trends would exacerbate existing health disparities is an urgent question begging to be studied.

Patient and provider relationships are only one factor that influences utilization patterns. Many others exist. For example, the 1993–1995 Asset of Health Dynamics (AHEAD) for the oldest old was analyzed to examine the effect of economic factors on disparities by gender, race, and ethnicity in the use of health care services (Dunlop, Manheim, Song, & Chang, 2002). Compared to non-Hispanic White men, the number of physician contacts and outpatient surgeries were lower for African American men; non-Hispanic White women had fewer outpatient surgeries, and Hispanic women were less inclined to seek post–acute care in a nursing home. Disparities in the use of medical services covered by Medicare were not associated with economic access for patients with similar categories of health needs. Cultural and attitudinal factors were not measured in the study, but were suggested as possible explanations for the results. In another study that used data from the 1998 National Research Corporation Healthcare Market Guide, ratings for their health plan were lower among non-White respondents than among Whites (Haviland, Morales, Reise, & Hays, 2003). Asian Americans/Pacific Islanders in particular were less satisfied with their medical care.

Attitude toward the use of long-term care services varies among older Japanese Americans and Whites according to prognosis and intensity of care (McCormick et al., 2002). More than half of the Japanese Americans (53%, $n = 1,244$) preferred nursing home care for a chronic debilitating disease compared to Whites (38%, $n = 1,354$), and an overwhelming high percentage of both groups preferred home care for a short-term condition. Japanese Americans would rely on family members for home care, whereas Whites preferred paid providers. However, in the event of a permanent disability, Japanese Americans intended to use nursing home care. In the Veteran's Administration health care system, preferences for and use of outpatient care were significantly associated with race and identity as a veteran, particularly for African Americans and Hispanics (Harada et al., 2002). These studies include qualitative methods—case scenarios and focus groups, respectively. These strategies provided useful qualitative information to define and differentiate access preferences between groups.

Although these approaches are complex and labor-intensive, the older person is able to expand on his or her experiences and perceptions using his or her own words and expressions. Connecting preferences and utilization to the cultural context of racial and ethnic minority patients requires the development and testing of ethnographic types of research designs. Centers for Excellence and nurse-managed health care programs are well positioned to move into this arena to reduce disparities in health care.

The decision by an African American or Asian American elder to access specific services depends also on adequate knowledge about a disease and appropriate treatment. Delayed treatment for diabetes may occur when the elder has limited understanding of the criteria being used in the diagnostic process. Advances in diabetes research have refined the criteria for diagnosis recommended by the World Health Organization (WHO) and the American Diabetes Association (ADA). It appears that both criteria have the potential for misdiagnosis, as reported in a study of Japanese Americans in Hawaii and Los Angeles (Okubo et al., 1999). Thus the researchers recommend combining the two criteria: the glucose tolerance test and fasting plasma glucose. African American and Asian American elders with limited English-language skills and formal education may be unable to advocate for the diagnostic protocol as recommended by the Okubo team to ensure an early and accurate diagnosis. Delayed treatment in this situation may be associated with a lack of access to culturally appropriate and understandable information.

In another study examining delays in treatment, acute care for myocardial infarction in inner-city hospitals was significantly delayed for ethnic minorities by an average of 44.3 hours (Asian Americans, 92 hours; Hispanic/Latinos, 41.5 hours; African Americans, 30.8 hours; Whites, 31.6 hours) (Henderson, Magana, Korn, Genna, & Bretsky, 2002). There were group differences in the mode of transportation to the emergency room, and the decision to seek care was complicated by an underutilization of emergency medical services.

Interventions are critical for racial and ethnic minority elders and health care providers to reduce delays to treatment. However, we were unable to locate studies that focused on culturally appropriate intervention models developed to reduce morbidity and mortality due to myocardial infarction. Furthermore, experiences with discrimination and blatant social injustice (Richardson, 1996), negative effects of historical events (Yeo et al., 1996), highly traditional support systems (Abe-Kim, Takeuchi, & Hwang, 2002), characteristics of health-seeking behaviors (Plowden & Miller, 2000), and other factors are rarely measured as they relate to seeking health care services. Incorporating these constructs in future research conveys the message that getting to the core etiologies of and interventions for health disparities involves the full participation of racial and ethnic minority communities in an environment of trust (Shavers, Lynch, & Burmeister, 2002).

CHARACTERISTICS OF PROVIDERS AND HEALTH CARE SETTINGS

The results of the above studies should also be examined in light of patient-provider relationships. Race was found to be a critical factor in trust relationships (Corbie-Smith, Thomas, & George, 2002). In telephone interviews with adult primary care patients (age 18–65), Cooper-Patrick et al. (1999) found that patients who were treated by physicians of their own race and ethnicity rated the providers' decision-making styles as more participatory than those of other race and ethnicity. Another study using data from the 1996 and 1997 Community Tracking Survey indicated that African American patients reported less positive perceptions of physician satisfaction and trust compared to Whites, particularly for those who lacked physician continuity on repeat clinic visits (Doescher, Saver, Franks, & Fiscella, 2000).

Physicians to a large extent control the ratio of available physicians to elders. This statement is supported by a study that explored acceptance of elders by specialists and primary care physicians who completed a questionnaire to ascertain their degree of acceptance of new Medicaid managed care patients into their practices (Backus et al., 2001). Specialists were more likely to accept new Medicaid patients, although this was limited to fee-for-service patients only. Many Medicare and Medicaid patients are now enrolled in managed care health plans, and the above results contribute to our understanding of access to primary care services by racial and ethnic minority older adults.

Teaching hospitals are commonly acknowledged to be at the forefront of providing the most current, scientific-based health care in the United States. One study described the influence of race, ethnicity, and affluence on the use of teaching hospitals by patients with a newly diagnosed serious illness who were insured by Medicare. Results indicated lower levels of use by Hispanics and Asian Americans than by their White counterparts (Iwashyna, Curlin, & Christakis, 2002). Hierarchical linear modeling was used to account for variation in the availability of teaching hospitals to members of racial and ethnic groups. Those who were most likely to seek care from teaching hospitals were patients who lived in the poorest and in the wealthiest communities. Herein lies a significant disparity in access to new treatment and new technology. Other variables, including attitude toward receiving care from trainees and environmental issues such as transportation, also influence utilization. Identifying alternative evidence-based explanations for the previously described results would not be possible from a preexisting dataset. Although the large sample would provide an adequate number of cases to analyze for effects, it would be difficult to draw culture-based inferences about utilization.

A difference in the treatment of racial and ethnic minority elders by hospitals has also been documented. A prospective study was conducted to assess the frequency of transfer and to determine nonmedical factors associated with it. Gurwitz et al. (2002) analyzed the National Registry of Myocardial Infarction data from June 1994 to March 1998. After adjustment for differences in clinical and hospital characteristics, factors associated most with transfers were older age (> 75 years) and being African American. The factors were especially relevant for patients who were initially admitted to hospitals with limited therapeutic capabilities, although this persisted to some degree for hospitals with full resources. There is a need for studies to examine other factors that might contribute to biases in treatment.

Similar studies need to be examined with regard to racial and ethnic minority participation in research studies. Enrollment in clinical trials by racial and ethnic minority older adults is beginning to gain attention. There is much to be learned about the enabling factors for participation. Sateren et al. (2002) analyzed the National Cancer Institute patient database of sponsored cancer treatment trials over a 12-month period, including information on the availability of an oncologist and the existence of a multidisciplinary cancer treatment program. African Americans, Asian Americans, and Hispanics were attracted to the clinical trials at much lower rates than Whites, and the highest level of participation was in the suburban areas. While factors such as being on Medicare, the presence of an oncologist, and the availability of a multidisciplinary team increased the likelihood of participation, this did not appear to influence participation for different groups of racial and ethnic minority older adults. Research on culturally appropriate messages to improve participation in clinical trials by these groups is needed to close the gap in cancer care.

HEALTH SCREENING AND INTERVENTION

Cancer screening rates vary across Asian groups. Taylor et al. (2002) found the rate of Pap testing for Chinese women (age 20 –79) is lower than the standard established by the National Cancer Institute's Year 2000 goals. Recent screening was associated with thinking the test is necessary for sexually inactive women, physician referral, having a consistent primary care provider, and having received obstetrical services in the United States. For the underutilizers in the sample, a subgroup was contacted by a trilingual, bicultural staff, and another subgroup received materials by mail. The first method yielded a 39% participation in Pap smears, and the second method yielded a 25% participation before the follow-up data collection period (Taylor et al., 2002). Although rates are still low, this method provides some promise in encouraging participation in screening.

Over the past 10 years, research on cancer screening for Asian Americans reached an unprecedented level. A summary of 17 descriptive studies in Table 8.2 shows efforts toward addressing the issues of group differences, small population size, cultural beliefs, English-language literacy, health literacy, and geographic location. The campaign against reproductive cancer in the racial and ethnic minority community is a useful model for problem identification and intervention research. Although sample sizes ranged from 45 to 1,090 participants, a pattern emerged showing that belief systems contributed to the health-seeking behavior of women from different racial and ethnic groups. Collectively, the results can inform the development of culturally appropriate intervention studies. Expertise in language translation highlights the value of applying a rigorous process to preserve internal cultural consistency.

Unfortunately, the research momentum about screening has slowed down. However, with the accumulated knowledge and lessons learned from Asian American groups, the next generation of investigations should include experimental studies, and the network of researchers in this field could collaborate to test these strategies.

To link beliefs with up-to-date status on annual Pap testing, a questionnaire was completed by African American and Hispanic women who were up-to-date with cervical screening (Jennings-Dozier, 1999). They were contacted through urban community agencies. Differences in beliefs were found. African Americans were more concerned about physician behavior and less with the Pap testing experience. Other concerns involved approval from family and friends, having a choice of provider, and access to free screening. Hispanic women were concerned with the benefits of the procedure and less with the testing experience. Other concerns were similar to African Americans, except that Hispanics were more likely to express preference for a female physician. Although the information was collected from a convenience sample, the study offers a window of opportunity to pursue screening-related behavioral, normative, and control beliefs, many of which may be rooted in the women's cultural beliefs.

Phillips, Cohen, and Tarzian (2001) describe a holistic approach to the experience of breast cancer screening in low-income African American women that includes relationships with family and friends. Future research efforts could combine these findings with the observations by O'Malley, Mandelblatt, Gold, Cagney, and Kerner (1997) that maintenance of breast and cervical cancer screening in a multiethnic population in the East Coast was associated with a consistent site of care. A linear trend in the rise of screening rates was found when a usual source of care and a regular physician at the site were available, especially for uninsured African American and Hispanic/Latino American women. Similar results were reported by Zhu et al. (2000), who found that African American women's repeat mammograms were influenced by access to a regular physician. Having a consistent provider correlates with high access rates. It is interesting to note that, to date, barriers to mammography use continue to differ between African Americans and Whites, and race has been reported to have no effect on these barriers (Han, Wells, & Primas, 2003). In contrast, Bibb (2001) found late-stage diagnosis of breast cancer in African American women, which could be explained by economic factors. The mixed observations suggest that research efforts should focus more on aggressive interventions for American women to reduce late-stage diagnosis and provide a positive breast cancer screening experience (Underwood, 1998). An emphasis on provider consistency (either a physician or a nurse practitioner) should be an important component of such efforts.

An awareness campaign was conducted consisting of an educational intervention and free screening for men targeted for prostate cancer in a Midwest urban community (Barber et al., 1998). A short questionnaire was administered before and after the videotape training and screening procedures to measure knowledge and attitude about prostate cancer. Results indicated that African American men had less knowledge about the disease, preferred private screening to mass screening, and were better reached by radio. In another study, Weinrich, Faison-Smith, Hudson-Priest, Royal, and Powell (2002) concluded that cancer education in the workplace is cost effective. These studies describe short-term results. To ensure a long-lasting effect, more experimental intervention models infused with ethnogeriatric content should be tested in multiethnic groups, especially for individuals with a family history of the disease.

Culture-based exploration of the patient's perception of diseases such as cancer is beginning to be done qualitatively (Cooley & Jennings-Dozier, 1998). Adapting the research methods of the pioneer studies on explanatory models of illness (Kleinman, 1982; Kleinman et al., 1978) could provide a strong foundation for these efforts.

TREATMENT OUTCOMES

A retrospective chart review showed significant differences between African Americans, Hispanics, and Whites with regard to hypertension and diabetes control (Baumann et al., 2002). African American patients were in poor control compared to the other groups. In a retrospective analysis of discharge data from 10 states, Gaskin and Hoffman (2000) found that African Americans and Hispanics were more likely to be admitted for preventable health conditions, and this was especially observed in the elderly from both groups. These patterns must now be studied beyond screening and monitoring programs in primary care services to clarify the interplay of cultural and language factors in clinical encounters.

Although African Americans, Hispanics, and Native Americans experience an exceptionally high rate of illness and mortality due to diabetes compared to Whites, the disease appears to be poorly managed in these groups (Smedly, Stith, & Nelson, 2003). Based on an analysis of close to 1,400 Medicare patients, Chin, Zhang, and Merrell (1998) found that African Americans tended to use hospital emergency service more, have fewer physician visits, and receive fewer preventive measures (glycosylated hemoglobin, lipids, vision check, and vaccination). Suggestions to increase knowledge through experiential education and access to resources were identified by participants in focus groups (Anderson-Loftin & Moneyham, 2000). These were viewed as critical elements of diabetes education programs. A diabetes intervention for urban African Americans is currently in progress (Phillips, Hertzberg, & Cook, 2003). It is the first comprehensive clinical trial with a large sample size, and this model could be a prototype for other ethnic groups.

In examining treatment patterns for breast cancer, differences in treatment have been noted between ethnic groups. For example, in one study Asian American and Pacific Islander (API) women, specifically Chinese American and Filipino American women, had significantly more mastectomies than White women (Prehn et al., 2002). Many API patients did not receive further adjuvant therapy, radiation therapy, and hormone therapy. Patients undergoing cancer treatment are expected to make repeated outpatient or inpatient visits. Perceived potential barriers to cancer treatment reported by African American and Hispanic patients include problems with distance, access to a car, and availability of a driver, which may cause them to forego needed treatment (Guidry, Aday, Zhang, & Winn, 1997).

In an equal-access health care system, African American women had better survival rates than those who were in the Surveillance, Epidemiology, and End Results (SEER) program (Wojcik, Spinks, & Optenberg, 1998). When individualized, comprehensive care was provided, older African Americans had a lower mortality rate and were more likely to experience improvement in activities of daily living (ADL) than White participants during the first year of intervention (Tan, Lui, Eng, Jha, & Covinsky, 2003). Older African American women with breast cancer cited assistance with coexisting conditions and with navigating the health care system as helpful case management services (Jennings-Sanders & Anderson, 2003). Such services provide aspects of a holistic approach in cancer care.

A successful and well-received model for long-term care of frail older adults called the Program of All-inclusive Care for the Elderly (PACE) is an excellent example of blending elder-focused needs and a culturally responsive health care service (Tan et al., 2003). Adaptation of the model to reduce health disparities may be an option for racial and ethnic older adults in the community. The outcomes of the PACE model represent a breakthrough in various levels of geriatric care. At the core of the program is an emphasis on quality of life as defined by the older person, translated into action plans that are accessible, available, acceptable, and appropriate.

ALTERNATE HEALTH CARE OPTIONS

Combining indigenous health care with Western medicine is becoming a common practice among Asians, particularly those in the immigrant community. A descriptive study of the health service utilization and health-seeking behavior of Korean Americans revealed utilization of traditional Korean medicine, *hanbang*, Western medicine, and a combination of both (Kim, Han, Kim, & Duong, 2002). Health insurance and the source of health care were also associated with the types of services chosen. Information from this type of study needs to be linked to efficacy and health status in order to provide the highest quality of care to Korean Americans and other racial and ethnic minorities.

Many older Koreans and other Asian groups continue to be attracted to traditional healing practices over the use of formal in-home or community long-term care services. It is important to assess the out-of-pocket costs of services by traditional healers along with the social benefits of this choice of care (Moon, Lubben, & Villa, 1998). Major predictors for the use of traditional Korean healers include having a medically diagnosed chronic health problem, having insurance, and having stronger social networks and higher social support (Pourat, Lubben, Wallace, & Moon, 1999). Research in this area would facilitate the development of strategies that blend both systems of care to allow a highly traditional ethnogeriatric patient to preserve his or her cultural preferences.

As an example, the Hmong community in the United States is gradually adapting to the host culture, and despite the acculturation experience over the past 25 years, the Hmong shaman or *tu txiv neeb* (pronounced too tse neng) or traditional healer continues to be a respected and effective health care resource. Many Hmongs concurrently receive care from a physician and a shaman. To better understand how shamanism could complement Western health care, 11 Hmong shamans and 32 Hmong patients were interviewed (Plotnikoff, Numrich, Wu, Yang, & Xiong, 2002). The shamans described their spiritual perspectives, training and skills, and professional activities, while the Hmong patients described their beliefs about spiritual healing and health care. This exploratory investigation suggests that shamanism is intimately integrated into the Hmong's belief about effective health practices. Further research in this area is necessary.

The data supporting a strong preference for traditional healers suggest a link to the holistic view of health and the belief in balance and harmony among many Asian groups. Furthermore, it should be noted that African American women indicated a strong preference for a holistic approach to cancer screening practices (Phillips et al., 2001). A descriptive study on management of chronic illness by African Americans, Filipino Americans, and Hispanics revealed social and cultural differences in self-care and level of knowledge about illness (Becker, Beyene, Newsom, & Rodgers, 1998). It underscored the importance of health promotion models that are comprehensive and inclusive of the ethnic elder's beliefs and cultural practices. A gap continues to exist in providing culturally compatible and acceptable services in the mainstream health care system, although selected health plans are beginning to offer health promotion services. For nurse researchers, the opportunity to develop a research plan on alternative health may represent a coming full circle to the values that the discipline supports. Having an ethnogeriatric focus would add another dimension to the research design.

RECOMMENDATIONS

Problem Identification

The discussion section of this chapter is organized using health status and access to health care and resources as a major topic, with subtopics consisting of utilization patterns, characteristics of providers and health care settings, health screening, treatment outcomes, and alternate health care options. Based on this framework, other related research questions can be formulated in connection with reducing health disparities from an ethnogeriatric context. The variability in utilization patterns of cancer screening services (see Table 8.2), diabetes care, and cardiovascular prevention programs by African American and Asian American groups help explain the multifaceted impediments to health care experienced by ethnic minority elders.

A large number of the studies are descriptive studies, which build substantial knowledge about general concepts and to some extent specific applications for a problem area. The cancer screening studies are examples of the scientific knowledge currently available on some Asian American groups regarding early detection of breast, cervical, and colorectal cancer. Although descriptive, formative studies should continue on other Asian American groups, behavioral intervention studies would take us closer to increasing screening and survival rates as well as productivity for older ethnic minority elders person. Education is by far the option most recommended by many researchers. Targeting research on specific ethnic groups may increase methodological challenges of sample size, language translation of questionnaires, and recruitment strategies. These challenges must be confronted because intragroup diversity must be understood to guide the development of effective, efficient, and culturally sensitive interventions. Therefore, experimental and quasi-experimental studies should be initiated with careful attention to threats to internal validity, random assignment, culturally appropriate teaching and learning protocols, data analysis, and community participation at the outset.

Studies have also demonstrated that some racial and ethnic minority elders present with increased functional decline or disabilities and with more target-organ damage from some chronic illnesses (Bibb, 2001; Cotter, Gern, Ho, & Chang, 2002; Ness et al., 1999); however, there is limited information on how minority elders present themselves to the health care system (Abe-Kim et al., 2002), their length of stay (LOS) in acute settings (Gurwitz et al., 2002; Henderson et al., 2002), and the outcomes when they return to the community. Postdischarge outcomes for older women in particular merit special attention, since 41% of African American elders live alone and 41.4% of Asian Americans live with a spouse. In addition, approximately one third of older women who are African American, Asian American/Pacific Islander, and Hispanic/Latino American live with relatives or nonrelatives compared to 15% of older White women (Federal Interagency Forum, 2000; Social Security Administration, 2000a, 2000b). This problem area is particularly important for nursing research in view of the practice of discharging patients to the care of family members, who may be ill-equipped to manage complicated treatment plans in a home environment. In the case of every geriatric patient, following through with treatment and management is seldom a simple process (Kane, Ouslander, & Abrass, 1989).

Culture-Based Perceptions of Health Needs and Health Care

The reports on the perceptions, attitudes, beliefs, values, and culture of racial and ethnic minority elders (Corbie-Smith et al., 2002; Doescher et al., 2000; Iwashyna et al., 2002; Moon et al., 1998) contribute to our insights about certain groups; however, the examination must be taken to the next step. Studies must be done on how factors such as cultural beliefs and values (McBride et al., 1998; Phillips et al., 2001), family relations (Abe-Kim et al., 2002), environmental variables (Guidry et al., 1997), patient-provider relationships (Backus et al., 2001; Doescher et al., 2000; Shavers et al., 2002), preference for traditional health practitioners (Kim et al., 2002; Plotnikoff et al., 2002; Pourat et al., 1999; Yu, Chen, Kim, & Abdulrahim, 2002), and the delivery system (Jennings-Sanders & Anderson, 2003; O'Malley et al., 1997; Tan et al., 2003) impact patient outcomes.

Language issues in clinical encounters can be overcome; however, to communicate effectively and create trust relationships, some knowledge of cultural factors influencing the ethnic elder's expectations of the provider is necessary. Experimental studies can begin to test communication models such as LEARN (Berlin & Fowkes, 1983), ETHNIC(S) (Kobylarz, Heath, & Like, 2002), and explanatory models (Kleinman, 1982; Kleinman et al., 1978). Eventually, how nursing translates the information to more evidence-based ethnogeriatric nursing practice will be an exciting area of research (Leininger & McFarland, 2002).

Method and Sampling

African American, Asian American, and Hispanic elders differ in how they gain access to health care services (Tables 8.1 and 8.2). Furthermore, demographic data have suggested health-compromising characteristics that provide reason for concern. In conjunction with limited education, poverty is high among divorced African American women age 65 to 74 years and older adults who are African American (26.4%) and Hispanic/Latino American (21%), compared to 10.5% of the total population of older adults (Department of Labor, 2003; Federal Interagency Forum, 2000). Many studies have found that racial and ethnic populations differ in the manifestation of symptoms and the severity of diseases; however, there is a gap in exploring the relationships between these factors in large representative cohort studies (De la Cruz, McBride, Compas, Calixto, & Van Derveer, 2002). Longitudinal studies with large representative samples as opposed to more cross-sectional studies must take priority for researchers. Without such data, Richardson (1996) states, "Future cohorts of . . . elders [will be] cloaked in . . . a maze of fortune telling" (p. 59).

The qualitative studies found in this review have been helpful not only in problem identification but also in giving suggestions about sampling (Cooley & Jennings-Dozier, 1998; Plowden & Miller, 2000) and more effective approaches to intervention studies for racial and ethnic minority elders (Anderson-Loftin & Moneyham, 2000; Liburd et al., 1999; Phillips et al., 2001; Schoengerg, 1998). Although these studies had small samples, findings are noteworthy and deserve further consideration in larger sample studies. Qualitative studies with inadequate numbers make it difficult to generalize to the population at large. One approach is to combine qualitative with quantitative methods in larger representative samples of racial and ethnic minority elder populations (McBride et al., 1998). Flaskerud (2002) suggests that more nursing research should focus on methodological approaches that involve participants in the research process, interventions that give real resources, and community-based problem areas. These priority areas apply also to ethnogeriatric research.

Large data sets such as SEER (Bibb, 2001; Klonoff-Cohen, Schaffroth, Edelstein, Molgaard, & Saltzsteen, 1998), the Behavioral Risk Factor

Surveillance System (BRFSS) (Coughlin & Uhler, 2000), the National Health and Nutrition Examination Survey III (NHANES III) (Sundquist et al., 2002), and the National Health Interview Survey (NHIS) (Kim et al., 1998) provide ample opportunity to raise post-facto questions after answers to the primary questions have been generated and disseminated; hence the term *secondary analysis*.

Based on the ethnogeriatric framework where health, aging, and ethnicity intersect (Figure 8.1), results and conclusions from spin-off studies serve to identify constructs and domains of interest that eventually must be linked to observable terms to discover or extend any empirical meaning for the ethnic minority group (Fawcett & Downs, 1986). They can become building blocks for theoretical formulations in nursing and ethnogeriatric research. However, the highest standards for scientific inquiry must be maintained to reduce health disparities. Collaboration among researchers, especially in Centers of Excellence, has been a successful model for an increase in sample size, cross-fertilization of perspectives, and theory building.

Theory Development and Alternate Models for Health Care

Several theoretical models were noted in the research studies. The Health Belief Model was used to define, explain, understand, and predict behavior as it relates to preventive health, thereby examining the relationships between perception and resultant behaviors (Plowden & Miller, 2000). The Transtheoretical Model guides research questions about readiness to adopt a health behavior involving cancer screening. The goal is to advance to higher stages of change until the behavior becomes a "habit" (McBride et al., 1998; Tu et al., 2002). The model continues to be a dominant model in health promotion research. Adopting healthy behavior is especially relevant in ethnogeriatric care when chronic illness requires the individual to change behavior in order to effectively manage his or her life with diabetes or hypertension. A theory is emerging that describes and explains the beliefs and behaviors of Chinese Americans. Conformity with nature has three interrelated constructs: harmonizing with the environment, following bliss, and listening to heaven (Chen, 1996). It resonates with the Taoist and Confucian philosophies, which guide the precepts of classical Chinese medicine (Lao, 1999; McBride et al., 1996). Investigations of health disparities and access issues require conceptual models to direct the questions toward precise definitions of culture-based problem areas. It is possible to apply these conceptual models and nursing models to study health disparities. A researcher might apply Roger's Life Process Model to study the availability of holistic care to ethnic seniors. The model can be a good fit since it proposes that the person and the environment are coexisting forces (Rogers, 1980). Because the individual is unique, according to this model, the single-case research design (Garmezy, 1982) may be useful to consider for initiating a Rogerian approach to theory development around health disparities and holistic health care.

Better understanding of the role served by traditional care providers could enable their inclusion into contemporary health services to address the unmet needs of the ethnically diverse population of older adults. Research must be done on the acceptability of elements of traditional healing practices, such as taking time to talk, including culture-based healing rituals in intervention programs, clarifying the role of social and family networks in the treatment process, and formally linking traditional healers to health delivery systems. These approaches may have potential for improving the older person's perceptions of well-being and outcomes of care (Cassidy, 1998a, 1998b).

SUMMARY AND CONCLUSION

The demographic imperative is a compelling rationale for ethnogeriatric research. Almost all of the studies reviewed for this chapter are descriptive, cross-sectional designs. The disparate group sizes and the diversity between and within groups continue to impact aspects of the research process, from allocation of research funds to meeting the standards for scientific rigor, such as sample sizes, data collection methods, data analysis, generalizability, and transforming culturally relevant results into practical use by policymakers, health professionals, and the ethnic communities. These far-reaching methodological issues are particularly difficult for researchers when population sizes of racial and ethnic groups are small and are scattered across the United States (e.g., Cambodians, Hmongs, and Vietnamese). Results from aggregated data are difficult to interpret when the data are presented as characteristics of a homogeneous racial and ethnic group.

Comparative intervention studies with intragroup samples are an urgent and critical goal for both the researchers and the ethnic minority communities. The ever-increasing body of knowledge used to identify the unmet needs of ethnic minority elders seems to lose momentum when the results and conclusions must move to the treatment phase. Researchers must find alternate sampling strategies without the traditional use of White American elders as the "gold standard" in order to peel off the layers of biases found in many well-designed studies due to lack of attention to the cultural context of the problem in question. Historical experiences have rendered many Asian groups vulnerable to psychological problems, and the level of satisfaction with health care may be interrelated with utilization of mental health services. Many issues about health disparities and ethnic minority elders are waiting to be explained or require intervention studies from their perspective. The effectiveness of interventions must be measured at different time periods to match the natural continuum of the elders' life processes and to track the dynamic influence of cultural beliefs on health status and access to health care. Therefore, combining qualitative and quantitative measures in longitudinal experimental studies is long overdue for the African American and Asian American older adults, as well as for other racial and ethnic groups. This chapter presented the state of evidence-based knowledge in health care for African American and Asian American older adults to highlight the gaps in which geriatric and ethnogeriatric research should play significant roles.

ACKNOWLEDGMENT

The preparation of the chapter was partially supported by the Bureau of Health Professions, Health Resources Administration, United States Department of Health and Human Services, and the Center for Education in Family and Community Medicine, Stanford University School of Medicine. We thank Jillian Dubman, Marlene Dominguez, and Tina Paterson for their assistance in the research and preparation of the manuscript.

REFERENCES

Abe-Kim, J., Takeuchi, D., & Hwang, W. (2002). Predictors of help-seeking for emotional distress among Chinese Americans: Family matters. *Journal of Consulting Clinical Psychology, 70,* 1186–1190.

Administration on Aging. (2001). *Older adults and mental health: Issues and opportunities.* Rockville, MD: U.S. Department of Health and Human Services.

Anderson-Loftin, W., & Moneyham, J. (2000). Long-term disease management needs of southern African Americans with diabetes. *Diabetes Education, 26,* 821–832.

Asian American Pacific Community Health Organizations (email communication, June 10, 2003).

Backus, L., Osmond, D., Grumbach, K., Vranizan, K., Phuong, L., & Bindman, A. (2001). Specialists' and primary care physicians' participation in medicaid managed care. *Journal of General Internal Medicine, 6,* 815–821.

Barber, K., Shaw, R., Folts, M., Taylor, D., Ryan, A., Hughes, M., Scott, V., & Abbott, R. (1998). Differences between African American and Caucasian men participating in a community-based prostate cancer screening program. *Journal of Community Health, 23,* 441–451.

Baumann, L. C., Chang, M., & Hoebeke, R. (2002). Clinical outcomes for low-income adults with hypertension and diabetes. *Nursing Research, 51,* 191–198.

Becker, G. (2001). Effects of being uninsured on ethnic minorities'management of chronic illness. *Western Journal of Medicine, 175,* 19–23.

Becker, G., Beyene, Y., Newsom, E., & Rodgers, D. (1998). Knowledge and care of chronic illness in three ethnic minority groups. *Family Medicine, 30,* 173–178.

Berlin, E., & Fowkes, W. (1983). A teaching framework for cross-cultural health care: Application in family practice. *Cross-Cultural Medicine. The Western Journal of Medicine, 136,* 934–938.

Bibb, S. C. (2001). The relationship between access and stage at diagnosis of breast cancer in African American and Caucasian women. *Oncology Nursing Forum, 28,* 711–719.

Carey Jackson, J., Taylor, V., Chitnarong, K., Mahloch, J., Fischer, M., Sam, R., & Seng, P. (2000). Development of a cervical cancer control intervention program for Cambodian American women. *Journal of Community Health, 25,* 359–375.

Carlisle, D., Leake, B., & Shapiro, M. (1997). Racial and ethnic disparities in the use of cardiovascular procedures: Associations with type of health insurance. *American Journal of Public Health, 87,* 263–267.

Carter, A., Borchardt, N., Cooney, M., & Greene, D. (2000). Dual test diabetes screening project: Screening for poor glycemic control in a large workplace population. *Diabetes Technology Therapy, 2,* 529–536.

Cassidy, C. (1998a). Chinese medicine users in the United States. Part I: Utilization, satisfaction, and medical plurality. *Journal of Complementary Medicine, 4,* 17–27.

Cassidy, C. (1998b). Chinese medicine users in the United States. Part II: Preferred aspects of care. *Journal of Complementary Medicine, 4,* 189–202.

Chen, Y. (1996). Conformity with nature: A theory of Chinese American elders' health promotion and illness prevention processes. *Advance Nursing Science, 19,* 17–26.

Chin, M., Zhang, J., & Merrell, K. (1998). Diabetes in the African American Medicare population: Morbidity, quality of care, and resource utilization. *Diabetes Care, 21,* 1090–1095.

Choi, E., McGandy, R., Dallal, G., Russell, R., Jacob, R., Schaeffer, R., & Sadowski, J. (1990). The prevalence of cardiovascular risk factors among elderly Schines Americans. *Archives of Internal Medicine, 150,* 413–418.

Collaborative on Ethnogeriatric Education. (2000). *Core curriculum in ethnogeriatrics*. Palo Alto, CA: Stanford Geriatric Education Center, Stanford University.

Collaborative on Ethnogeriatric Education. (2001). *Ethnic specific modules of the curriculum in ethnogeriatrics*. Palo Alto, CA: Stanford Geriatric Education Center, Stanford University.

Cooley, M., & Jennings-Dozier, K. (1998). Cultural assessment of Black American men treated for prostate cancer: Clinical case studies. *Oncology Nursing Forum, 25*, 1729–1735.

Cooper-Patrick, L., Gallo, J., Gonzales, J., Powe, N., Nelson, C., & Ford, D. (1999). Race, gender, and partnership in the patient-physician relationship. *Journal of the American Medical Association, 282*, 583–589.

Corbie-Smith, G., Thomas, S., & George, D. (2002). Distrust, race and research. *Archives of Internal Medicine, 21*, 2458–2463.

Cotter, M., Gern, R., Ho, G., & Chang, R. (2002). Role of family history and ethnicity on the mode and age of prostate cancer presentation. *Prostate, 50*, 216–221.

Coughlin, S., & Uhler, R. (2000). Breast and cervical cancer screening practices among Asian and Pacific Islander women in the United States, 1994–1997. *Cancer Epidemiology, Biomarkers, and Prevention, 9*, 597–603.

De la Cruz, F., McBride, M., Compas, L., Calixto, P., & Van Derveer, C. (2002). White paper on the health status of Filipino Americans and recommendations for research. *Nursing Outlook, 50*, 7–15.

Department of Labor. (2003). *Bureau of Labor census*. Retrieved March 10, 2003, from http://www.bls.census.gov/cps/cpsmain.htm

Doescher, M., Saver, B., Franks, P., & Fiscella, K. (2000). Racial and ethnic disparities in perception of physician style and trust. *Archives of Family Medicine, 9*, 1156–1163.

Dunlop, D., Manheim, L., Song, J., & Chang, R. (2002). Gender and ethnic/racial disparities in health care utilization among older adults. *Journal of Gerontology, Behavioral Psychology, and Social Sciences, 57*, S221–233.

El-kebbi, I., Cook, C., & Ziemer, D. (2003). Association of younger age with poor glycemic control and obesity in urban African Americans with type 2 diabetes. *Archives of Internal Medicine, 163*, 69–75.

Facione, N., Giancarlo, C., & Chan, L. (2000). Perceived risk and help-seeking behavior for breast cancer. A Chinese-American perspective. *Cancer Nursing, 23*, 258–267.

Fawcett, J., & Downs, F. (1986). *The relationship of theory and research*. Norwalk, CT: Appleton-Century Crofts.

Federal Interagency Forum on Aging-Related Statistics. (August, 2000). *Older Americans 2000: Key indicators of well-being*. Federal Interagency Forum on Aging-Related Statistics, Washington, DC: U.S. Government Printing Office (http://agingstats.gov).

Flaskerud, J. (2002). Health disparities among vulnerable populations: Evolution of knowledge over 5 decades in Nursing Research publications. *Nursing Research, 51*, 74–85.

Garmezy, N. (1982). The case for the single case in research. In A. Kazdin & A. H. Tuma (Eds.), *Single-case research design*. San Francisco, CA: Jossey-Bass.

Gaskin, D. J., & Hoffman, C. (2000). Racial and ethnic differences in preventable hospitalizations across 10 states. *Medical Care Research Review, 57*(Suppl. 1), 85–107.

Guidry, J., Aday, L., Zhang, D., & Winn, R. (1997). Transportation as a barrier to treatment. *Cancer Practice, 5*, 361–366.

Gurwitz, J., Goldberg, R., Malmgren, J., Barron, H., Tiefendrum, A., Frederick, P., & Gore, J. (2002). Hospital transfer of patients with acute myocardial infarction: The effects of age, race, and insurance type. *American Journal of Medicine, 112*, 528–534.

Han, B., Wells, B., & Primas, M. (2003). Comparison of mammography use by older Black and White women. *Journal of the American Geriatrics Society, 51*, 203–212.

Harada, N., Damron-Rodriguez, J., Villa, M., Washington, D., Dhanani, S., Shon, H., Chattopadhyay, M., Fishbein, H., Lee, M., Makinodan, T., & Andersen, R. (2002). Veteran identity and race/ethnicity: Influences on VA outpatient utilization. *Medical Care, 40*(Suppl. 1), 1117–1128.

Harper, M. (1990). *Minority aging: Essential curriculum for selected health and allied health professions.* Washington, DC: HRSA, USDHHS, Health Resources and Service Administration, U.S. Dept. of Health and Human Services, U.S. Public Health Service.

Haviland, M., Morales, L., Reise, S., & Hays, R. (2003). Do health care ratings differ by race and ethnicity? *Journal of Community and Joint Quality Safety, 29*, 134–145.

Henderson, S., Magana, R., Korn, C., Genna, T., & Bretsky, P. (2002). Delayed presentation for care during acute myocardial infarction in a Hispanic population of Los Angeles county. *Ethnic Diseases, 12*, 3–7.

Hislop, G. (2002). Cervical cancer screening among Chinese Americans. *Cancer Detection and Prevention, 26*, 139–145.

Iwashyna, T., Curlin, F., & Christakis, N. (2002). Racial, ethnic, and affluence difference in elderly patients' use of teaching hospitals. *Journal of General Internal Medicine, 17*, 696–703.

Jennings-Dozier, K. (1999). Perceptual determinants of Pap test up-to-date status among minority women. *Oncology Nursing Forum, 26*, 1327–1333.

Jennings-Sanders, A., & Anderson, E. (2003). Older women with breast cancer: Perception of the effectiveness of nurse case-managers. *Nursing Outlook, 51*, 108–114.

Juon, H., Choi, Y., & Kim, M. (2000). Cancer screening behaviors among Korean-American women. *Cancer Detection and Prevention, 24*, 589–601.

Kane, R., Ouslander, J., & Abrass, I. (1989). *Essentials of clinical geriatrics* (2nd ed.). New York: McGraw-Hill.

Kelly, A., Fores Chacori, M., Wollan, P., Trapp, M., Weaver, A., Barrier, P., Franz, W., & Kottke, T. (1996). A program to increase breast and cervical cancer screening for Cambodian women in a midwestern community. *Mayo Clinic Proceedings, 71*, 437–444.

Kim, K., Yu, E., Chen, E., Kim, J., & Brintnall, R. (1998). Colorectal cancer screening. Knowledge and practices among Korean Americans. *Cancer Practice, 6*, 167–175.

Kim, K., Yu, E., Chen, E., Kim, J., Kaufman, M., & Purkiss, J. (1999). Cervical cancer screening knowledge and practices among Korean-American women. *Cancer Nursing, 22*, 297–302.

Kim, M., Han, H., Kim, K., & Duong, D. (2002). The use of traditional and Western medicine among Korean American elderly. *Journal of Community Health, 27*, 109–120.

Kleinman, A. (1982). Neurasthenia and depression: A study of somatization and culture in China. *Culture, Medicine, and Psychiatry, 6*, 117–119.

Kleinman, A., Eisenberg, L., & Good, B. (1978). Culture, illness, and care: Clinical lessons from anthropologic and cross-cultural research. *Annals of Internal Medicine, 88*, 251–258.

Klonoff-Cohen, H., Schaffroth, L., Edelstein, S., Molgaard, C., & Saltzstein, S. (1998). Breast cancer histology in Caucasians, African Americans, Hispanics, Asians, and Pacific Islanders. *Ethnicity and Health, 3*, 189–198.

Kobylarz, F., Heath, J., & Like, R. (2002). The ETHNIC(S) mnemonic: A clinical tool for ethnogeriatric education. *Journal of the American Geriatric Society, 50*, 1582–1589.

Lao, L. (1999). Traditional Chinese medicine. In W. B. Jonas & J. S. Levin (Eds.), *Essentials of complementary and alternative medicine*. New York: Lippincott Williams and Wilkins.

Lauderdale, D., & Goldberg, J. (1996). The expanded racial and ethnic codes in the Medicare data files: Their completeness of coverage and accuracy. *American Journal of Public Health, 86*, 712–716.

Leininger, M., & McFarland, M. (2002). *Transcultural nursing: Concepts, theories, research, and practice* (3rd ed.). New York: McGraw-Hill.

Liburd, L., Anderson, L., Edgar, T., & Jack, L. (1999). Body size and body shape: Perceptions of Black women with diabetes. *Diabetes Education, 25*, 382–388.

Ma, G., Tan, Y., Feeley, R., & Thomas, P. (2002). Perceived risks of certain types of cancer and heart disease among Asian American smokers and non-smokers. *Journal of Community Health, 27*, 233–246.

Markides, K., & Black, S. (1996). Race, ethnicity, and aging. In R. H. Binstock & L. K. George (Eds.), *Handbook of aging and the social sciences*. San Diego: Academic.

Martin, J., Engle, V., & Graney, M. (1999). Determinants of health-related hardiness among urban older African-American women with chronic illnesses. *Holistic Nursing Practitioner, 13*, 62–70.

Maxwell, A., Bastani, R., & Warda, U. (2000). Demographic predictors of cancer screening among Filipino and Korean immigrants in the United States. *American Journal of Preventive Medicine, 18*, 62–68.

McBride, M., Morioka-Douglas, N., & Yeo, G. (1996). *Aging and health: Asian and Pacific Islander American elders* (Working Paper Series No. 3, 2nd ed.). Palo Alto, CA: Stanford Geriatric Education Center, Stanford University.

McBride, M., Pasick, R., Stewart, S., Tuason, N., Sabogal, F., & Duenas, G. (1998). Factors associated with cervical cancer screening among Filipino women in California. *Asian American and Pacific Islander Journal of Health, 6*, 358–367.

McCabe, M., & Cuellar, J. (1994). *Aging and health: American Indian/Alaska Native elder* (Working Paper Series No. 6, 2nd ed.). Palo Alto, CA: Ethnogeriatric Reviews, Stanford Geriatric Education Center, Stanford University.

McCormick, W., Ohata, C., Uomoto, J., Young, H., Graves, A., Kukull, W., Teri, L., Vitaliano, P., Mortimer, J., McCurry, S., Bowen, J., & Larson, E. (2002). Similarities and differences in attitudes toward long-term care between Japanese Americans and Caucasian Americans. *Journal of the American Geriatrics Society, 50,* 1149–1155.

Minniefield, W., Yang, J., & Muti, P. (2001). Differences in attitudes toward donation among African Americans and Whites in the United States. *Journal of the National Medical Association, 93,* 372–379.

Moon, A., Lubben, J. E., & Villa, V. (1998). Awareness and utilization of community long-term care services by elderly Korean and nonHispanic White Americans. *The Gerontologist, 38,* 309–316.

Nakemata, T., Moore, D., Knopp, R., Marcovina, S., Perrin, E., Hughes, D., Suzuki, K., Mori, M., Sempos, C., Hatano, S., Hayashi, C., & Hasegawa, M. (1996). Cholesterol levels among Japanese Americans and other populations: Seattle Nikkei Health Study. *Journal of Atherosclerosis and Thrombosis, 3,* 103–113.

National Institute of Health, Working Group on Health Disparities. (2003). *Addressing health disparities: The NIH program of action.* Accessed March 10, 2003, from http://healthdisparities/nih.gov/whatare.html

National Institute on Diabetes and Digestive and Kidney Diseases. (2003). *Diabetes in Asian and Pacific Islander Americans.* Accessed March, 10, 2003, from http: diabetes.niddk.nih.gov/dm/pubs/asianam/asianam.htm

Ness, J., Nassimiha, D., Feria, M., & Aronow, W. (1999). Diabetes mellitus in older African-Americans, Hispanics, and Whites in an academic hospital-based geriatrics practice. *Coronary Artery Diseases, 10,* 343–346.

Northouse, L., Caffey, M., Deichelbohrer, L., Schmidt, L., Guziatek-Trojniak, L., West, S., Kershaw, T., & Mood, D. (1999). The quality of life of African American women with breast cancer. *Research in Nursing Health, 22,* 449–460.

Office of Management and Budget. (2001, January 16). Provisional guidance on the implementation of the 1997 Standards for Federal Data on Race and Ethnicity. *Federal Register, 66*(10), 3829–3831.

Okubo, M., Watanabe, H., Fujikawa, R., Kawamura, T., Egusa, G., & Yamakido, M. (1999). Reduced prevalence of diabetes according to 1997 American Diabetes Association criteria. *Diabetologia, 42,* 1168–1170.

O'Malley, A., Mandelblatt, J., Gold, K., Cagney, K., & Kerner, J. (1997). Continuity of care affects the use of breast and cervical cancer screening in a multiethnic population. *Archive of Internal Medicine, 157,* 1462–1470.

Pastor, P., Makuc, D., Reuben, C., & Xia, H. (2002). Chartbook on trends in the health of Americans. *Health, United States, 2002.* Hyattsville, MD: National Center for Health Statistics.

Phillips, J., Cohen, M., & Tarzian, A. (2001). African American women's experiences with breast cancer screening. *Journal of Nursing Scholarship, 33,* 135–140.

Phillips, L., Hertzberg, V., & Cook, C. (2003). The improving primary care of African Americans with diabetes (IPCAAD) project: Rationale and design. *Controlled Clinical Trials, 23*, 554–569.

Plotnikoff, G., Numrich, C., Wu, C., Yang, D., & Xiong, P. (2002). Hmong shamanism. Animist spiritual healing in Minnesota. *Minnesota Medicine, 85*, 29–24.

Plowden, K., & Miller, J. (2000). Motivators of health-seeking behaviors in urban African-American men: An exploration of triggers and barriers. *Journal of the National Black Nurses Association, 11*, 15–20.

Pourat, N., Lubben, J., Wallace, S., & Moon, A. (1999). Predictors of use of traditional Korean healers among elderly Koreans in Los Angeles. *The Gerontologist, 39*, 711–719.

Prehn, A., Topol, B., Stewart, A., Glaser, S., O'Connor, L., & West, D. (2002). Differences in treatment patterns for localized breast carcinoma among Asian/ Pacific Islander women. *Cancer, 95*, 2268–2275.

Richardson, J. (1996). *Aging and health: African American elders* (2nd ed.). Working Paper Series No. 4. Ethnogeriatric Reviews, Stanford Geriatric Education Center, Stanford University, Palo Alto, CA.

Rogers, M. (1980). Nursing: A science of unitary man. In J. Riehl & C. Roy (Eds.), *Conceptual models for nursing practice* (2nd ed., pp. 329–337). New York: Appleton-Century-Crofts.

Rooks, R., Simonsick, E., Miles, T., Newman, A., Kritchevsky, S., Schulz, R., & Harris, T. (2002). The association of race and socioeconomic status with cardiovascular disease indicators among older adults in the health, aging, and body composition study. *Journal of Gerontology: Psychological Sciences/Social Sciences, 57*, 5247–5256.

Sadler, G., Dhanjal, S., Shah, N., Shah, R., Ko, C., Anghel, M., & Harshburger, R. (2001). Asian Indian women: Knowledge, attitudes and behaviors toward breast cancer early detection. *Public Health Nursing, 18*, 357–363.

Sateren, M., Trimble, E., Abrams, J., Brawley, O., Breen, N., Ford, L., McCabe, M., Kaplan, R., Smith, M., Ungerleider, R., & Christian, M. (2002). How sociodemo- graphics, presence of oncology specialists, and hospital cancer programs affect accrual to cancer treatment trials. *Journal of Clinical Oncology, 20*, 2109–2117.

Schoengerg, N. (1998). The relationship between perceptions of social support and adherence to dietary recommendations among African-American elders with hy- pertension. *International Journal of Aging and Human Development, 47*, 279–297.

Schulmeister, L., & Lifsey, D. (1999). Cervical cancer screening knowledge, behaviors, and beliefs of Vietnamese women. *Oncology Nursing Forum, 26*, 879–887.

Shakoor-Abdullah, B., Kotchen, J., Walker, W., Chelius, T., & Hoffman, R. (1997). Incorporating socio-economic and risk factor diversity into the development of an African-American community blood pressure control program. *Ethnicity and Diseases, 7*, 175–183.

Shavers, V., Lynch, C., & Burmeister, L. (2002). Racial differences in factors that influence the willingness to participate in medical research studies. *Annals of Epidemiology, 12*, 248–256.

Smedley, B., Stith, A., & Nelson, A. (Eds.). (2003). *Unequal treatment: Confronting racial and ethnic disparities in healthcare.* Institute of Medicine, Washington, DC: National Academies Press.

Social Security Administration. (2000a). *Income of the population 55 or older, 1998.* Tables VIII.4 and VIII.11. Washington, DC: U.S. Government Printing Office.

Social Security Administration. (2000b). *Income of the Population 55 or older, 1998.* Washington, DC: U.S. Government Printing Office.

Sundquist, J., Winkleby, M., & Pudaric, S. (2002). Cardiovascular risk factors among Black, Mexican American, and White women and men: An analysis of NHANES III, 1988–1994. Third National Health and Nutrition Survey. *Journal of the American Geriatrics Society, 49,* 109–116.

Tan, E., Lui, L., Eng, C., Jha, A., & Covinsky, K. (2003). Differences in mortality of Black and White patients enrolled in the program of all-inclusive care for the elderly. *Journal of the American Geriatrics Society, 51,* 246–251.

Tang, T., Solomon, L., & McCracken, L. (2000). Cultural barriers to mammography, clinical breast exam, and breast self-exam among Chinese-American women 60 and older. *Preventive Medicine, 31,* 575–583.

Tang, T., Solomon, L., & McCracken, L. (2001). Barriers to fecal occult blood testing and sigmoidoscopy among older Chinese-American women. *Cancer Practice, 9,* 277–282.

Taylor, V., Hislop, G., Jackson, J., Tu, S., Yasui, Y., Schwartz, S., Teh, C., Kuniyuki, A., Acorda, E., Marchand, A., & Thompson, B. (2002). A randomized control trial of interventions to promote cervical cancer screening among Chinese women in North America. *Journal of the National Cancer Institute, 94,* 670–677.

Taylor, V., Jackson, J., Tu, S., Yasui, Y., Schwartz, S., Kuniyuki, A., Acorda, E., Lin, K., & Hislop, G. (2002). Cervical cancer screening among Chinese Americans. *Cancer Detection Prevention, 26,* 136–145.

Tu, S., Yasui, Y., Kuniyuki, A., Schwartz, S., Jackson, J., & Taylor, V. (2002). Breast cancer screening: Stages of adoption among Cambodian American women. *Cancer Detection and Prevention, 26,* 33–41.

Tu, S., Yasui, Y., Kuniyuki, A., Thompson, B., Schwartz, S., Jackson, J., & Taylor, V. (2000). Breast cancer screening among Cambodian American women. *Cancer Detection and Prevention, 24,* 549–563.

Underwood, S. (1998). Reducing the cancer burden among African Americans: A call to arms. *Cancer, 83*(Suppl. 8), 1877–1884.

United States Census Bureau. (2000). *Population projections of the United States by age, sex, race, Hispanic origin and nativity.* Retrieved January 2000 from htt://www.aoa.gov/minorityaccess/intro.html

U.S. Department of Health and Human Services. (2000, November). *Healthy People 2010, Understanding and improving health and objectives for improving health* (Vols. 1 and 2). Washington, DC: U.S. Government Printing Office. Accessed March 10, 2003, from http://www.healthypeople.giv

U.S. Department of Health and Human Services. (2001). *Mental health: Culture, race, and ethnicity—a supplement to mental health: A report to the Surgeon General—executive summary.* Rockville, MD: Author.

Utsey, S., Chae, M., Brown, C., & Kelly, D. (2002). Effect of group membership on ethnic identity, race-related stress, and quality of life. *Cultural Diversity and Ethnic Minority Psychology, 8,* 366–377.

Vaccarino, V., Gahbauer, E., Kasl, S., Charpentier, P., Acampora, D., & Krumholz, H. (2002). Differences between African Americans and Whites in the outcome of heart failure: Evidence for a greater functional decline in African Americans. *American Heart Journal, 143,* 1058–1067.

Villa, M., Cuellar, J., Gamel, N., & Yeo, G. (1993). *Aging and health: Hispanic American elders* (Working Paper Series No. 5, 2nd ed.). Palo Alto, CA: Ethnogeriatric Reviews, Stanford Geriatric Education Center, Stanford University.

Weinrich, S., Faison-Smith, L., Hudson-Priest, J., Royal, C., & Powell, I. (2002). Stability of self-reported family history of prostate cancer among African American men. *Journal of Nursing Measures, 10,* 39–46.

Weinrich, S., Weinrich, M., Atwood, J., Cobb, M., & Anderson, R. (1999). Contrasting costs of a prostate cancer educational program by race and educational method. *American Journal of Health Behavior, 23,* 144–156.

Wismer, B., Moskowitz, J., Chen, A., Kang, S., Novotny, T., Min, K., Lew, R., & Tager, I. (1998). Mammography and clinical breast examination among Korean American women in two California counties. *Preventive Medicine, 27,* 144–151.

Wojcik, B., Spinks, M., & Optenberg, S. (1998). Breast carcinoma survival analysis for African American and White women in an equal-access health care system. *Cancer, 82,* 1310–1318.

Wright, P., Fortinsky, R., Covinsky, K., Anderson, P., & Landefeld, C. (2000). Delivery of preventive services to older Black patients using neighborhood health centers. *Journal of the American Geriatrics Society, 48,* 124–130.

Yeo, G., David, D., & Llorens, L. (1996). Faculty development in ethnogeriatrics. *Educational Gerontology, 22,* 79–91

Yeo, G., Hikoyeda, N., McBride, M., Chin, S-Y., Edmonds, M., & Hendrix, L. (1998). *Cohort analysis as a tool in ethnogeriatrics: Historical profiles of elders from eight ethnic populations in the United States* (Working Paper Series No. 12, 2nd ed.). Palo Alto, CA: Ethnogeriatric Reviews, Stanford Geriatric Education Center, Stanford University.

Yu, E., Chen, E., Kim, K., & Abdulrahim, S. (2002). Smoking among Chinese Americans: Behaviors, knowledge, and beliefs. *American Journal of Public Health, 92,* 1007–1012.

Zhu, K., Hunter, S., Bernard, L., Payne-Wilks, K., Roland, C., & Levin, R. (2000). Mammography screening in single older African-Americans: A study of related factors. *Ethnic Diseases, 10,* 395–405.

PART III

Special Conditions

Chapter 9

Cancer in U.S. Ethnic and
Racial Minority Populations

Sandra Millon Underwood, Barbara Powe, Mary Canales,
Cathy D. Meade, and Eun-Ok Im

ABSTRACT

Discoveries, breakthroughs, and advances made in the area of cancer prevention
and cancer control over the last 2 decades have led to declines in the rates of
cancer incidence and mortality and increases in life expectancy and survival for
many cancer patients. However, although the trends relative to cancer incidence,
mortality, and 5-year survival for the nation as a whole have significantly
improved, data reveal that there are significant disparities in the degree to
which the burden of cancer that remains is borne by racial and ethnic minority
population groups. As a practice-oriented discipline grounded in research, nursing could have a dominant role in efforts aimed toward eliminating the cancer
disparities experienced by racial and ethnic population groups. Several reports
of nursing studies have been published in the peer-reviewed literature that
address factors associated with the cancer disparities experienced between and
among U.S. racial and ethnic minority groups. However, given that few efforts
have been undertaken to comprehensively review and critique this body of
research, little is known about the scope, quality, and potential impact of this
body of nursing science. This report presents the results of one of the first
comprehensive reviews of nursing research undertaken to explore and address
factors associated with the evolution of the cancer-related health disparities in
ethnic and racial minority population groups within the United States. The
findings reveal that, while the body of nursing research has contributed much
to the identification and understanding of factors associated with the excess
cancer morbidity and mortality of minority populations, in order for the profes-

sion to more fully contribute to the elimination of cancer-related disparities, there is a need for nurses to further expand and strengthen this base of knowledge.

Keywords: cancer prevention, cancer treatment, health disparities

REVIEW AND CRITIQUE OF THE STATE OF THE SCIENCE

Cancer is the second leading cause of disease and mortality in the United States, exceeded only by cardiovascular disease. According to estimates reported by the American Cancer Society (ACS), in the year 2003, approximately 1.3 million Americans will be diagnosed with invasive cancer, more than 1 million Americans will be diagnosed with basal or squamous cell skin cancer, and approximately 556,500 Americans will die from the disease (ACS, 2003). The most common form of cancer experienced by American men is cancer of the prostate, followed by cancer of the lung and bronchus, colon and rectum, and urinary bladder; melanoma of the skin; and non-Hodgkin's lymphoma. The most common form of cancer experienced by American women is cancer of the breast, followed by cancer of the lung and bronchus, colon and rectum, uterus, non-Hodgkin's lymphoma, and melanoma. And the most common form of cancer experienced by children is leukemia, followed by brain and spinal cancer, neuroblastoma, and Wilms tumor (Ries et al., 2002).

Advances made over the last 2 decades relative to cancer risk reduction, early detection, screening, diagnosis, and treatment have led to declines in the rates of cancer incidence and mortality and increases in life expectancy and survival for many cancer patients. However, although the national trends in cancer incidence, mortality, and 5-year survival for the nation as a whole have significantly improved, data from the National Cancer Institute, American Cancer Society, Institutes of Medicine, and Centers for Disease Control and Prevention reveal that, when compared to the majority non-Hispanic White population, there are significant disparities in the degree to which the burden of cancer that remains is borne by racial and ethnic minority population groups (Clegg, Li, Hankey, Chu, & Edwards, 2002; Ries et al., 2002).

CANCER IN U.S. RACIAL/ETHNIC MINORITY POPULATIONS

A cancer disparity occurs when one segment of the population suffers disproportionately from cancer. The cancer disparities borne by racial and ethnic minority population groups in the United States, measured in terms of overall cancer incidence, mortality, and 5-year relative survival, are profound (Table 9.1). The National Cancer Institute Surveillance, Epidemiology and End Results (SEER) Program, the most authoritative source of information on cancer incidence, mortality, and survival in the United States, reports that African Americans, Native Americans and Alaska Natives, Asian Americans and Pacific Islanders, and Hispanics generally experience higher cancer incidence, higher cancer mortality, and lower 5-year relative cancer survival rates when compared to the non-Hispanic White population. Similar disparities are often observed among racial and ethnic minority subpopulation groups relative to many site-specific cancers (ACS, 2003; Clegg et al., 2002; Ries et al., 2002).

When compared with other racial and ethnic population groups in the United States, data reveal that African American populations experience the highest overall cancer incidence and the highest overall cancer mortality, whereas American Indian and Alaska Native populations experience the lowest cancer 5-year relative survival. According to SEER Program reports, the incidence rates of stomach and liver cancer among Asian Americans and Pacific Islanders, cervical cancer among Hispanics, uterine cancer among Native Hawaiians, and prostate cancer among African Americans are substantially higher than in any other racial and ethnic population group in the United States (Ries et al., 2002).

The mortality rate of stomach cancer among Asian Americans and Pacific Islanders, cervical cancer among African Americans, and prostate cancer among African Americans is substantially higher than in any other racial and ethnic population group in the United States. And the 5-year relative survival rates of lung and bronchial cancer among American Indians and Alaskan Natives men and women, the 5-year relative survival rates of colon and rectum cancer among African American men and American Indian and Alaska Native women, the 5-year relative survival rates of prostate cancer among American Indian and Alaska Native men, and the 5-year relative survival rates of breast cancer among African American women are noted to be the substantially lower than in any other racial and ethnic population group in the United States (Ries et al., 2002).

Subgroup analysis of trends in cancer incidence and mortality among Hispanic, Asian American, and Pacific Islander population groups reveals similar disparities. In general, the rate of cancer incidence and cancer mortality among Hispanics is generally lower than the cancer incidence and mortality rates of non-Hispanics. However, Hispanics, especially first-generation migrants, experience a heavy burden of cancer of the stomach,

TABLE 9.1   Cancer Incidence and Mortality Rates by Site, Race, and Ethnicity, United States, 1992–1999*

Incidence	White	Black	Asian/ Pacific Islander	American Indian/Alas- kan Native	Hispanic†
All sites					
Males	568.2	703.6	408.9	277.7	393.1
Females	424.4	404.8	306.5	224.2	290.5
Total	480.4	526.6	348.6	244.6	329.6
Breast (female)	137.0	120.7	93.4	59.4	82.6
Colon & rectum					
Males	64.4	70.7	58.7	40.7	43.9
Females	46.1	55.8	39.5	30.8	29.7
Total	53.9	61.9	47.9	35.2	35.7
Lung & bronchus					
Males	82.9	124.1	63.8	51.4	44.1
Females	51.1	53.2	28.5	23.3	22.8
Total	64.3	82.6	44.0	35.4	31.5
Prostate	172.9	275.3	107.2	60.7	127.6

Mortality	White	Black	Asian/ Pacific Islander	American Indian/Alas- kan Native	Hispanic†
All sites					
Males	258.1	369.0	160.6	154.5	163.7
Females	171.2	204.5	104.4	110.4	105.7
Total	205.1	267.3	128.6	128.6	129.2
Breast (female)	29.3	37.3	13.1	14.8	17.5
Colon & rectum					
Males	26.7	34.8	16.5	14.6	16.6
Females	18.4	25.4	11.6	11.3	10.6
Total	21.9	29.1	13.7	12.8	13.2
Lung & bronchus					
Males	81.7	113.0	42.3	49.3	38.2
Females	41.1	39.6	19.3	24.9	13.8
Total	57.9	68.9	29.3	35.5	24.1
Prostate	32.9	75.1	15.1	18.8	22.6

*Per 100,000, age-adjusted to the 2000 U.S. standard population. Incidence rates obtained from SEER registries covering 10%–15% of the U.S. population. Mortality data are from all states.
†Hispanics are not mutually exclusive from Whites, African Americans, Asian/Pacific Islanders, and American Indian/Alaskan Natives.
Source: Ries, L., et al. (2002). Reprinted with permission from the National Cancer Institute. Surveillance, Epidemiology and End Results Program.

liver, and cervix (ACS, 2001; Canto & Chu, 2000; Modiano, Villar-Werstler, Meister, & Figueroa-Valles, 1995; Trapido et al., 1995). For example, data reveal that Hispanic American women have twice the incidence of cervical cancer than non-Hispanic American women. Cervical cancer incidence is higher in Mexican American and Puerto Rican American women than in non-Hispanic White women. With the exception of those living in the Southeast, the incidence rates of stomach cancer are at least 1.5 times higher among Hispanics than among non-Hispanics. Hispanics experience a 60% higher mortality rate from stomach cancer and liver cancer than non-Hispanic populations. In addition, the mortality rate from cervical cancer is 40% higher among Hispanic women than among non-Hispanic American women.

Within the Asian American and Pacific Islander population, Filipino Americans and Korean Americans have the lowest cancer incidence and lowest cancer mortality rates (Miller et al., 1996). However, Native Hawaiians have the highest overall cancer incidence rate and the highest overall cancer mortality rate. Japanese Americans have the highest incidence rate for stomach and colorectal cancer. Chinese Americans have the highest incidence rates of nasopharyngeal and liver cancer. And Filipino Americans have the highest incidence rates of thyroid cancer. Vietnamese American women have the highest incidence rates of liver and intrahepatic bile duct cancers (Miller et al., 1996).

REDUCING CANCER-RELATED HEALTH DISPARITIES THROUGH EVIDENCE-BASED NURSING PRACTICE

Cancer was once thought to result from viral, chemical, and/or hereditary causes. However, discoveries in the fields of cancer epidemiology, biology, and genetics have broadened the knowledge and understanding of the factors and mechanisms associated with the genesis and prevention of cancer. Decades of research suggest that the cancer disparities experienced by racial and ethnic minority population groups are not the result of race in the biological and genetic sense but rather the result of a host of complex interactions of environmental conditions, personal lifestyles, socioeconomic status, and factors associated with access, utilization, and delivery of care within the health care system that may vary or be influenced by race and ethnicity. Included among them are environmental exposures to carcinogenic substances; lifestyle choices and behaviors that result in tobacco use, poor diets and nutritional habits, physical inactivity, and obesity; language, linguistics, and literacy; culture; religion; education; socioeconomic status; personal decisions that result in delays in cancer screening, diagnosis, treatment, and follow-up; and barriers to access to quality cancer care. Reports drafted and disseminated by the National Academy of Sciences, Institute of Medicine, and others also indicate that health care professionals within the health care system often deliver differential and substandard primary, secondary, and tertiary cancer care to racial and ethnic minority population groups (Smedley, Stite, & Nelson, 2002).

As a practice-oriented discipline guided by theory, grounded in research, and dedicated to improving the health state of individuals, families, groups, communities, and the public, nursing could have a dominant role in efforts aimed toward eliminating the cancer disparities experienced by racial and ethnic population groups within its patient care, education, research, and administrative domains of practice. Several nursing research reports have been published in the peer-reviewed literature that address factors associated with the cancer disparities experienced between and among U.S. racial and ethnic minority groups. The same is true of reports of research that aim toward the design, evaluation, and application of nursing interventions to reduce and/or eliminate them. However, given that few efforts have been undertaken to comprehensively review and critique this body of research, little is known about the scope, quality, and potential impact of this body of nursing practice. This report presents the results of one of the first comprehensive reviews, analyses, and critiques of nursing research undertaken to explore and address factors associated with the evolution of the cancer-related health disparities in ethnic and racial minority population groups within the United States.

METHODS FOR SELECTION AND ANALYSIS OF THE LITERATURE

Using the mechanisms prescribed by Cooper (1982), a review was done of peer-reviewed nursing research published from 1986 to 2002 and focused on cancer among ethnic and racial minority population groups in the United States. The year 1986 was set as the starting point for this review, since it was at this time that the secretary of the Department of

Health and Human Services released a task force report on Black and minority health that documented disparities in key health indicators among racially and ethnically defined groups in the United States (Heckler, 1985).

The review process was conducted in four phases. During Phase I a literature search was conducted using the MEDLINE and CINAHL (Cumulative Index to Nursing and Allied Health Literature) databases. The MEDLINE database was searched using four categories of search terms: cancer (*cancer, oncology, neoplasm*), ethnic/racial population group (*Mexican American, Asian American, Hispanic American, Black, Indian, North American, ethnic group, minority group, racial stock*), disparities (*vulnerable population, rural populations, farm workers, migrants, transients, disparities, disparity*), and nursing (*nurse, nurses, nursing, nursing education*). The online CINAHL database was searched using three categories of search terms: neoplasms, ethnic/racial population group (*ethnicgroups, Native American, minority groups*), and nursing (*nurse, nurses, nursing*). During Phase II a literature search in a selected group of peer-reviewed oncology nursing journals, clinical nursing journals, research journals, and journals published by national ethnic and minority nursing organizations was conducted. Included among the selected nursing journals were *Oncology Nursing Forum, Cancer Nursing, Seminars in Oncology Nursing, Journal of Pediatric Oncology Nursing, Nursing Outlook, Nursing Research, Research in Nursing and Health, Advances in Nursing Science, Image: the Journal of Nursing Scholarship, Nursing Clinics of North America, Journal of the National Black Nurses Association,* and *Journal of the Association of Black Nursing Faculty.* The authors recognized that the outcomes of oncology nursing research studies are published in a variety of multidisciplinary peer-reviewed journals. However, for the purpose of this report, the authors chose to limit the search, review, and critique to the aforementioned peer-reviewed professional nursing journals, which have nurses as their primary audience. These literature searches yielded a total of 163 citations or articles.

During Phase III each of the articles was evaluated and marked for inclusion (or exclusion) in the final review and analysis. The four criteria used for selecting research reports for review and analysis were as follows: (1) the reports were summaries of qualitative or quantitative research studies; (2) the reports addressed cancer among U.S. ethnic and racial minority populations; (3) the studies were undertaken in the United States; and (4) the primary author of the report was a registered nurse. Reports summarizing nursing research focused on cancer conducted outside the

United States, reports with foreign subjects or participants; reports authored by nonnurses as the first author; literature reviews; concept analyses; and theoretical and conceptual reports were not included in this research review and analysis. The final review included 56 research reports.

The dimensions of the cancer continuum (prevention/risk reduction, detection, diagnosis, treatment, symptom management, survivorship, palliative care/end of life) were used as a framework for thematically sorting the reports marked for inclusion in this review (Phase IV). During the analysis, emphasis was placed on U.S. ethnic and racial minority populations as defined by the United States Department of Commerce (1978) and the core components of the research process (problem, purpose, conceptual/theoretical framework, study population, research design/sampling, instrumentation, findings, implications). Following the initial review and sorting of the reports by the authors, 10 content areas emerged as the major foci of nursing research focused on cancer among racial and ethnic minority groups: cancer knowledge, attitudes, and beliefs; cancer risk factors; cancer screening; cancer diagnosis; cancer treatment; cancer survivorship; outreach and community partnership; intervention; research participation; and instrumentation (see Table 9.2).

RESULTS

Knowledge, Attitudes, and Beliefs About Cancer and Cancer Screening

Twenty articles included in this review examined knowledge, attitudes, and beliefs about cancer and cancer screening. Fourteen of the articles focused on knowledge, attitudes, and beliefs about cancer and cancer screening of a specific organ site, whereas six articles were nonsite-specific.

Six articles focused on breast cancer and breast cancer screening in different racial and ethnic minority samples. The Transactional Model of Stress and Coping guided research by Kinney et al. (2002), who examined the relationship between beliefs about God as a controlling force in health and adherence to breast cancer screening among African American women. A cross-sectional design was used to collect data from a nonrandom sample of 52 African American females who were members of a larger study of African American kindred with a BRCA1 mutation. Women in the sample

TABLE 9.2 Nursing Research Focused on Cancer Among U.S. Ethnic/Racial Minority Population Groups, 1986–2002

Citation	Race and ethnicity	Gender	Sampling method	Cancer type	Cancer continuum	Study design	Explicit framework
Knowledge, attitudes, and beliefs							
Douglass et al. (1995)	AA	F	R	Breast	Screening	Quant	N
Fearing et al. (2000)	AA	F	NR	Prostate	Screening	Quant	Y
Foxall et al. (2001)	AA, H, NA	F	NR	Breast, uterine	Screening	Quant	N
Han et al. (2000)	AS	F	NR	Breast	Screening	Quant	Y
Kinney et al. (2002)	AA	F	NR	Breast	Screening	Quant	Y
Lee (2000)	AS	F	NR	Uterine	Screening	Qual	Y
Powe (1995a)	AA, C	M, F	R	Colorectal	Screening	Quant	Y
Powe (1995b)	AA, C	M, F	R	Colorectal	Screening	Quant	Y
Powe (1995c)	AA, C	M, F	R	Colorectal	Screening	Quant	Y
Rashidi & Rajaram (2000)	AS	F	NR	Breast	Screening	Quant	N
Salazar (1996)	H	F	NR	Breast	Screening	Qual	Y

Race/ethnicity: AA = African American, A = Asian, C = Caucasian, H = Hispanic, NA = Native American, NR = not reported.
Gender: M = male, F = female, NR = not reported.
Sampling method: R = random, NR = nonrandom.
Study design: Quant = quantitative, Qual = qualitative.
Instrumentation: R = reliability reported, V = validity reported, R/V = reliability and validity reported, N = no psychometrics reported, N/A = not applicable.
Explicit framework: Y = yes, N = no.

(continued)

TABLE 9.2 *(continued)*

Citation	Race and ethnicity	Gender	Sampling method	Cancer type	Cancer continuum	Study design	Explicit framework
Schulmeister & Lifsey (1999)	AS	F	NR	Uterine	Screening	Quant	Y
Smiley et al. (2000)	H, AS	F	NR	Breast	Screening	Quant	Y
Sugarek et al. (1988)	AA, H, C	F	R	Nonspecific	Screening	Quant	Y
Swinney (2002)	AA	M, F	NR	Nonspecific	Screening	Quant	N
Underwood (1990a)	AA	M	NR	Nonspecific	Screening	Quant	Y
Underwood (1990b)	AA	M	NR	Nonspecific	Screening	Quant	Y
Underwood (1992)	AA	M	NR	Nonspecific	Screening	Quant	Y
Underwood & Sanders (1990)	AA	M	NR	Nonspecific	Screening	Quant	Y
Underwood & Sanders (1991)	AA	M	NR	Testicular	Screening	Quant	Y
Risk factors							
Weinrich et al. (2002)	AA	M	NR	Prostate	Genetic risk	Quant	N
Screening							
Burnett et al. (1995)	AA, C	F	NR	Breast, uterine	Screening	Quant	Y
Champion & Menon (1997)	AA, C	F	NR	Breast	Screening	Quant	Y
Jennings (1997)	AA, H	F	NR	Uterine	Screening	Qual	N
Jennings-Dozier (1999a)	AA, H	F	NR	Uterine	Screening	Quant	N

TABLE 9.2 *(continued)*

Citation	Race and ethnicity	Gender	Sampling method	Cancer type	Cancer continuum	Study design	Explicit framework
Jennings-Dozier & Lawrence (2000)	AA, H	F	NR	Uterine	Screening	Quant	N
Katapodi et al. (2002)	AA, C, H	F	NR	Breast	Screening	Quant	Y
Nemcek (1989)	AA	F	NR	Breast	Screening	Quant	Y
Phillips & Wilbur (1995)	AA	F	NR	Breast	Screening	Quant	Y
Shelton et al. (1999)	AA	M	NR	Prostate	Screening	Quant	Y
Underwood (1999)	AA	F	NR	Breast	Screening	Quant	N
Zimmerman (1997)	H	M	NR	Prostate	Screening	Quant	Y
Diagnosis							
Bibb (2001)	AA, C	F	NR	Breast	Diagnosis	Quant	Y
Facione & Katapodi (1998)	AA, C, H	F	NR	Breast	Diagnosis	Qual	N
Lauver (1992)	AA, C	F	NR	Breast	Diagnosis	Quant	Y
Lauver (1994)	AA, C	F	NR	Breast	Diagnosis	Quant	Y
Tomaino-Brunner et al. (1996)	AA, C, H	F	NR	Uterine	Diagnosis	Qual	Y

(continued)

TABLE 9.2 *(continued)*

Citation	Race and ethnicity	Gender	Sampling method	Cancer type	Cancer continuum	Study design	Explicit framework
Treatment							
O'Hare et al. (1993)	AA	M, F	NR	Nonspecific	Treatment	Quant	N
Survivorship							
Dirksen & Erickson (2002)	C, H	F	NR	Breast	Survivorship	Quant	Y
Mellon (2002)	AA, C	M, F	NR	Nonspecific	Survivorship	Qual Quant	Y
Moore (2001)	AA, C	F	NR	Breast	Survivorship	Qual	N
Northouse et al. (1999)	AA	F	NR	Breast	Survivorship	Quant	Y
Wilmoth & Sanders (2001)	AA	F	NR	Breast	Survivorship	Qual	N
Intervention							
Adderley-Kelly & Green (1997)	AA	F	NR	Breast	Screening	Quant	Y
Baldwin (1996)	AA	F	NR	Breast, uterine	Screening	Qual	N
Ehmann (1993)	NR	F	NR	Breast	Screening	Qual	N
Lauver & Rubin (1990)	AA	F	NR	Uterine	Diagnosis	Quant	Y
Powe & Weinrich (1999)	AA, C	M, F	R	Colorectal	Screening	Quant	Y
Weinrich et al. (1994)	AA, C	M, F	NR	Colorectal	Screening	Quant	N
Willis et al. (1989)	AA	F	NR	Breast	Screening	Quant	N

TABLE 9.2 *(continued)*

Citation	Race and ethnicity	Gender	Sampling method	Cancer type	Cancer continuum	Study design	Explicit framework
Research							
Millon-Underwood et al. (1993)	AA	M, F	NR	Nonspecific	Nonspecific	Quant	N
Outlaw et al. (2000)	AA	M, F	NR	Nonspecific	Nonspecific	Quant	N
Instrumentation							
Adams et al. (1997)	H	F	NR	Uterine	Prevention	Quant	Y
Champion & Scott (1997)	AA	F	NR	Breast	Screening	Quant	Y
Ford et al. (2002)	AA	F	R	Breast	Risk Assessment	Qual	N
Jennings-Dozier (1999b)	AA, H	F	NR	Uterine	Screening	Quant	Y

had a low adherence to breast cancer screening. Low GLHC scores and the presence of a primary care provider were associated with participation in mammography and clinical breast examination among this high-risk group of African American women.

In a study with rural Hispanic women, Salazar (1996) explored facilitators and barriers that influence mammography utilization patterns. Guided by a Multi-attribute Utility Model, this qualitative study employed a two-stage exploratory design. In the first stage, interview data were collected from a nonrandom sample of 29 women to identify positive and negative factors affecting the mammography screening decision. In the second stage, women completed a survey to determine the importance of those factors in mammography decisions. Data revealed that there was misinformation about risk factors associated with the breast. The majority of women in the study had never had a mammogram. The barriers to mammography screening included embarrassment, access issues, poverty, family responsibilities, and a lack of support from their husbands.

Similar barriers to breast cancer screening were identified in a cross-sectional study by Han, Williams, and Harrison (2000) with a convenience sample of 133 Korean women. Bivariate analysis revealed that Korean women who never had a clinical breast examination had lower knowledge and higher perceived barriers to breast cancer screening. Logistic regression revealed that their husband's nationality, having regular checkups, and having encouragement from their family and physicians were predictors of participation in breast cancer screening.

Finally, Rashidi and Rajaram (2000) examined frequency of breast self-examination (BSE) and knowledge among Middle Eastern Islamic immigrant women. Data revealed that although the majority of the women involved in the study had heard of BSE, they had not performed BSE monthly during the previous year. The majority had not learned about BSE from a health care professional and had not had a clinical breast examination (CBE).

Several studies reported differences in health beliefs and screening practices between racial and ethnic minority and non-Hispanic populations. Smiley, McMillan, Johnson, and Ojeda (2000) used the Health Belief Model and the Health Locus of Control Model in an exploratory, comparative design to compare beliefs about breast cancer and health locus of control (LOC) in Hispanic and non-Hispanic White women. Findings showed that Hispanic and non-Hispanic women differed significantly in health beliefs and LOC. The Hispanic women viewed health as a matter of luck and displayed more worry about cancer, while the non-Hispanic White women had higher perceived susceptibility to breast cancer.

Differences in health beliefs and breast cancer screening were also explored in a study by Foxall, Barron, and Houfek (2001). In an examination of secondary data, findings revealed that Hispanic and American Indian women had higher rates of BSE and greater perceived risk for gynecological cancer. Caucasian and African American women had higher rates of participation in mammography. Increased body awareness was related to fewer gynecologic exams for American Indian women. In contrast, Douglass, Bartolucci, Waterbor, and Sirles (1995) reported that Caucasian women had a significantly higher mean score for barriers to mammography than did African American women. African Americans in the sample performed breast self-examination more frequently than Caucasian women. However, there were no significant differences in frequency of use of mammography and clinical breast examination between the two groups.

Three articles focused on knowledge, attitudes, and beliefs about cervical cancer and cervical cancer screening. Lee (2000) used the Health Belief Model to describe knowledge about cervical cancer and to identify barriers and motivators for screening among Korean American women. Findings revealed misinformation and a lack of knowledge about causative factors and preventive strategies among the women. Barriers to cervical cancer screening included economic and time factors, language issues, fear, fatalism, denial, and Confucian thinking. Similar findings were reported by Schulmeister and Lifsey (1999) in a study to describe knowledge, beliefs, and cervical cancer screening among Vietnamese women who migrated to the United States. Findings revealed that most of the women involved in the study had never had a Pap test, did not know what a Pap test was, and were not aware of their risk for cervical cancer. Barriers to participation in cervical cancer screening for these women were fear, cost, and lack of a physician. Finally, in a secondary data analysis, Foxall et al. (2001) reported that increased body awareness was related to fewer gynecologic exams for American Indian women.

Three articles included in this analysis addressed knowledge, attitudes, and beliefs associated with colorectal cancer screening. These articles by Powe (1995a, 1995b, 1995c) used the Fatalism Model and the Powe Fatalism Inventory (PFI; Powe, 1995c) to determine the relationships between education, income, ethnicity, gender, age, cancer fatalism (the belief that death is inevitable when cancer is present), and cancer screening.

In a descriptive correlational study with 118 African American and 74 Caucasian men and women, results revealed that African American women had the highest cancer fatalism scores compared to Caucasians. Participants with lower levels of formal education and lower annual incomes also had higher cancer fatalism scores. Age was not related to cancer fatalism scores. In a second article, by Powe (1995a), findings revealed that higher cancer fatalism scores were associated with lower levels of colorectal cancer knowledge. Finally, Powe (1995b) described the relationship between cancer fatalism and participation in fecal occult blood testing using the same sample as the first study (1995c). In this study participants viewed an educational video produced by the American Cancer Society that provided general information on colorectal cancer and the importance of participating in colorectal cancer screening. Immediately after the video, free fecal occult blood testing (FOBT) kits were provided. Participants then completed the PFI and were instructed to use the FOBT kits and return them to their center within 7 days. Findings revealed that African Americans had higher cancer fatalism scores and lower rates of participation in FOBT than Caucasians. Cancer fatalism was noted to be the only significant predictor of participation in FOBT for this sample when demographic factors such as age, income, and education were controlled.

One article included in this analysis addressed knowledge, attitudes, and beliefs of men about prostate cancer and prostate cancer screening, and one addressed knowledge, attitudes, and beliefs of men about testicular cancer and testicular cancer screening. Fearing, Bell, Newton, and Lambert (2000) used Pender's Health Promotion Model to investigate health beliefs and prostate cancer screening among African American men. A quantitative, descriptive design was used, and data were collected from a nonrandom sample of 59 African American men using a self-administered questionnaire adapted from a breast cancer survey by Lambert, Newton, and deMeneses (1998). There was a high level of prostate cancer knowledge and early detection and screening practices among the men. Men reported that good health contributed to the prevention of prostate cancer and that faith was important to staying healthy. The men believed prostate cancer was not preventable and that treatment would be painful and impair sexual functioning.

In another study, Millon-Underwood and Sanders (1991a) used the Health Belief Model to investigate knowledge, health beliefs, and practice of testicular self-examination (TSE) among African American men. In this quantitative, descriptive study, data were collected from a nonrandom sample of 211 African American men participating in intramural sporting activities using a three-part inventory designed by the authors. Findings revealed that the majority of men involved in the study had not heard of TSE. However, knowledge relative to the testicular cancer and testicular cancer screening was shown to be predictive of TSE.

Six of the articles included in this analysis addressed cancer knowledge, attitudes, and beliefs not specific to an organ site. In a quantitative, descriptive study, Sugarek, Deyo, and Holmes (1988) used the Health Belief Model and the Health Locus of Control Model to explore beliefs, attitudes, and locus of control among Mexican Americans, African Americans, and Caucasians. Data were collected from a randomly selected sample of 37 Mexican American, 32 African American, and 32 Caucasian women. The authors found that Mexican Americans in the sample were less educated, valued early detection least, and were the most fatalistic (external locus of control) about cancer. However, fatalism was significantly greater among participants with less than six years of formal education.

Swinney (2002) undertook a quantitative, descriptive study to describe and examine the relationships among self-esteem, locus of control, and perceived health status in African Americans with cancer and to identify predictors of perceived health status. The author reported that participants with normal to high levels of self-esteem and an internal health locus of control perceived their state of health and well-being positively. There was a positive relationship between self-esteem and powerful other locus of control. Further, participants tended to view God as the powerful other capable of influencing their health and well-being.

Underwood (1991), Millon-Underwood and Sanders (1990), and Millon-Underwood and Sanders (1991b) used the Health Belief Model to describe and explore relations among perceptions, health maintenance, cancer screening, cancer risk factors, cancer prevention, and early cancer detection and risk reduction among African American men. In a descriptive study Millon-Underwood and Sanders (1990) collected data from a nonrandom sample of 171 African American men using an investigator-designed Health Behaviors Inventory with reported validity and reliability. Data analyses revealed significant relationships between knowledge of early cancer warning signs and attitudes related to perceptions about screening, seriousness of cancer, cancer risk detection, and early detection practices. In Underwood (1991) findings revealed that perceptions significantly contribute to the health behavior of African American men, especially with regard to early cancer detection. In a third study by Underwood (1992), a learned helplessness framework was used to evaluate the extent to which perceptions of helplessness affect cancer risk reduction and early detection behaviors among a self-selected sample of 236 African American men. Findings revealed that the perceptions of helplessness related to control of health greatly influenced the utilization of cancer risk reduction and early detection behaviors of the men.

Finally, Millon-Underwood and Sanders (1991b) examined the relationship between knowledge of cancer warning signs, risk factors, and screening procedures, cancer related activities, perceptions of susceptibility to cancer, and value of early cancer detection practices among a convenience sample of 177 African American men. Findings revealed that the majority of men were not aware of the warning signs of cancer. There were significant relationships between knowledge of early warning signs of cancer, attitudes related to screening procedures, perceptions of seriousness of cancer, and cancer risk reduction and early detection health promotion behaviors.

In summary, the majority of the knowledge, attitudes, and beliefs (KAB) research conducted by nurse investigators targeted breast cancer, with fewer studies addressing these issues for colorectal, prostate, testicular, and uterine cancer. None of the studies that met criteria for inclusion in this review addressed these issues for patients with oral or lung cancers, which are also quite prevalent among racial and ethnic minority groups. This body of nursing KAB research has furthered our understanding of the complexity of these phenomena among racial and ethnic minority groups and the influence on outcome measures across the cancer continuum. The research has shown that knowledge, attitudes, and beliefs such as internal versus external locus of control factors, fear, cancer fatalism, and low self-efficacy frequently result in lower levels of participation in cancer screening behaviors among these populations. In addition, the research has shown that demographic factors such as lower income and lower levels of education were highly correlated with KAB and rates of participation in cancer screening. These studies provide direction for designing interventions by providers and clients that incorporate specific cultural beliefs about cancer and cancer screening, such as fatalism, as well as strategies to overcome barriers to screening. These studies also support the need for outreach to racial and ethnic minority populations.

Cancer Risk Factors

Only one article included in the review addressed cancer risk factors. Weinrich et al. (2002) conducted a correlational study aimed toward measuring demographic predictors for interest in prostate cancer susceptibility testing among African American men involved in the African American Hereditary Prostate Cancer Study and the South Carolina Prostate Cancer Education and Screening Study. Questions drafted by the investigators were posed to 320 African American men following the completion of the protocol of the original study. The researchers found that most men expressed an interest in genetic prostate cancer susceptibility testing. This interest did not vary by family history, age, or education. Marital status was noted to be the only significant demographic predictor. Interest in genetic prostate cancer susceptibility testing did, however, vary by marital status. Men who were married were significantly more likely to indicate an interest in prostate cancer susceptibility testing than were men who were not married. However, it was also noted that there was a significant degree of confusion among the men relative to genetic prostate cancer susceptibility testing and prostate cancer screening. The authors noted that given the risks associated with job and insurance discrimination, there is a need for public education relative to genetic testing.

Cancer Screening

Twelve of the articles included in this review focused on cancer screening. Ten of these addressed cancer screening in women, of which five focused on breast cancer, four on cervical cancer, and one on both breast and cervical cancer. Two of articles addressed prostate cancer screening for men.

Champion and Menon (1997) undertook a study aimed toward identifying variables associated with mammography utilization and BSE among African American women. Data were collected from a convenience sample of 328 low-income African American women during an in-home interview using existing instruments modified to measure perceived susceptibility to breast cancer, benefits and barriers to BSE and mammography, and self-reported confidence in BSE performance. Focus groups were held with members of the target population to determine the content validity of the scales. There were fairly high levels of compliance with mammography and BSE, with the recommendation of a health care provider for screening mammography identified as a significant factor. Other variables that significantly predicted mammography utilization included perceived barriers, recent thoughts about mammography, and a regular medical provider.

Similar findings about the importance of providers in influencing screening behaviors were reported. Phillips and Wilbur (1995) examined adherence to breast cancer screening guidelines in a sample of 154 African American women. Findings indicated that the majority of women reported adherence to recommendations for monthly BSE practice and yearly clinical breast exam, with mammography screening lower than recommended. Provider recommendation was an important factor in women's screening behavior. Underwood (1999) conducted an exploratory study to examine the breast cancer screening behaviors of African American women with known and no known risk factors. The American Cancer Society (ACTS) guidelines for breast cancer screening were used as the compliance standard. A purposeful sample of 197 African American women was surveyed. The findings indicated that the majority of women were not in compliance with recommendations for breast cancer screening. Age (> 50 years) and discussions with provider regarding breast cancer risk were significantly related to compliance with the recommended breast cancer screening guidelines.

The influence of others and social support have also been reported as significant factors influencing cancer screening. Nemcek (1989) investigated the relationship between BSE practice, health locus of control, and breast cancer knowledge among a convenience sample of 95 African American women. Findings indicated that age (> 50 years) and prior exposure to breast disease were significantly associated with frequency of BSE practice. The influence of "powerful others" was also significantly associated with breast cancer practices. Similarly, Katapodi, Facione, Miaskowski, Dodd, and Waters (2002) conducted a descriptive, cross-sectional survey to examine the relationship between women's reported social support and their adherence to recommended breast cancer screening guidelines. A convenience sample of 833 Latina, Caucasian, and African American women without breast cancer were recruited and stratified by income, age, and education. Higher levels of self-reported social support were related to higher income and higher education, and women who adhered to recommended screening guidelines reported higher social support. Comparisons in self-reported social support and adherence screening guidelines among women were not reported.

Three studies focused on cervical cancer screening practices among African American and Latina women. It is important to note that these studies reflect the program of research of the first author; each study builds upon the preceding study or expands the findings through additional analysis (Jennings, 1997; Jennings-Dozier, 1999b; Jennings-Dozier & Lawrence, 2000). The overall purpose of the studies was to identify barriers and facilitating factors associated with Papanicolaou (Pap) smear use among African American and Latina women, using the Theory of Planned Behavior as the theoretical framework.

The initial Jennings (1997) study, which used an exploratory design and focus group methodology, was aimed to develop a population-specific questionnaire. Snowball sampling techniques were used to recruit a total of 32 African American and 20 Latina women. False-negative results, financial burden, and the role of the physician were the most salient beliefs for the African American women, whereas embarrassment, use of a cold or unclean speculum, and discomfort were the most salient for the Latina participants. These findings were the basis for the development of methods to enhance Pap smear usage among the target populations.

Two of the studies in this program of research were quantitative; one used a descriptive correlational design (Jennings-Dozier, 1999a), while one was a secondary data analysis (Jennings-Dozier & Lawrence, 2000). Convenience sampling was used to recruit a sample of 204 women that included 108 African American and 96 Latina subjects. Data were collected using an investigator-developed questionnaire (Jennings-Dozier, 1999b), and a demographic assessment survey was used to measure up-to-date status, which was based on a self-reported Pap smear within 14 months of study enrollment. Outcome variables focused on specific beliefs that supported adherence to annual Pap tests for women who were up-to-date compared to those who were not. Implications for nursing practice suggested that future cancer prevention and early detection education programs consider those beliefs identified by women who were not up-to-date and focus on promoting those beliefs that are held by women who were up-to-date.

Jennings-Dozier and Lawrence (2000) conducted a secondary data analysis to test whether age, income, insurance coverage, marital status, level of education, and number of persons living at home were predictive of adherence to annual Pap testing. Insurance coverage and level of education (high school) were significant predictors of adherence for Black women in the sample, while age (younger than 40 years) and place of birth (born in the United States mainland) were significant predictors of adherence for Hispanic women.

Burnett, Steakley, and Tefft (1995) used a cross-sectional, correlational design to identify barriers to breast and cervical cancer screening among medically underserved women of the District of Columbia. The Theory of Reasoned Action provided the theoretical framework for the study. The convenience sample included 305 African American and 27 Caucasian women. The demographic characteristics of the sample were not reported by race. The authors found that intention to have a mammogram was positively related to the influence of significant others and negatively related to uncaring health care professionals. Intention to have a Pap test was positively related to one's attitude toward the test and the influence of significant others; intention to perform BSE was positively related to attitude toward BSE and previous performance of BSE. There were no significant relationships between intention to perform screening behaviors and demographic variables. Level of education, alone, was not sufficient to influence intentionality toward cancer screening practices.

Two articles focused on cancer screening practices among men. Zimmerman (1997) conducted a descriptive quantitative study with a convenience sample of 51 Hispanic men to identify factors that influence Hispanic males' decisions to participate in prostate cancer screening. Face-to-face interviews were conducted in either Spanish or English. Factors that influenced participants' attendance at a prostate screening clinic included availability of screening services during evening and weekend hours, convenience of screening sites, and cost. The men suggested strategies for promoting prostrate screening among Hispanic men.

Shelton, Weinrich, and Reynolds (1999) conducted a descriptive, correlational study based on the Theory of Planned Behavior to identify the relationship between perceived barriers and participation in a free prostate cancer screening program. A purposive sample of 1,395 African American men was recruited. Shelton and colleagues reported that, only one barrier—"would be embarrassed"—was statistically significant for the target population. Further investigation related to the meaning of "embarrassment" for African American men and its relationship to prostate cancer screening is warranted.

In summary, the majority of cancer screening research conducted by nurses has focused on African American women, with breast and cervical cancer screening studies predominant. Of note is the lack of research focused on men and other types of cancer in which screening has been available, particularly colorectal cancer. Although theoretical frameworks guided the majority of studies, nursing theory was not the basis for any of the research reviewed.

Of concern methodologically was the lack of experimental or quasi-experimental study designs. All of the studies used compliance or adherence to cancer screening guidelines as outcome variables. Although a variety of factors were identified that influenced screening behaviors, the role of the health care provider was salient among many of the studies reviewed. Aspects of the provider role that were highlighted included the importance of a provider recommendation for screening, consistent or regular care, and the relationship between provider and patient. Common influential patient factors were socioeconomic status, age, social support, and embarrassment. Recommendations for outreach efforts focused on the development of educational strategies for providers regarding their role in improving patients' knowledge of and participation in screening, and the development of culturally appropriate educational programs for specific minority populations, especially those at high risk for cancer.

Cancer Diagnosis

Five of the articles included in this review addressed cancer diagnosis in women. Four of the studies focused on the diagnosis of breast cancer, and one focused on the diagnosis of cervical cancer. Two of the studies focused on the diagnosis of breast cancer focused on the impact of psychosocial variables on breast care-seeking behaviors (Lauver, 1992, 1994). One was a study undertaken to examine the impact of access to health care on breast cancer screening and the stage of breast cancer diagnosis (Bibb, 2001). One was a study aimed toward understanding how women decide whether and when to seek an evaluation for self-discovered breast symptoms (Facione & Giancarlo, 1998). Finally, one study focused on cervical cancer diagnosis and knowledge of women regarding a cervical cancer diagnostic procedure (Tomaino-Brunner, Freda, & Runowicz, 1996).

The two studies focused on the breast cancer care-seeking behaviors of African American and Caucasian women were conduced by Lauver (1992, 1994). One of these aimed to assess the impact of psychosocial variables and race on the intention to seek care for breast symptoms (Lauver, 1992), and one aimed to assess the influence of anxiety, utility beliefs, norms, and habit on care-seeking behaviors of a group of 64 Caucasian and 71 African American women seeking care for a self-identified breast cancer symptom (Lauver, 1994). Both of these studies used a descriptive design and were based on the theory of care seeking. Data were collected using a set of standardized tools and participant interviews. The researcher noted a positive and significant influence of social norms on the intention to seek care for breast cancer symptoms among Caucasian women, but not among the African American women (Lauver, 1992). However, among women seeking care for a self-identified breast cancer symptom, race was noted to have neither a direct nor interactive effect on care seeking.

The study conducted by Bibb (2001) involved the secondary analysis of tumor registry records of a Department of Defense Military health system, aimed toward identifying relationships between access and the stage of breast cancer diagnosis. This descriptive-comparative study was based on the Aday/Andersen Study of Access Framework and involved the review of the tumor registry records of 62 African American and 573 Caucasian women diagnosed with breast cancer over a 10-year period. The study findings demonstrated that when compared to White Caucasian women, even when economic access to medical care was available, African American women were less likely to participate in breast cancer screening and were diagnosed at later stages.

The study undertaken by Facione and Giancarlo (1998) sought to gain understanding of how women decide whether and when to seek an evaluation for self-discovered symptoms. This qualitative study used the narrative accounts of focus groups conducted with 23 Caucasian, 31 Latino, and 26 African American women. It explained their personal experiences with self-discovered breast symptoms and experiences of friends, acquaintances, and family members. Nine themes emerged from the analysis of the narrative accounts: the symptom discovery, disclosing the symptom to another person, interpreting the potential threat of the breast symptom, reliance on alternative and complementary therapies, deciding not to lose the breast, feelings about the symptom discovery, feeling about the provider visit, anticipating abandonment by others, and economic influences.

Multiple factors were identified that could increase the likelihood of advanced disease at diagnosis. Included among them were narrative comments suggesting incorrect symptom attributions and risk estimations; reluctance to consider the threat posed by the symptom; failure to tell another person about the symptom; and expectations of abandonment by male partners, deportation, prejudice, and refusal of treatment due to poverty. Personal accounts of advanced breast cancer also suggested a reliance on alternative healing, concerns about overwhelming family resources, and extreme modesty that inhibited obtaining a physical examination. Several of the predictors of the timing of breast symptom diagnosis were noted to be common among the Latino, African American, and Caucasian women. The authors suggested that the design of interventions aimed at earlier detection of breast cancer must connect with the person's beliefs and assumptions, provide pragmatic solutions for perceived constraints on seeking evaluations of self-discovered symptoms, and explore the use of community narratives to confirm the value of early detection of breast cancer.

To determine what women scheduled for colposcopy knew about the procedure and to understand their concerns, Tomaino-Brunner et al. (1996) conducted a descriptive, exploratory, qualitative study about the test and its implications. A total of 29 women, all of whom were scheduled for colposcopy during a 3-month period at an inner-city academic center, participated in the study. The sample consisted of 19 African American, 9 Hispanic, and 1 White woman ranging in age from 17 to 59 years. Four themes emerged from the open-ended interview data: fear about their health, apprehension about the colposcopy, uncertainty about the meaning of the Pap test and why the appointment was necessary, and pervasive lack of knowledge about all aspects of the referral appointment. Further, a great majority of women reported having "no idea" why they were scheduled for the appointment or what could be found through the colposcopy. Findings supported the need for intervention studies focused on examining the effect of anticipatory counseling and education for this group of women.

Treatment

Only one article included in this review addressed cancer treatment. O'Hare, Malone, Lusk, and McCorkle (1993) undertook a descriptive study aimed toward examining the unmet needs of 63 low-income urban-dwelling African American patients with cancer after hospitalization. They collected data using standardized instruments, and an investigator designed a checklist to measure functional distress and symptom distress. Data revealed that among the study sample the personal and home activity needs were not being met adequately; there was significant symptom distress related to nausea, intensity of pain, and difficulty breathing; among those with breast and gynecological cancers, there were high levels of symptom distress; and elderly African American women who were poor, alone, and chronically ill were likely to have unmet needs and high levels of symptom distress. The authors suggested that further study be undertaken to better understand the unmet needs and their effect on patient outcomes from the perspective of both patients and providers.

Cancer Survivorship

Five of the articles included in this review related to cancer survivorship. Two were qualitative studies describing the lived experiences of African American survivors of breast cancer (Moore, 2001; Wilmoth & Sanders, 2001), one was a qualitative study focused on the meaning of illness and quality of life for African American and Caucasian survivors of breast, colon, prostate, and uterine cancer and their family (Mellen, 2002), one was a descriptive study aimed toward testing a conceptual model of well-being among Hispanic and non-Hispanic White survivors of breast cancer (Dirksen & Erickson, 2002), and one was an exploratory cross-sectional study aimed toward testing a stress and coping framework among African American survivors of breast cancer (Northouse et al., 1999).

The study conducted by Moore (2001) explored the reception of messages about breast cancer by African American breast cancer survivors. During the course of the study, narrative accounts of the breast cancer experience were collected from 23 African American survivors of stage I to stage IV breast cancer. The narrative accounts, gathered during interviews and informal discussions with survivors and their family members, were used to retrospectively examine the impact that receiving messages about breast cancer had on the women involved in the study and to evaluate how the images that evolved from the messages affected their perceived breast cancer risk and their illness experience. Three themes emerged from the interviews. African American breast cancer survivors perceived that: (1) breast cancer was a White woman's disease; (2) breast cancer was caused by stress from affairs of the heart, heartbreak, social life, racism, and the experience of loss; and (3) there was a lack of social support and understanding within the health care system for African American survivors of breast cancer. Analysis of the narrative accounts of the Caucasian survivors of breast cancer involved in the study was not reported.

Similarly, Wilmoth and Sanders (2001) conducted an exploratory study to identify personal issues and concerns of African American women breast cancer survivors after their treatment. The study sample included 16 African American survivors of breast cancer recruited from churches and the community. Focus groups were used, and data were analyzed using principles of content analysis as described by Morgan (1997). Five themes highlighting concerns similar to those expressed by Caucasian survivors of breast cancer and three themes highlighting concerns unique to African American survivors of breast cancer emerged. Concerns common to Caucasian and African American women were concerns about body appearance, social support, health activism, menopause, and the challenge of learning to live with a chronic illness. Concerns unique to African American women were the predisposition to keloid formation, the lack of a prosthesis readily available in their skin tones, and the sense of urgency in educating other African American women about the risk for breast cancer. Given the identification of unique concerns and needs of African American women relative to cancer care, there was a need for further research to identify mechanisms to ensure the delivery of culturally appropriate care.

The descriptive qualitative study conducted by Mellon (2002) aimed to explain and compare the meaning of cancer to the family and family quality of life among cancer survivors and family members of cancer survivors. The study involved 62 Caucasian and 61 African American survivors of breast, colon, prostate, and uterine cancer and their family members. After completing a series of standardized questionnaires, study participants were asked how they would describe the meaning of the illness to their family and how they thought the illness had affected their family quality of life. The questions were derived from the Family Survivorship Model of McCubbin and McCubbin (1996). Content analysis of the responses to the questions revealed that there were more similarities than differences in meaning, and quality of life (QOL) was noted between survivors and family members. For the cancer survivors and their family members, the meaning of the illness was expressed as personal perceptions, emotional reactions, and intense feelings felt at the time of diagnosis. Both also reported positive and negative effects of the cancer on the quality of life of the family and long-term stressors. However, cancer survivors noted the importance of receiving support from others, whereas family members mentioned the importance of showing concern and giving support to their family member. Cancer survivors openly expressed concern that their families were distressed and worried about the cancer, whereas family members expressed that they kept their feeling to themselves while attempting to present and maintain a positive attitude. Comparisons between African American and Caucasian participants and their families were not reported.

Dirksen and Erickson (2002) conducted a descriptive and comparative study to test the Well-being Among Survivors of Breast Cancer Conceptual Model with Hispanic and non-Hispanic White survivors of breast cancer. A convenience sample of 50 Hispanic and 50 non-Hispanic White women who had completed treatment for breast cancer and were disease-free completed a series of standardized instruments. Both groups of women reported high levels of well-being. However, unlike other reports in the literature, older Hispanic women in this study had higher levels of well-being than non-Hispanic White women. No other statistically significant differences in well-being or other study variables were found between groups, and demographic characteristics were not related significantly to well-being.

The study conducted by Northouse et al. (1999) used a stress and coping framework to examine how person-, resource-, and illness-related factors affected the quality of life of African American women ($N = 98$) who were at least 1 month post breast cancer. The overall goal of this descriptive correlational cross-sectional study was to assess the influence of appraisal of illness on person-, social-, and illness-related antecedents (optimism, current concerns, family functioning, and symptom distress) and quality of life. Contrary to reports of other research studies, the women reported a fairly high quality of life, were generally optimistic, and had effective family functioning. Data analysis revealed that the model explained 75% of the variance in quality of life, with appraisal, family functioning, symptom distress, and recurrence status explaining a significant amount of the variance. Although the quality of life of the African American survivors of breast cancer in this study was found to be relatively high, the authors concluded that future research was needed to test interventions that will ultimately assist this group of women to decrease or resolve their concerns, maintain their family support, and reduce symptom distress so that they can maintain a high quality in their lives in spite of their disease.

Intervention

A total of seven articles included in this analysis focused on the evaluation of interventions. Willis, Davis, Cairns, and Janiszewski (1989) reported the steps of a descriptive pilot project to increase Black women's knowledge about breast cancer and use of BSE and other screening methods. This project was based upon a collaborative effort between the Illinois Cancer Council and the Chicago Chapter of the National Black Nurses Association. Nurses were trained to deliver the intervention, which included materials from the NCI Breast Examination in Hospital Program. Ten nurses were trained in the core content of the program, and they recruited women ($N = 148$) from their respective hospitalized units. Methods included delivering the pretest, demonstrating BSE, providing literature, and then posttest and follow-up within 90 days. Results indicated that the overall difference in reported BSE frequency after BSE instruction was not statistically significant. Although this pilot program demonstrated feasibility, several problems were encountered, including unexpected staff changes and difficulties with the questionnaire. The results strongly suggest that evaluation activities should be simple and straightforward and that collaboration among organizations is a productive strategy for reaching Black communities.

In another study aimed at breast cancer detection, Ehmann (1993) described the development and implementation of a breast health awareness educational strategy among minority and low-income adolescent females; however, the specific racial and ethnic breakdown of participants was not reported. The rationale behind the use of a BSE rap, a lively music-video presentation, was to motivate teens to share information with their mothers and grandmothers, thus promoting intergenerational messages for saving lives from breast cancer. No theoretical framework was identified to support the study.

Although the content of the video focused on myths of breast cancer, risk, mammography, breast cancer diagnosis, and treatment, no formative data were provided to support the specific processes or decisions used for the content intended to motivate adolescents. The author developed a participant evaluation tool to assess certain features of the music video among 109 inner-city middle and high school students. A total of 78% stated they would encourage their mothers and grandmothers to get a mammogram, and 63% agreed that a music video made them feel comfortable discussing BSE. Although the creation of a music video as a communication strategy for teens is valuable, the efficacy of such tools needs to be verified with more formalized evaluation methods and long-term studies.

Baldwin (1996) reported on data from two qualitative studies that were conducted to gain a better understanding of the lived experiences of African American women engaging in health-seeking behaviors such as Pap smear testing, breast self-examination, and mammography. In the first study, three focus groups ($N = 30$) were held with African American women to pilot-test a teaching module on breast and cervical health for low-income African American women. In the second study, which used nine individual interviews, the aim was to illuminate the lived experiences of low-income African American women who participated in breast and cervical cancer early detection and screening services. Using recognized thematic analysis procedures, four themes emerged from the focus groups: (1) I value my beliefs; (2) I am proud of being Black; (3) I am struggling to survive; and (4) I am a human being. Several themes emerged from the interviews: (1) surviving; (2) experiencing cancer from a family or friend's perspective; (3) wanting to know that my body is healthy; and (4) wanting information. Data were then infused into a model in which phenomena were explained from the perspective of the low-income African American women and their worldview and lived experiences. The authors concluded that such constructs should be further tested and recommended that the Afrocentric model could serve as a basis for culture-specific tools for assessing decisions relating to breast and cervical cancer, for designing community-based educational programs, and for integrating these results into nursing curricula.

In a study by Lauver and Rubin (1990), the effects of alternatively framed messages and dispositional optimism on follow-up for abnormal PAP tests were explored in a sample of primarily Black (67%) low-income women. Messages were randomly provided in two ways. One message was a loss-framed message that focused on the losses that women would incur in not following-up an abnormal cervical cancer screening with colposcopy. The other was a gain-framed message that focused on the gains that women would incur in following-up an abnormal cervical cancer screening with colposcopy. The researchers hypothesized that loss-framed messages about follow-up of abnormal screening would promote greater attendance for colposcopy more than gain-framed messages and that dispositional optimism would be positively associated with colposcopy follow-up. The findings did not support the hypothesized impact of message framing. The authors suggested that advantaged versus disadvantaged groups may hold different cultural values on losses and gains and that message framing may not explain behavior in certain health care settings. The authors concluded that more practical explanations related to attendance might be barriers of childcare, time, menstruation, and money. They suggested that future research should specify sociocultural variables that may interact with message framing.

One study pilot tested an educational intervention for increasing BSE and breast cancer screening among older African American women (Adderley-Kelly & Green, 1997). Bandura's social learning theory guided the pilot study. A convenience sample of 25 African American women, ages 60–84 years, was recruited from a mid-Atlantic housing facility. A

control group (12) and an intervention group (13) received a group education session with one-to-one guided BSE practice. A pretest-posttest experimental design was used to evaluate the effectiveness of the intervention.
Subjects who increased their BSE self-efficacy scores were more likely
to have made an appointment for a clinical breast examination one month
following treatment. The results indicated that self-efficacy may be enhanced through group teaching and one-to-one guided practice that fosters
mastery of BSE.

Two studies in this review addressed interventions to reach elderly
populations with colorectal screening messages. Weinrich, Weinrich,
Boyd, Atwood, and Cervenka (1994) conducted a pilot study to measure
the effect of the Adaptation for Changes (AAC) methods for fecal-occult
blood screening (FOBS). The study was conducted at meal sites in the
South, and the sample included 135 subjects (82% female and 56% African
American). A quasi-experimental pretest-posttest design was used to evaluate the effects of three educational interventions for FOBS: FOBS using
the Adaptation for Aging Changes with Practice (AACP) method; FOBS
using the ACS method (traditional); and FOBS taught by Adaptation for
Aging Changes (without practice). The traditional method involved a nurse
presenting an ACTS slide tape presentation and distributing hemoccult
kits and dietary instruction for testing of the stool. The AAC method
modified the traditional presentation by accommodating for normal aging
changes by allowing for increased time for learning, demonstrating the
procedure for memory retention, and adapting materials at the fifth-grade
reading level. Other educational techniques included using peanut butter
to demonstrate the technique, giving self-stick notes for reminders, and
using posters at the meal sites. The AACP was identical to the AAC
method, with the addition of practice for the procedure of FOBS with
feedback.

Results indicated that a greater percentage of participants taught by
AACP took part in the FOBS than those taught by AAC or the traditional
method. This significant difference supports the premise of increased
participation in FOBS taught by AACP. However, there were no significant
differences between the AAC and traditional methods. The authors suggested that this might have been due to the positive relationships established
between interviewers and the participants. They concluded that this study
supports the need to adapt teaching and to tailor the intervention for normal
changes, including time for actually practicing the desired techniques.

In a study previously described, Powe and Weinrich (1999) evaluated
the effectiveness of a video intervention in decreasing cancer fatalism,

increasing knowledge of colorectal cancer, and increasing participation in fecal-occult blood testing (FOBT) among African American elders. Using a repeated measures pretest-posttest experimental design, a total of 70 subjects were enrolled in this study ($n = 42$ experimental; $n = 28$ control). The control group viewed the ACTS video entitled "Colorectal Cancer: The Cancer That No One Talks About" while the intervention group viewed the video entitled "Telling the Story . . . to Live Is God's Will," which included techniques of storytelling and role modeling. Analysis of covariance indicated that the intervention group showed a greater decrease in cancer fatalism scores and a greater increase in knowledge of colorectal cancer scores than the control group. There was no significant difference in the rate of FOBT participation. The majority of both groups took part in the screening. Both videos were effective in increasing participation in FOBT. However, the authors suggested that the control group might have inadvertently received an additional intervention that may have contributed to the high rates of participation in FOBT. The authors concluded that intervention video was successful in increasing knowledge of colorectal cancer and decreasing perceptions of cancer fatalism.

In summary, the majority of these studies focus on the design of interventions among African Americans relating to the areas of breast/ cervical or colon cancer. Additional efforts by nurse researchers should address other at-risk populations in light of the growing diversity and multicultural nature of the United States. Nurses should also conduct investigations of promising interventions relating to other common cancers such as prostate and lung. Similar to the other reviews in this chapter, there persists a need for more experimental studies such as that of Powe and Weinrich (1999). Although the value of descriptive and formative research is widely recognized and appropriate for many nursing research questions, information gained from exploratory and pilot investigations should lead to experimental studies. Although most of the studies reviewed did employ some form of evaluation, the rigor and methods used for such evaluations was not reported consistently in sufficient detail to ensure confidence in results (Ehman, 1993; Willis et al., 1989).

Of the studies reported here, several themes were noted. First, there was an uneven reporting of the psychometric properties of instruments across studies and specifically how interventions were developed for in-tended racial and ethnic groups in consideration of culture and literacy and other psychographic characteristics. Such methodological issues are critical to ensuring reliability and validity of results. Future studies should rigorously address instrumentation issues and detail processes used to ensure that interventions are culturally acceptable, efficacious and understandable. With this said, several studies reviewed did suggest that culturally specific tools or tailored interventions may hold promise in health disparities research (Baldwin, 1996; Lauver & Rubin, 1990; Weinrich et al., 1994). This line of research should be further explored.

Research Participation

Two of the studies included in this review addressed research participation (Millon-Underwood, Sanders, & Davis, 1993; Outlaw, Bourjolly, & Barg, 2000). Both studies were descriptive in design and focused on research participation by African Americans. The study conducted by Outlaw et al. (2000) involved 37 physicians and 17 data managers in the identification of factors that prevent African Americans from participating in clinical trials. The study conducted by Millon-Underwood et al. (1993) involved 220 African American men and women from the community in the identification of factors that contributed to participation in investigational cancer programs and/or trials.

In each of these studies, data were collected with investigator-designed instruments that included items deemed to be conceptually and empirically relevant to participation in clinical research. The study findings indicated that among the physicians and data managers the three most common factors believed to prevent African Americans from participating in research were the complexity of clinical trials, their trouble seeing the value of research, and their fear of the health care system. Among the community men and women, the factor having the greatest influence on their willingness to participate in clinical research was their perceived efficacy of the research program. Future research is needed to identify determinants of participation of African American in clinical cancer trials and the design of interventions that may be used by nurses and other medical providers during the recruitment process.

Instrumentation

A total of four articles included in this review focused on the development and/or psychometric validation of instruments. Champion and Scott (1997) aimed to describe the psychometric properties of culturally sensitive scales designed to measure beliefs about mammography and breast self-examination screening in African American women. Guided by the Health Belief Model, the instrument included questions on perceived breast cancer susceptibility, benefits of breast self-exam, barriers to breast self-exam, self-efficacy, benefits of mammography, and barriers to mammography. The findings indicated that Cronbach's alpha reliability coefficients ranged from 0.65 to 0.90. Test–retest reliability of the instrument ranged from 0.40 to 0.68, and construct validity was confirmed.

Adams, DeJesus, Trujillo, and Cole (1997) examined psychometric properties by the Sexual Dimensions Instrument for Hispanic Women, a culturally sensitive sexual functioning instrument. A physiologic, psychological, and interpersonal perspective on sexual functioning served as the framework for this study.

Ford et al. (2002) used a qualitative approach to evaluate the Breast Cancer Risk Factor Survey for its appropriateness for African American women. The authors also assessed the perceptions of breast cancer risk factors among these women using the instrument. A randomly selected sample of 20 African American women (total) participated in two focus groups. Prior to the focus groups, the women were asked to complete the Breast Cancer Risk Factor Survey, which included items on the woman's health history (contraceptives, hormone replacement, menstruation, menopause, medical data). Women who were younger lacked awareness regarding breast cancer risk factors, whereas older women reported they did not know their family histories. The authors modified the survey substantially based on the results of the focus groups.

Jennings-Dozier (1999b), previously described, used a qualitative approach to determine the empirical adequacy of the Theory of Planned Behavior in explaining African American and Latina women's intentions to have a Pap test. Focus groups were conducted among a sample of African American and Latina women to establish the content validity of the belief-based measures of attitude, subjective norm, and perceived behavioral control scales (Jennings, 1997). The 75-item Pap Smear Questionnaire (PSQ) and Demographic Assessment Survey (DAS) were pilot-tested with a representative sample of 60 African American and 60 Latina women. The study findings did not support the empirical adequacy of the Theory of Planned Behavior for either group of minority women. The investigator recommended continued refinement of the PSQ instrument and future testing of a modified version that includes additional measures of social support and subjective norms.

This review and analysis revealed that very few nursing studies have been conducted in the area of "instrumentation" that consider issues associated with the cancer-related health disparities of racially and ethnic minority groups. Of these, few have been conducted among multiracial and multiethnic groups. All of the instrumentation studies selected for inclusion in this review focused on the development and/or psychometric validation of new instruments for use among African American women and Hispanic women. None of the instrumentation studies focused on the development and/or psychometric validation of instruments for use among Native American or Asian American women, or for minority men. The same was true of instrumentation studies focused on the development and/or psychometric validation of instruments for use among multiracial and multiethnic groups.

This group of nurse researchers aimed toward developing new instruments to answer research questions for the targeted population group rather than refining available instruments through validation and/or evaluation for use among multiethnic groups. Efforts to develop culturally competent instruments for use among racial and ethnic population groups need to be continued. However, the same is true of efforts to validate and test currently available instruments for use among ethnic minority populations.

PROGRAMMATIC REVIEW AND METHODOLOGICAL CRITIQUE OF THE NURSING RESEARCH

This review gave the authors an opportunity to analyze and critique the scope, quality, and potential impact of the body of nursing research focused on cancer in U.S. ethnic and racial minority populations. The review revealed that the body of nursing research undertaken to explore and address cancer in racially and ethnically defined populations has contributed much to the identification and understanding of the individual, familial, institutional, and societal factors associated with the excess cancer morbidity and mortality of minority populations.

However, several gaps and limitations were noted within this body of nursing research. Included among them were gaps relative to research that focused on the cancer experiences of many U.S. racially and ethnically defined minority population groups; cancers commonly experienced by minority population groups; cancer prevention, risk reduction, treatment, symptom management, palliative care, and end-of-life issues; cancer screening; limitations relative to research design, sampling, and instrumentation; and the development of programs of nursing research directed toward the prevention and control of cancer among racial and ethnic minority populations. In addition, the paucity of studies reported in the nursing literature was somewhat surprising, especially in light of the national attention to health disparities as outlined by the Department of Health and Human Services (USDHHS, 1990, 2000), the Institute of Medicine (Haynes & Smedley, 1999), and the American Public Health Association (APHA, HHS join forces, 2000).

One might reasonably expect that this body of research would have been used as the foundation for the development of research aimed toward addressing correlates and predictors of cancer-related health disparities and for the design and evaluation of interventions to reduce or eliminate them. However, the review revealed that this overall body of nursing research has produced few evidence-based interventions that can be used to reduce or eliminate cancer disparities in racial and ethnic minority populations. Of the sample of 56 articles included in this review, 49 articles (85.7%) focused on defining the perspectives and concerns of racial and ethnic minority population groups relative to cancer, cancer prevention, and cancer control, whereas only 7 articles (12.57%) focused on the design and evaluation of mechanisms and/or interventions for addressing them.

All of the studies included in the review involved racially and ethnically defined minority populations as subjects or participants. However, data analyses revealed that there was not reasonable representation of all of the major racially and ethnically defined minority population groups. Forty-six of the studies involved African Americans (82.1%), 14 involved Hispanics (25.0%), 16 involved non-Hispanic Whites (28.6%), 5 involved Asian Americans (8.9%), and 1 involved Native Americans (1.8%). Twenty-three of the studies involved participants from two or more racially and ethnically defined population groups. However, of these, only 13 (54.2%) reported and/or compared the study findings within and between the ethnic and racial groups.

The most common forms of cancer experienced by African American, Hispanic, Asian American, and Native American men are cancers of the prostate, lung and/or bronchus, and colon and/or rectum. The most common forms of cancer experienced by African American, Hispanic, Asian American, and Native American women are cancer of the breast, lung and/or bronchus, colon and/or rectum, and uterus. Nurse scientists have undertaken a number of efforts focused on the examination of issues and concerns related to breast, uterine, colorectal, and prostate cancer among ethnic and racial minority populations. Among the 46 studies included in this review that focused on a site-specific cancer, 26 studies (56.6%) focused on cancer of the breast, 12 studies (26.1%) focused on cancer of the uterus, 4 studies (7.1%) focused on cancer of the colon and/or rectum, 4 studies (8.7%) focused on cancer of the prostate, and 1 study (2.2%) focused on cancer of testicles. However, surprisingly and conspicuously absent were studies focused on cancer of the lung and/or bronchus.

A significant proportion of the studies examined the cancer experiences of women and/or issues and concerns associated with cancers that occur more often or only in women. However, few focused on the cancer experiences of men and/or issues and concerns associated with cancers that occur in men. Of the 56 studies included in this review, 38 studies (67.9%) examined the cancer experiences of women, and 8 studies (14.3%) examined the cancer experiences of men. Thirty-six studies (64.3%) of the studies examined issues and concerns associated with cancers of the breast and uterus, whereas 5 studies (8.9%) examined issues and concerns associated with cancers of the prostate and testicles.

The continuum of cancer care, although often conceived as involving the care of individuals who have a definitive diagnosis of cancer, can be more broadly conceptualized as involving the provision of care relative to prevention and risk reduction, cancer screening, cancer diagnosis, cancer treatment, symptom management, survivorship, and palliative and end-of-life care. Among the studies included in this review, one study focused on the assessment of genetic risks. Thirty-seven studies (66.1%) examined issues, concerns, and experiences associated with cancer screening. Six (10.7%) studies examined issues and concerns associated with cancer diagnosis. One study (1.8%) examined issues and concerns associated with cancer treatment. Five studies (8.9%) examined the overall lived experience of survivors of cancer. However, none of the nursing studies included in this review examined experiences associated with cancer prevention, risk reduction, symptom management, or palliative or end-of-life care.

Lifestyle choices and personal behavior, including tobacco use, diet and nutrition, physical inactivity, overweight status or obesity, and alcohol consumption, are known to account for the initiation of most new cancers and cause most cancer deaths. It is generally believed that if concerted efforts toward cancer prevention and risk reduction among African American, Hispanic, Asian American, and Native American populations were undertaken by nurses and other health care providers within the practice and community setting, cancer morbidity, cancer mortality, and cancer disparities would be significantly reduced. Culturally relevant and evidence-based cancer prevention and risk reduction interventions for use are sorely needed. Yet none of the studies in this review addressed tobacco use, diet and nutrition, physical inactivity, overweight status or obesity, or alcohol consumption. The same is true of the design of interventions focused on cancer prevention or the reduction of any one of these modifiable risk factors.

The American Cancer Society estimates that the 5-year relative cancer survival for the screening-accessible sites would increase significantly if more men and women participated in timely cancer screenings (ACTS, 2003). Recommended screening tests for cancer of the breast, colon, rectum, cervix, and prostate can detect cancer early when it is most curable and thereby save lives and improve cancer survival. Trends in cancer screening and early detection are known to significantly impact cancer morbidity and mortality of minority population groups. Although a significant proportion of the research reviewed examined issues associated with breast and cervical cancer screening among racial and ethnic minorities, fewer studies of issues associated with prostate and colorectal cancer among this population group were noted. Seventeen of the nursing studies (45.9%) that focused on screening addressed breast cancer screening (mammography, clinical breast examination and self-breast examination). Eight of the studies (21.6%) addressed cervical cancer screening (Pap smear and pelvic examination). Five of the studies (13.5%) addressed colorectal cancer screening. Three studies (8.1%) addressed prostate cancer screening (digital rectal examination and analyses of prostate specific antigen). One of the studies (2.7%) addressed screening for testicular cancer. However, although the discipline subscribes to the notion of the holistic nature of man/woman and holistic care, none of the studies conceptualized and assessed screening from a holistic perspective.

A variety of research methods and designs were used in the conduct of this body of nursing research. Following peer-review all of the studies were deemed to be scientifically sound, however, the review revealed that most of the studies were constructed using minimally rigorous designs, and that the procedures and methodologies used resulted in collection of lower levels of evidence. Ten of the studies (17.9%) included in this review was undertaken using qualitative methodologies; 45 of the studies (80.4%) used quantitative methodologies; and 1 study (1.8%) was undertaken using both qualitative and quantitative methodologies. Fifty-one of the studies (91.1%) were constructed using nonexperimental descriptive, exploratory, correlational designs. Five of the studies (8.9%) were constructed using experimental or quasi-experimental control group designs.

Research conducted within any discipline should be consistent with the philosophical orientation and theories of that discipline (Burns & Grove, 2003). Theories, conceptual models, and frameworks are the mechanisms through which researchers organize and interpret research findings. Most of the studies in this review did not report the use of a theoretical or conceptual framework based on nursing theory. The theoretical, conceptual, or philosophical underpinnings guiding the research were explicitly described in 36 of the studies (64.3%). Of these, 7 studies (19.4%) used nursing frameworks to explain and/or predict the influence of culture, cultural competency, and culture care on the cancer experience of population groups. The remaining studies were designed using frameworks derived from the fields of education, social science, and management.

The sample sizes of the studies included in this review varied with the research design. The methods of sample size determination and power analyses, while a critical determinant of the generalizability of the study results, in most instances were not reported. The sample sizes of the studies using qualitative methods ranged from 16 to 635. The sample sizes of the studies using quantitative methods ranged from 51 to 831. Nonprobability, convenience, and purposeful samplings were used in 50 of the studies (89.3%). Six (10.7%) reported the use of probability sampling by random selection.

A variety of data collection instruments and investigator-designed instruments were used in the studies reviewed. However, reports describing if and/or how the psychometric properties of reliability, validity, or cultural appropriateness of the data collection instruments used in this body of research were most often not reported.

Finally, the review suggests that there is a need to develop programs of nursing research directed toward the prevention and control of cancer among racial and ethnic minority populations. Programs of nursing research that progressively incorporate the phases of the cancer control research continuum, such as the implementation of studies focused on the development of hypotheses and methods, the conduct of controlled intervention studies with defined populations, and the evaluation of demonstration projects directed toward the elimination of cancer related health disparities, are essential to the development of knowledge relative to the prevention and control of cancer among racially and ethnic minority populations. Among the reports analyzed in this review, 13 exemplified how a theoretically based research agenda focused on cancer prevention and control can be implemented with minority populations to explore and address factors associated with the evolution of cancer-related health disparities (Jennings, 1997; Jennings-Dozier, 1999a, 1999b; Jennings-Dozier & Lawrence, 2000; Millon-Underwood & Sanders, 1990, 1991; Millon-Underwood et al., 1993; Powe, 1995a, 1995b, 1995c; Powe & Weinrich, 1999; Underwood, 1991, 1999). The approaches undertaken by these researchers could serve as models for the design of research programs for expanding this body of nursing science.

SUMMARY

Nursing is well positioned to contribute much to efforts aimed toward eliminating the cancer disparities experienced by racial and ethnic population groups. Nurses number 2.7 million and rank as the nation's largest and most highly regarded health care professional group (NCHS, 2002; Gallup, 2002). Nurses engage in virtually all health care–related settings across the country. Whether nursing generalists or oncology nursing specialists in primary, secondary, or tertiary care, the services nurses provide contribute to the promotion and maintenance of health; the prevention of illness; the care of men, women, and children during acute phases of illness; the rehabilitation or restoration of optimum functioning during the process of recovery from illness, injury, or infirmity; and the achievement of a dignified death. And, regardless of the setting, the clinical focus, the intended population, or the domain of practice, there are opportunities to introduce evidence-based nursing interventions that promote cancer prevention, cancer risk reduction, and cancer control.

Research is essential to the development of the scientific base of knowledge that will enable nurses to help reduce the cancer-related health disparities experienced among and between racial and ethnic minority population groups. A substantive body of knowledge has been acquired. However, in order for the profession to more fully contribute to the elimination of cancer-related disparities, there is a need for nurses to further expand this base of knowledge. The review suggests that there is a need for nursing research which:

- more fully addresses cancer and cancer care among and between Native American, Asian American, Hispanic, and African American population groups;

- examines issues and concerns commonly associated with lung, prostate, breast, colorectal, uterine, esophageal, gastrointestinal, and other cancers with the greatest morbidity and mortality among Native American, Asian American, Hispanic, and African American populations;
- addresses cancer prevention, risk reduction, screening, diagnosis, treatment, symptom management, palliative care, and end-of life dimensions of the cancer care continuum among and between Native American, Asian American, Hispanic, and African American populations;
- aims toward the design and evaluation of interventions designed to reduce risk and impede the adoption of lifestyle behaviors among Native American, Asian American, Hispanic, and African American populations that are known to be associated with the initiation of cancers and cause cancer death;
- aims toward the design and evaluation of interventions capable of allaying fears, correcting misperceptions, enhancing knowledge, and overcoming barriers identified by Native American, Asian American, Hispanic, and African American population groups relative to cancer risk reduction, prevention, early detection, and cancer control;
- further expands the current base of knowledge, beyond that of hypothesis generation and hypothesis testing, to include methods development, controlled intervention trials, defined population studies, and the evaluation of nurse-facilitated cancer prevention and control demonstration projects; and
- encourages the development of programs of research directed toward the prevention and control of cancer among racial and ethnic minority populations.

For nursing research to impact cancer-related health disparities of racial and ethnic minority populations, it must be based on sound scientific principles and have the methodological rigor to allow generalizability. All of the studies included in this review were deemed to be scientifically sound. However, results of this review suggest that attempts should also be made to:

- evaluate the role and feasibility of nursing theory relative to cancer among racial and ethnic minority populations; and

- strengthen the design and methodologies used in the conduct of future research focused on cancer in racial and ethnic minority populations.

As this body of research is further developed, it is recommended that investigators direct greater attention to the construction of theoretically based and methodologically rigorous designs when attempting to answer questions and test hypotheses related to the cancer experience of racial and ethnic minority population groups. It is believed that these efforts must be undertaken immediately if the science that directs nursing practice is to significantly contribute to the elimination of cancer disparities among racial and ethnic minority population groups.

ACKNOWLEDGMENTS

The authors would like to acknowledge Sue Felber, M.S.L.S., A.H.I.P., Coordinator—Medical Library, H. Lee Moffitt Cancer Center & Research Institute for her valuable contributions during the process of database research and literature review.

REFERENCES

*Adams, J., DeJesus, Y., Trujillo, M., & Cole, F. (1997). Assessing sexual dimensions in Hispanic women. Development of an instrument. *Cancer Nursing, 20*(4), 251–259.

*Adderley-Kelly, B., & Green, P. M. (1997). Breast cancer education, self-efficacy, and screening in older African American women. *Journal of National Black Nurses Association, 9*(1), 45–57.

American Cancer Society. (2001). *Cancer facts and figures for Hispanics, 2000–2001.* Atlanta, GA: American Cancer Society.

APHA, HHS join forces to combat health disparities. (2000, May). *The Nation's Health*, p. 1.

*Baldwin, D. (1996). A model for describing low-income African American women's participation in breast and cervical cancer early detection and screening. *Advances in Nursing Science, 19*(2), 27–42.

*Bibb, S. C. (2001). The relationship between access and stage at diagnosis of breast cancer in African American and Caucasian women. *Oncology Nursing Forum, 28*(4), 711–719.

---

*Indicates studies included in the analysis.

*Burnett, C. B., Steakley, C. S., & Tefft, M. C. (1995). Barriers to breast and cervical cancer screening in underserved women of the District of Columbia. *Oncology Nursing Forum, 22*(10), 1551–1557.

Burns, N., & Grove, S. (2003). *Understanding nursing research.* Philadelphia: W. B. Saunders.

Canto, M. T., & Chu, K. C. (2000). Annual cancer incidence rates for Hispanics in the United States. *Cancer, 88,* 2642–2652.

*Champion, V., & Menon, U. (1997). Predicting mammography and breast self-examination in African American women. *Cancer Nursing, 20*(5), 315–322.

*Champion, V. L., & Scott, C. R. (1997). Reliability and validity of breast cancer screening belief scales in African American women. *Nursing Research, 46*(6), 331–337.

Clegg, L. X., Li, F. P., Hankey, B. F., Chu, K., & Edwards, B. K. (2002). Cancer survival among U.S. Whites and minorities: A SEER Program population-based study. *Archives of Internal Medicine, 162,* 1985–1989.

Cooper, H. M. (1982). Scientific guidelines for conducting integrative research reviews. *Review of Educational Research, 52,* 291–302.

*Dirksen, S. R., & Erickson, J. R. (2002). Well-being in Hispanic and non-Hispanic white survivors of breast cancer. *Oncology Nursing Forum, 29*(5), 820–826.

*Douglass, M., Bartolucci, A., Waterbor, J., & Sirles, A. (1995). Breast cancer early detection: Differences between African American and White women's health beliefs and detection practices. *Oncology Nursing Forum, 22*(5), 835–837.

*Ehmann, J. L. (1993). BSE Rap: Intergenerational ties to save lives. *Oncology Nursing Forum, 20*(8), 1255–1259.

*Facione, N. C., & Giancarlo, C. A. (1998). Narratives of breast symptom discovery and cancer diagnosis: Psychologic risk for advanced cancer at diagnosis. *Cancer Nursing, 21,* 430–440.

Facione, N. C., & Katapodi, M. (2000). Culture as an influence on breast cancer screening and early detection. *Seminars in Oncology Nursing, 16,* 238–247.

*Fearing, A., Bell, D., Newton, M., & Lambert, S. (2000). Prostate screening health beliefs and practices of African American men. *Journal of the Association of Black Nursing Faculty, 11*(6), 141–144.

*Ford, M. E., Hill, D. D., Blount, A., Morrison, J., Worsham, M., Havstad, S. L., & Johnson, C. C. (2002). Modifying a breast cancer risk factor survey for African American women. *Oncology Nursing Forum, 29*(5), 827–834.

*Foxall, M. J., Barron, C. R., & Houfek, J. F. (2001). Ethnic influences on body awareness, trait anxiety, perceived risk, and breast and gynecologic cancer screening practices. *Oncology Nursing Forum, 28*(4), 727–738.

Gallup Organization. (2003). *Public rates nursing as most honest and ethical profession.* Washington, DC: The Gallup Organization.

*Han, Y., Williams, R. D., & Harrison, R. A. (2000). Breast cancer screening knowledge, attitudes, and practices among Korean American women. *Oncology Nursing Forum, 27*(10), 1585–1591.

Haynes, M. A., & Smedley, B. D. (1999). The unequal burden of cancer: An assessment of NIH research and programs for ethnic minorities and the medically underserved.

In M. A. Haynes & B. D. Smedley (Eds.), *The unequal burden of cancer*. Washington, DC: National Academy Press.

Heckler, M. (1985). Report of the Secretary's Task Force on Black and Minority Health. Washington, DC: U.S. Department of Health and Human Services.

*Jennings, K. M. (1997). Getting a Pap smear: Focus group responses of African American and Latina women. *Oncology Nursing Forum, 24,* 827–385.

*Jennings-Dozier, K. (1999a). Perceptual determinants of Pap test up-to-date status among minority women. *Oncology Nursing Forum, 26,* 1587.

*Jennings-Dozier, K. (1999b). Predicting intentions to obtain a pap smear among African American and Latina women: Testing the Theory of Planned Behavior. *Nursing Research, 48*(4), 198–205.

*Jennings-Dozier, K., & Lawrence, D. (2000). Sociodemographic predictors of adherence to annual cervical cancer screening in minority women. *Cancer Nursing, 23,* 350–356.

*Katapodi, M. C., Facione, N. C., Miaskowski, C., Dodd, M. J., & Waters, C. (2002). The influence of social support on breast cancer screening in a multicultural community sample. *Oncology Nursing Forum, 29* 845–852.

*Kinney, A. Y., Emery, G., Dudley, W. N., & Croyle, R. T. (2002). Screening behaviors among African American women at high risk for breast cancer: Do beliefs about god matter? *Oncology Nursing Forum, 29,* 835–843.

Lambert, S., Newton, M., & deMeneses, M. (1998). Barriers to mammography in older, low-income African American women. *Journal of Ministry in Addiction and Recovery, 4*(2), 16–19.

*Lauver, D. (1992). Psychosocial variables, race, and intention to seek care for breast cancer symptoms. *Nursing Research, 41,* 236–241.

*Lauver, D. (1994). Care-seeking behavior with breast cancer symptoms in Caucasian and African American women. *Research in Nursing and Health, 17,* 421–431.

*Lauver, D., & Rubin, M. (1990). Message framing, dispositional optimism, and follow-up for abnormal Papanicolaou tests. *Research in Nursing and Health, 13,* 199–207.

*Lee, M. C. (2000). Knowledge, barriers, and motivators related to cervical cancer screening among Korean-American women. A focus group approach. *Cancer Nursing, 23,* 168–175.

McCubbin, M. A., & McCubbin, H. I. (1996). Resiliency in families: A conceptual model of family adjustment and adaptation in response to stress and crises. In H. I. McCubbin, A. L. Thompson, & M. A. McCubbin (Eds.), *Family assessment: Resiliency, coping, and adaptation—Inventories for research and practice* (pp. 1–64). Madison, WI: University of Wisconsin System.

*Mellon, S. (2002). Comparisons between cancer survivors and family members on meaning of the illness and family quality of life. *Oncology Nursing Forum, 29,* 1117–1125.

Miller, B. A., Kolonel, L. N., Bernstein, L., Young, Jr, J. L., Swanson, G. M., West, D., Key, C. R., Liff, J. M., Glover, C. S., Alexander, G. A., et al. (Eds.). (1996). Racial and ethnic patterns of cancer in the United States 1988–1992. NIH Pub.

No. 96-4104. Bethesda, MD: National Cancer Institute. Available from: *http:// www-seer.ims.nci.nih.gov/Publications/REPoC.*

*Millon-Underwood, S., & Sanders, E. (1990). Factors contributing to health promotion behaviors among African-American men. *Oncology Nursing Forum, 17,* 707–712.

*Millon-Underwood, S., & Sanders, E. (1991a). Testicular self-examination among African-American men. *Journal of the National Black Nurses Association, 5*(1), 18–28.

Millon-Underwood, S., & Sanders, E. (1991b). Factors contributing to health promotion behaviors among African-American men. *Oncology Nursing Forum, 17,* 707–712.

*Millon-Underwood, S., Sanders, E., & Davis, M. (1993). Determinants of participation in state-of-the-art cancer prevention, early detection/screening, and treatment trials among African-Americans. *Cancer Nursing, 16*(1), 25–33.

Modiano, M. R., Villar-Werstler, P., Meister, J., & Figueroa-Valles, N. (1995). Cancer in Hispanics: Issues of concern. *Monographs of the National Cancer Institute, 18,* 57–63.

*Moore, R. J. (2001). African American women and breast cancer: Notes from a study of narrative. *Cancer Nursing, 24*(1), 35–42.

Morgan, D. L. (1997). *Focus groups as qualitative research* (2nd ed.). Thousand Oaks, CA: Sage.

National Center for Health Statistics. (2002). *Health United States, 2002, with chartbook on trends in the health of Americans.* Hyattsville, MD: United States Department of Health and Human Services, Centers for Disease Control and Prevention, National Center for Health Statistics.

*Nemcek, M. A. (1989). Factors influencing Black women's breast self-examination practice. *Cancer Nursing, 12*(6), 339–343.

Nichols, B. S., Misra, R., & Alexy, B. (1996). Cancer detection: How effective is public education? *Cancer Nursing, 19*(2), 98–103.

*Northouse, L. L., Caffey, M., Deichelbohrer, L., Schmidt, L., Guziatek-Trojniak, L., West, S., Kershaw, T., & Mood, D. (1999). The quality of life of African American women with breast cancer. *Research in Nursing and Health, 22*(6), 449–460.

*O'Hare, P. A., Malone, D., Lusk, E., & McCorkle, R. (1993). Unmet needs of Black patients with cancer posthospitalization: A descriptive study. *Oncology Nursing Forum, 20*(4), 659–664.

*Outlaw, F. H., Bourjolly, J. N., & Barg, F. K. (2000). A study on recruitment of Black Americans into clinical trials through a cultural competence lens. *Cancer Nursing, 23*(6), 444–451.

*Phillips, J. M., & Wilbur, J. (1995). Adherence to breast cancer screening guidelines among African-American women of differing employment status. *Cancer Nursing, 18*(4), 258–269.

*Powe, B. D., & Weinrich, S. (1999). An intervention to decrease cancer fatalism among rural elders. *Oncology Nursing Forum, 26*(3), 583–588.

*Powe, B. D. (1995a). Cancer fatalism among elderly Caucasians and African Americans. *Oncology Nursing Forum, 22*(9), 1355–1359.

Powe, B. D. (1995b). Fatalism among elderly African Americans: Effects on colorectal cancer screening. *Cancer Nursing, 18*(5), 385–392.

*Powe, B. D. (1995c). Perceptions of cancer fatalism among African Americans: The influence of education, income, and cancer knowledge. *Journal of the National Black Nurses Association, 7*(2), 41–48.

*Rashidi, A., & Rajaram, S. S. (2000). Middle Eastern Asian Islamic women and breast self-examination. Needs assessment. *Cancer Nursing, 23*(1), 64–70.

Ries, L. A. G., Eisner, M., Kosary, C., Hankey, B., Miller, B., Clegg, L., & Edwards, B. (Eds.). (2002). Cancer facts and figures. *SEER cancer statistics review, 1973–1999.* Bethesda, MD: National Cancer Institute. Retrieved March 2, 2004 from http://seer.cancer.gov/csr/1973_1999/

*Salazar, M. K. (1996). Hispanic women's beliefs about breast cancer and mammography. *Cancer Nursing, 19*(6), 437–446.

*Schulmeister, L., & Lifsey, D. S. (1999). Cervical cancer screening knowledge, behaviors, and beliefs of Vietnamese women. *Oncology Nursing Forum, 26*(5), 879–887.

*Shelton, P., Weinrich, S., & Reynolds, W. A., Jr. (1999). Barriers to prostate cancer screening in African American men. *Journal of the National Black Nurses Association, 10*(2), 14–28.

Smedley, B. D., Stite, A. Y., & Nelson, A. R. (2002). *Unequal treatment: Confronting racial and ethnic disparities in health care.* Washington, DC: National Academy Press.

*Smiley, M. R., McMillan, S. C., Johnson, S., & Ojeda, M. (2000). Comparison of Florida Hispanic and non-Hispanic Caucasian women in their health beliefs related to breast cancer and health locus of control. *Oncology Nursing Forum, 27*(6), 975–984.

*Sugarek, N. J., Deyo, R. A., & Holmes, B. C. (1988). Locus of control and beliefs about cancer in a multi-ethnic clinic population. *Oncology Nursing Forum, 15*(4), 481–486.

*Swinney, J. E. (2002). African Americans with cancer: The relationships among self-esteem, locus of control, and health perception. *Research in Nursing and Health, 25*(5), 371–382.

*Tomaino-Brunner, C., Freda, M. C., & Runowicz, C. D. (1996). "I hope I don't have cancer": Colposcopy and minority women. *Oncology Nursing Forum, 23*(1), 39–44.

Trapido, E. J., Valdez, R. B., Obeso, J. L., Strickman-Stein, N., Rotger, A., & Perez-Stable, E. J. (1995). Epidemiology of cancer among Hispanics in the United States. *Monographs of the National Cancer Institute, 18*, 17–28.

*Underwood, S. M. (1991). African-American men. Perceptual determinants of early cancer detection and cancer risk reduction. *Cancer Nursing, 14*, 281–288.

Underwood, S. (1991). Cancer risk reduction behavior among African American men. Focus on learned helplessness. *Journal of Community Health Nursing, 9*, 21–31.

*Underwood, S. M. (1999). Breast cancer screening among African American women: Addressing the needs of African American women with known and no known risk factors. *Journal of the National Black Nurses Association, 10*(1), 46–55.

United States Department of Commerce. (1978). Directive No.15. Race and ethnic standards for Federal statistics and administrative reporting. In *Statistical policy handbook.* Washington, DC: U.S. Department of Commerce, Office of Federal Statistical Policy and Standards.

United States Department of Health and Human Services. (1990). *Healthy people 2000: National health promotion and disease prevention objectives.* Washington, DC: U.S. Government Printing Office.

United States Department of Health and Human Services. (2000). *Healthy people 2010: Understanding and improving health.* Washington, DC: U.S. Government Printing Office.

Weinrich, S. P. (1994). *Interventions to increase prostate cancer screening.* Bethesda, MD: National Cancer Institute, National Institutes of Health, CA60561-01.

*Weinrich, S., Royal, C., Pettaway, C. A., Dunston, G., Faison-Smith, L., Priest, J. H., Roberson-Smith, P., Frost, J., Jenkins, J., Brooks, K. A., & Powell, I. (2002). Interest in genetic prostate cancer susceptibility testing among African American men. *Cancer Nursing, 25*(1), 28–34.

*Weinrich, S. P., Weinrich, M. C., Boyd, M. D., Atwood, J., & Cervenka, B. (1994). Teaching older adults by adapting for aging changes. *Cancer Nursing, 17*(6), 494–500.

Weinrich, S., Weinrich, M., Boyd, M., Johnson, E., & Frank-Stromborg, M. (1992). Knowledge of colorectal cancer among older persons. *Cancer Nursing, 15*(5), 322–330.

*Willis, M. A., Davis, M., Cairns, N. U., & Janiszewski, R. (1989). Inter-agency collaboration: Teaching breast self-examination to Black women. *Oncology Nursing Forum, 16*(2), 171–177.

*Wilmoth, M. C., & Sanders, L. D. (2001). Accept me for myself: African American women's issues after breast cancer. *Oncology Nursing Forum, 28*(5), 875–879.

*Zimmerman, S. M. (1997). Factors influencing Hispanic participation in prostate cancer screening. *Oncology Nursing Forum, 24*(3), 499–504.

Chapter 10

Mental Health and Disabilities: What We Know About Racial and Ethnic Minority Children

MARY LOU DE LEON SIANTZ AND BETTE RUSK KELTNER

ABSTRACT

The recognition that children and adolescents suffer from mental health problems and disabilities is a recent phenomenon, not arising until the late 19th century. Because of the increasing numbers and importance of ethnic minority children and youth to the vitality of the United States, their mental health and disabilities can no longer be overlooked. Mental health is paramount for fostering social integration, unity, and inclusiveness within and between ethnic groups. Thus the significance of changing demographics and the disparity in mental health indicators make this a key issue for the future. Nursing research in this area has been limited, in spite of the fact that mental health problems and disabilities exert a disproportionate negative effect on racial and ethnic minority children (NIMH, 2001a). The purpose of this chapter is to critique the available nursing research on mental health and disabilities in racial and ethnic minority children, including how such research has been conceptualized, conducted, and interpreted.

Keywords: children, disabilities, health disparities, mental health

Knowledge about the treatments and prevention of mental health problems or disabilities among children and adolescents has only begun to develop during the last two decades, and little attention has been given to the mental health and disabilities of racial and ethnic minority children (NIMH, 2001a). Nursing research in this area has been especially limited, in spite of the fact that mental health problems and disabilities exert a disproportionate negative effect on racial and ethnic minority children (NIMH, 2001a). The purpose of this chapter is to critique the available nursing research on mental health and disabilities in racial and ethnic minority children, including how such research has been conceptualized, conducted, and interpreted.

In 1978, the President's Commission of Mental Health commented that low-income minority children and adolescents were especially at risk for psychological disorders and behavioral problems because of their socioeconomic status, social isolation, stressful environments, and lack of access to mental health services. More than 2 decades later, these conditions have not changed in the United States (NIMH, 2000; USPHS, 1999). Research in the prevention and treatment of disabilities and mental health problems in ethnic minority children remains a priority. Such research has never been more critically needed, because the numbers of ethnic minority children are growing. There are serious consequences associated with the paucity of nursing, as the phenomenon of mental health disabilities among children has become increasingly recognized as a priority in the United States in the President's New Freedom Commission on Mental Health. Preliminary recommendations from this commission emphasize the "need to identify policies that could be implemented by federal, state and local governments to maximize the utility of existing resources, improve coordination of treatments and services, and promote successful community integration for adults and children with mental illness." Evidence-based practice must account for underlying social conditions as well as biologic vulnerabilities that exist for many minority children (Algeria, Perez, & Williams, 2003) and nursing research could add significantly to this need.

The 2000 U.S. Census cited that there were 12,342,259 Hispanics, 10,885,696 African Americans, 840,312 American Indians and Alaska Natives, and 2,464,999 Asians and 127,179 Pacific Islanders under 18 years of age (U.S. Census Bureau, 2001). Racial and ethnic minority children comprise an increasing proportion of the American population, and they bear a greater burden of mental health needs and physical or developmental disabilities (NIMH, 2001b; USDHHS, 2001).

METHOD

Using keywords that included *child/adolescent psychiatric nursing, acculturation*, and *mental health and psychiatric research*, MEDLINE and

PsychINFO databases from 1980 to 2002 were searched; they yielded 100 citations. Additional keywords that were added included *ethnic/minority children and adolescent mental health/disabilities,* and *special education,* with ethnic descriptors of *African American, Asian Hispanic/Latino, Native American, American Indian, Pacific Islander,* and *Filipino.* Titles and abstracts were reviewed that matched keywords, resulting in 20 articles. Among these, 9 nursing studies were identified in three specific categories: descriptive, longitudinal, and intervention research.

In these 20 studies researchers described the disparities in child and adolescent mental health and the inaccessible mental health services among ethnic and minority children, including inadequate referral to appropriate care and an inadequate diagnostic process. Researchers reported an association between culture, race, and ethnicity and the inability to express mental health problems or identify treatment needs. The overall effects of poverty on child and adolescent mental health among ethnic/minority children were particularly highlighted (McLeod & Shanahan, 1996; Samaan, 2000). Several researchers (Buriel, 1994; Garcia-Coll et al., 1996; Laosa, 1989, 1990; McLoyd, 1998; Slaughter-Defoe, Nakagawa, Takanishi, & Johnson, 1990) discussed culturally appropriate models to guide the needed research. These research models focused on investigating protective factors as well as risk factors.

Other researchers described the growing incidence of specific mental health problems like depression among adolescent immigrants (Rumbaut & Portes, 2001), access to health services (Newacheck & Nung, 2002), or help-seeking behavior by ethnic minority adolescents. For example, Cauce, Domenech-Rodriguez, Paradise, Cochran, and Shea (2002), in an ethnographic study, determined that cultural factors affected treatment selection among ethnic minority adolescents. This research team underscored the importance of understanding how adolescents and their families identify problems, seek help, and engage in treatment. Samples included both within-group comparisons of a specific minority group and cross-comparisons of two or more groups.

The nine nursing studies identified for this review are presented according to the type of design used: descriptive, longitudinal, or intervention. In each of these categories, the strengths and weaknesses of the research are summarized.

Descriptive Research

Keltner's study of children in a Head Start program (1990) identified positive family factors associated with competence in preschool Black children. Keltner examined family characteristics that could potentially mediate the negative effects of poverty. The sample included 93 African American preschool children (48 males and 45 females) enrolled at two different metropolitan Head Start programs. It was found that families that engaged in predictable routine interactions were more likely to have children who demonstrated interest and participation in preschool. Family routines were also associated with cooperative and compliant behaviors among preschoolers. Older fathers had children who were more cooperative and compliant.

In another descriptive study that considered parental correlates of social and behavioral competence among Mexican migrant preschool children, Siantz and Smith (1994) found within-group differences among the parents and children. Subjects in this study included 60 randomly selected, primarily Spanish-speaking, Mexican migrant, 3- to 8-year-old children (48% male, 40% female), their parents, and teachers registered with the Texas Migrant Council's Migrant Head Start program in the Lower Rio Grande Valley of Texas, a population that was considered representative of the Mexican migrant population of the United States. The study used within-group analysis to understand the variance among the Mexican migrant children and their parents without comparing them to a non-Mexican sample. Parental social support was found to directly influence parents, and indirectly their preschool children. Siantz and Smith (1994) focused not only on maladjustment and negative outcomes associated with risk, but also on the importance of identifying competence and positive child outcomes and the protective factors that support such outcomes.

Because of the heterogeneity among racial and ethnic minority subgroups and the lack of knowledge and understanding about individual subgroups, it is important to study individual subgroups before making comparisons within or between minority and majority groups. Keltner's research with Native American children also underscores the importance of investigating within-group characteristics. With American Indians, variations not only exist among the many tribes, but also within particular tribes (Keltner, 1993).

In an ethnographic study of Native American children, Keltner (1993) identified family and community values that served as protective sources of support in the presence of environmental risk in two diverse Indian communities: the Lakota Sioux Indians on the Pine Ridge Reservation in South Dakota and the Alabama Indian Commission, which represents seven tribes. Leaders from the two Indian groups collaborated with Keltner and the research team to ensure that family strengths were identified and understood. Qualities of self-sufficiency, group identity, and reserve were identified as cultural markers of strength. Personal harmony with nature was particularly associated with mental health. Illness among Indians was considered a lack of harmony with nature. Signs and symptoms may overlap with conventional medical diagnoses.

In other ethnographic research, Keltner and Ramey (1994) studied the traditional values, beliefs, and cultural responses of American Indians to mental retardation. Most native Indian languages do not even have a word for *disability*. For some Indian groups, however, particular conditions have powerful meanings. For example, among Southwest tribes, epilepsy is by tradition considered a sign of sibling incest, thought to be harmful to the community as well as the individual.

Indian culture and community influence responses to mental retardation. For some parents, concern about the condition is focused on potential instead of limitation. For example, in one family's response, Keltner and Ramey (1994) described parents asking if their child will be able to "feed the chickens." Others may contest accepting a mental health label. Keltner reported that a well-educated professional family that adopted a Lakota Sioux boy with fetal alcohol syndrome resisted the label of *mental retardation*, believing that it was a purely cultural and misapplied term. Harmony for this family was only restored when the father accepted his child's biologically based condition and began to find ways to support his child's growth and development.

Keltner's research underscores the importance of investigating the variations that exist among tribes as well as within tribes. The ability to adapt and sometimes flourish under duress and extreme circumstances is a phenomenon under study in the Native American community. Resilience theory has been particularly relevant to the identification of cultural protective factors thought to mediate risks.

Far less is known about protective factors than about risks among racial and ethnic minority children. Research utilizing resilience theory, as these studies have shown, needs to conceptualize, study, and consider the behavioral problems, emotional problems, and disabilities of ethnic minority children with a new outlook. Such views need to consider positive outcomes and not just focus on disorders, deficits, risks, and vulnerabilities.

SUMMARY

The strengths of some of the studies by Keltner and Siantz is that they used within-group analyses to understand variance within the subgroups under study and identified specific protective cultural factors in their samples. Samples were not compared with a different minority or nonminority subgroup. Until recently, research on the mental health and disabilities of racial and ethnic minority children has been guided by inappropriate theoretical models such as the "deficit model." These models have been based on assumptions of deficiencies, and they have not considered culture or context. White middle-class norms have been the standard. Models that show promise of understanding the mental health and disabilities among ethnic minority children consider race, culture, context, ethnicity (Garcia Coll et al., 1996), risk, and resilience (Garmezy, 1993; Garmezy, Masten, & Tellegen, 1984).

Longitudinal Research

Two researchers have conducted longitudinal research on the mental health of ethnic minority children and families (Gross & Tucker, 1994; Gross, Conrad, Fogg, Willis, & Garvey, 1995; Gross, Wrenetha, & Fogg, 2001; Siantz, 2003).

Gross et al. (1995) conducted a prospective longitudinal study concerning the relationship between maternal depression and the mental health of two cohorts of preschool children in a community sample. Two cohorts of children and their mothers were followed over a 1-year period. Daycare providers completed two instruments measuring the children's social competence and behavior problems at the end of the year. Preschool mental health was rated by the day-care or preschool teacher. The Social Competence Scale (Kohn, 1977) and the Kohn Symptom Checklist (Kohn, 1977) were used. The maternal sample of Cohort 1 included 49% Whites, 41% African Americans, and 6% Hispanics, with an average of 2 children per mother. In cohort 2, 29% of the mothers were White, 49% were African American, and 19% were Hispanic. Gross et al. (1995) found that Cohort 1 mothers reported more depressive symptoms than Cohort 2 mothers. No significant differences were found in preschool mental health or maternal depression by race.

Results indicated that maternal depression was significantly related to lower social competence and more behavior problems in the children. Although there were no significant differences in child mental health scores by gender, boys of more depressed mothers were more likely to have poorer social competence and more behavior problems than girls. Item analyses suggested that the boys' behavior might have been especially aversive for depressed mothers, increasing the likelihood that these mothers would respond to and reinforce their son's challenging behavior.

In this study, little cultural information was provided besides the ethnic and racial composition of the sample. Within-group differences were not explored. The rationale for comparing three ethnic subgroups with a White nonminority sample was not described. The ethnicity of the day-care provider or of the day-care environment was not described. It may be that differences between the ethnicities of the day-care providers, the individual day-care environments, and the child may influence the child's behavior as well as the perception of a child's behavior. This is especially true if a second language is involved. There is ample evidence that those who lack familiarity with particular cultural subgroups may be more likely to incorrectly interpret what they see (Wallen, 1992). This may have been especially true if the day-care provider who rated a child was from a different racial or ethnic minority group than the child. While income levels for the sample were included, years of education were not.

This study did not provide any details of the ethnic minority participants, in spite of the fact that they made up more than half the sample. Given the significance of the association between maternal depression and preschool children's social competence and behavior problems, prevention is indicated. However, replication of this study or development of a culturally sensitive preventive intervention tailored to the race and ethnicity of the mothers and children included in this study would be a challenge to the design, based on the available data included in this study.

Siantz (2003) conducted a study to identify risk and protective factors that support the preschool child's social, language, and cognitive competence at two points in time. The sample included 220 Mexican migrant preschoolers enrolled in the Texas Migrant Council's Migrant Head Start program and their parents. This report was part of a larger study (Siantz & Smith, 1994). Parents were interviewed, and children were tested twice. The first time occurred during the fall after they had returned from their seasonal migration during the harvest season. The second time occurred the following fall. Parents were interviewed in either Spanish or English at home or at the migrant Head Start Center. Children were also given the choice of being tested in English or Spanish and frequently went back and forth. They were tested at the local Migrant Head Start Center. Examiners were bilingual and reliable in their testing after training. Many of them were former migrant farm workers themselves and were now working in the local community.

In this sample, fathers were more depressed than mothers, although both parents were at higher risk for depression than the general population at both data collection periods. Children's cognitive abilities were two standard deviations below the general population. Their motor skills were better than the general population's. At preschool, their language abilities were below the general population's in both Spanish and English. At the second point of data collection, language abilities improved. This may have been due to their preschool experience. Social competence was associated with parental mental health and parenting behavior. If parents felt supported, they were more likely to be warm and nurturing to their children. This in turn was associated with social competence among peers at the preschool.

Limitations of the study included the fact that it was done in the migrant home base and not during the seasonal migration. Responses were subject to recall of experiences during the previous harvest season just completed. Retention was also a challenge. Several of the participants returned to Mexico, while others moved to other parts of Texas and found permanent employment, leaving the migrant stream.

Intervention Research

Several intervention studies on parent training to promote positive parenting and prevent conduct disorder were reported by Gross (Gross & Tucker, 1994; Gross et al., 1995) and Webster-Stratton. However, with the exception of Gross et al. (1995), Gross, Wrenetha, and Fogg (2001), and Webster-Stratton (1998a, 1998b) nursing intervention studies on mental health and disabilities among racial and ethnic minority children were limited.

Researchers have found that certain family characteristics place children at risk for developing conduct problems. These characteristics include low income, low education, teen pregnancy, isolation, high levels of stress, single parenthood, parental psychiatric illness, parental criminal history or substance abuse, and high levels of marital discord (Webster-Stratton, 1990). A child's risk of developing conduct problems increases exponentially with the child's exposure to each additional risk factor (Coi et al., 1993). Children in Head Start populations are at higher than average risk for developing conduct problems because risk factors are present at higher than average rates in the families served (McLoyd, 1990).

To examine the efficacy of a parent intervention to prevent conduct disorders, a clinical trial was designed (Webster-Stratton, 1998b). Nine

Head Start centers were randomly assigned (by lottery) to either an experimental condition in which parents, teachers, and family service workers participated in the intervention (PARTNERS) or to a control group in which parents, teachers, and family service workers participated in the regular center-based Head Start program (CONTROL). These nine centers were chosen on the basis of their similarity in terms of ethnic minority percentages, teachers' and family service worker qualifications and education, number of classrooms, number of children, children's enrollment age, and length of Head Start class (4 hours/day). Centers were also chosen on the basis of their willingness to participate. This study illustrates the extra effort that is sometimes needed to ensure adequate numbers of ethnic and minority parents and children in both the control and experimental groups. In this study, three of the centers that were assigned to the intervention condition remained in that condition during the second year. As a result, there were more families in the experimental than in the control condition, making comparisons difficult.

The short-term and long-term findings of this study suggested that the parenting program was successful because it strengthened parenting competence and reduced an inconsistent, harsh, or overly critical parenting style. The intervention also increased parental involvement in the school as reported by the teachers. Finally, when observed in the home, experimental children in the study demonstrated significant drops in negative behaviors, noncompliance, and negative affect and significant increases in positive affect in their interactions with mothers compared with control children, whose behaviors remained stable. One year later, experimental children continued to have significant increases in their levels of positive affect and decreases in negative affect in their interactions with their mothers at home, compared to control children.

A major limitation reported in this study was the significant difference between the intervention and control condition in regard to minority status. The control group had a higher percentage (47%) of minorities than the intervention group (33%). Webster-Stratton reported an effort to match for ethnicity when selecting centers. However, some neighborhoods were more populated by certain ethnic groups than others. Although all other demographic and family risk factors were comparable across the two conditions, it was unclear how this difference in minority status may have influenced the results.

Another reported limitation was that the question remained whether the parenting program worked differently for minority families in the intervention condition. Since there were six different Asian groups, in addition to Hispanic, African American, Native American, and various combinations, there was not a large enough sample of any one minority group to conduct analyses by groups. Furthermore, there was no justification to combine all of the various minority groups.

Based on the findings, it is not possible to identify implications for preventive intervention with racial and ethnic minority children. Without targeting racial and ethnic minority families in their own right, the numbers remain small. However, in the following section, factors that facilitate the participation of low-income parents are described. These factors provide effective strategies that can be generalized to recruit and retain racial and ethnic minority populations. It is important to understand that it is the program characteristics, not the clients, that determine the success of parent training with low-income populations.

Webster-Stratton (1998b) identified important strategies to engage and maintain low-income parents from the previous study that can be used with racial and ethnic minority parents who overwhelmingly are low income. Parents were engaged in the intervention study in collaborative training groups, which were also used as a support system for the parents.

According to Webster-Stratton (1998b), successful parenting intervention studies need to be community-based first and involve parents in the planning and recruitment. Parents should also be involved as co-group leaders and help to set priorities for program content. Intervention studies need to be realistic and consider the constraints of low-income parents, providing child care, transportation, food, and evening groups as well as daytime groups. Program delivery should build on collaboration with parents for developing solutions alongside with the trainer. Training methods should be responsive to a variety of learning styles and use performance-based training methods such as videotape modeling, role playing, and home assignments. Content needs to be relevant and sensitive to individual parent needs and family circumstances. Group formats are not only cost effective but also strengthen social networks within the family and the community, leading to parental empowerment. Such intervention research strategies will lead to the engagement of parents, with such involvement helping parents to learn the content and gain the control and competence they need to cope with the stresses of parenting under the conditions of poverty (Webster-Stratton, 1998b).

In an intervention study that sought to determine what motivated participation or dropout among low-income racial and ethnic minority families, Gross et al. (2001) recruited 155 families into a parent training group. This study is an example of research that is trying to apply a community partnership model to sustain participant interest and motivation. Of particular interest was the response of the participants when asked about their reaction to incentives and motivations to participate after they had already made the commitment to participate. The purpose of the training was to reduce child behavior problems and coercive disciplinary strategies and to promote positive parent-child relationships and children's social competence. The investigator used 11 licensed day-care centers serving low-income families of toddlers in Chicago. About 60.5% of the population were African American families, and 33.1% were Latino. The 12-week intervention was planned as an intervention for families who might not have the opportunity to participate in such a program. The program was developed by Webster-Stratton (1990) and has been previously demonstrated to be effective in reducing child behavior problems and promoting positive parenting strategies, primarily in Caucasian families of older children with a history of conduct disorder.

Parents who completed baseline measures and enrolled in one of the parent training groups were interviewed by telephone or in person about their decision to enroll. Average attendance was 5.45 sessions among the 155 parents who enrolled in the intervention and 7.4 sessions among the 108 parents who did not drop out of the program. Of the 155 enrolled parents, 26.5% attended 0 or 1 of the parent group sessions, 26.5% attended only 2–5 sessions, and 47% attended 6 or more sessions. Thirty percent of the parents ($n = 47$) dropped out because of low attendance or failure to complete the postintervention assessment. Attrition was not related to education, employment status, income, race, relationship of the participating parent to the target child, parental age, child gender, childbirth order, parity, or parent immigration status. Unmarried parents with partners were more likely to drop out of the group than parents who were married, single, or foster parents.

A particularly important outcome for the investigator was insight into the need to conceptualize low-income research participants as consumers rather than subjects. The researcher noted the need to ask participants whether recruitment and retention strategies were meaningful to them. Of special note is Gross's recommendation to consider that participant reactions to recruitment and retention strategies may be specific to certain developmental periods, neighborhoods, or cultures. By considering participant reaction subgroup by subgroup, researchers will be more likely to construct intervention research that can be effectively offered and attended by minority participants, with implications for specific minority populations. Subjects may be more likely to participate because others around them will be more like them. In turn, participants will feel like a partner instead of a subject.

Another important finding from this study was the fact that parents participated in this study because the intervention also gave them personal support. It helped strengthen their parenting skills in spite of the fact that the intervention focused on their child's behavior, and not theirs.

SUMMARY

The nine nursing studies included in the review were relatively recent, having been conducted during the 1990s. Developmental periods ranged from preschool through adolescence. Multiple sources of data were used, including institutional records, parents, day-care providers, teachers, as well as child self-reports. Data collection methods used included observations, interviews, home and school visits, and focus groups. Findings focused primarily on African Americans, Hispanic/Latinos, and Native Americans. Parents were studied as well as children, with parents identified as critical resources for children. Research included both urban and rural samples and community environments like day-care centers, family homes, and schools. Studies ranged from single descriptions at one point in time ($N = 5$), to descriptions over time ($N = 2$), and interventions ($N = 2$).

Two researchers (Keltner, 1990; Siantz, 1997) identified the importance of focusing on cultural strengths and protective factors, not just risks. African American family qualities associated with the social competence of preschool children were investigated (Keltner, 1990). The cultural characteristics of Native American children and adolescents and their mental health needs (Keltner, 1993), and the cultural beliefs concerning mental retardation of two diverse American Indian communities (Keltner & Ramey, 1994) using ethnographic methodology were described. Correlates of developmental outcomes among Mexican migrant children were also studied at one point in time (Siantz & Smith, 1994) and at two points in time (Siantz, 2003). Others sought to examine the relationship between maternal depression and preschool children's mental health in a community sample of low-income African American and Hispanic mothers.

The only intervention study of the prevention of conduct problems in low-income children (Webster-Stratton, 1998a) included diverse minority groups in its sample, but not a large enough sample of any one group to conduct analyses by groups and too diverse to combine minority groups. In separate papers based on this study, Webster-Stratton (1998b) and Gross et al. (2001) discussed critical features of the intervention that promoted low-income parental engagement in the study. Neither study focused on one ethnic minority subgroup. Of particular note was Gross's recommendation to construct recruitment and retention strategies for intervention studies on a case-by-case basis with low-income subjects taking into consideration the uniqueness of the population being studied.

Research with racial and ethnic minority children and families has usually relied on two-group studies to demonstrate the manner in which culture explains differences between the minority group and Euro-Americans. In Gross et al.'s study (1995), little cultural information was provided besides the ethnic or racial category. Differences within each group were not explored. The rationale for comparing three ethnic subgroups with a White nonminority sample was not described.

Typically, two-group comparison studies draw random samples of Euro-American and minority children and parents, compare the two groups on a parent or child variable, and then conclude that any difference between the two groups is the result of culture. Often the results are discussed in terms of how the minority parents and children are different from the Euro-American parents and children.

Drawing random samples of ethnic minority subgroups and then using the means to make conclusions about culture is misleading, because it assumes that the minority groups are homogeneous. In reality, for example, a random sample of Mexican American children and parents will produce a sample with individuals who differ on a variety of culturally related characteristics, such as proficiency of language spoken, generation status, length of time in the United States, and level of acculturation (Buriel & DeMent, 1997).

RECOMMENDATIONS FOR FUTURE RESEARCH

A need exists for longitudinal research that will follow developmental trajectories and provide new knowledge about prevention of mental health problems and disability over time. Gross and Webster-Stratton's research provides a start toward the controlled clinical trials that are needed to prevent and eliminate disparities in mental health and disabilities.

More within-group research, such as Keltner's and Siantz's work, is needed, with eventual cross-comparison once the body of knowledge of specific subgroups is established. Even more than adults, children need to be studied in the context of their social environments and their families and peers, as all of the studies reviewed have done.

Learning about other cultures requires intensive study, time, expertise, and commitment. A side effect of superficial attention to culture is trivializing serious mental illness or disability as a culturally distinct characteristic. Researchers need to consider why racial and ethnic minority parents may not adhere to protocols that may benefit their children. Is a reserved manner an indicator of inadequate social interaction or a cultural strength, as Keltner and Ramey (1994) point out? What unique protective factors exist to support the family that will indirectly promote the social competence and resilience of ethnic minority children?

Despite the fact that research on mental health and disabilities among ethnic minority children is challenging, child and adolescent nurse researchers must continue to develop and test nursing interventions that are sensitive to the developmental and cultural needs of infants, preschoolers, school-aged children, and adolescents at risk or experiencing mental health problems to establish their reliability and validity (Siantz, 1992). A need exists to remove the stigma of mental and physical handicaps that ethnic minority children experience by producing partnerships that will educate nurses in mental health and disabilities and promote research that will reduce the disparities that racial and ethnic minority children and their families are currently experiencing.

REFERENCES

Alegria, M., Perez, D., & Williams, S. (2003). The role of public policies in reducing mental health status disparities for people of color. *Health Affairs, 22*(5), 51–64.

Buriel, R. (1994). Acculturation, respect for cultural differences, and biculturalism among three generations of Mexican-Americans and European-American school children. *Journal of Genetic Psychology, 154,* 531–543.

Buriel, R., & De Ment, T. (1997). Immigration and sociocultual change in Mexican, Chinese, and Vietnamese American families. In A. Booth, A. C. Croutre, & N. Landale (Eds.), *Immigration and the family: Research and policy on U.S. Immigrants* (pp. 165–200), Mahwah, NJ: Lawrence Erlbaum.

Cauce, A. M., Domenech-Rodriguez, M., Paradise, M., Cochran, B. N., & Shea, J. M. (2002). Cultural and contextual influences in mental health help seeking: A focus on ethnic minority youth. *Journal of Consulting and Clinical Psychology,* *70*(1), 44–55.

Coi, J. D., Watt, N. F., West, S. G., Hawkins, D., Asarnow, J. R., Markman, H. J., Ramey, S. L., Shure, M. B., & Long, B. (1993). The science of prevention: A conceptual framework and some directions for a national research program. *American Psychologist, 48,* 1013–1022.

Garcia Coll, C. T., Lambert, G., Jenkins, R., McAdoo, H. P., Crnic, K., Wasik, B. H., & Vasquez Garcia, H. G. (1996). An integrative model for the study of developmental competencies in minority children. *Child Development, 67,* 1891–1914.

Garmezy, N. (1993). Children in poverty: Resilience despite risk. *Psychiatry, 56,* 127–136.

Garmezy, N., Masten, A. S., & Tellegen, A. (1984). The study of stress and competence in children: A building block for developmental psychopathology. *Child Development, 55,* 97–111.

Gross, D., Conrad, B., Fogg, L., Willis, L., & Garvey, C. (1995). A longitudinal model of maternal depression and preschool children's mental health. *Nursing Research, 44,* 96–101.

Gross, D., & Tucker, S. (1994). Parenting confidence during toddlerhood: A comparison of mothers and fathers. *Nurse Practitioner, 19,* 29–34.

Gross, D., Wrenetha, J., & Fogg, L. (2001). What motivates participation and dropout among low-income urban families of color in a prevention intervention? *Family Relations, 50,* 246–254.

Institute of Medicine (IOM). (1989). *Research on children and adolescents with mental, behavioral, and developmental disorders: Mobilizing a national initiative. Report of a study by a committee of the Institute of Medicine.* Washington, DC: National Academy Press.

Keltner, B. (1990). Family characteristics of preschool social competence among Black children in a Head Start program. *Child Psychiatry and Human Development, 21*(2), 95–108.

Keltner, B. (1993). Native American children and adolescents: Cultural distinctiveness and mental health needs. *Journal of Child and Adolescent Psychiatric and Mental Health Nursing, 6*(4), 18–23.

Keltner, B., & Ramey, S. (1994). Mental retardation in the Indian culture. *Civitan Magazine, 74,* 16–17.

Kohn, M. (1977). The Kohn Social Competence Scale and Kohn Symptom Checklist for the preschool child: A follow-up report. *Journal of Abnormal Child Psychology, 5,* 249–263.

Laosa, L. (1989). Social competence in childhood: Toward a developmental, socioculturally relativistic paradigm. *Journal of Applied Developmental Psychology, 10,* 447–468.

Laosa, L. (1990). Psychosocial stress, coping, and development of Hispanic immigrant children. In F. C. Seraafica, A. I. Schwebel, R. K. Russell, P. D. Isaac, & L. B. Myers (Eds.), *Mental health of ethnic minorities* (pp. 227–251). Norwood, NJ: Ablex.

McLeod, J. D., & Shanahan, M. J. (1996). Trajectories of poverty and children's mental health. *Journal of Health and Social Behavior, 37*, 207–220.

McLoyd, V. (1990). The impact of economic hardship on Black families and children: Psychological distress, parenting, and socioemotional development. *Child Development, 61*, 311–346.

McLoyd, V. (1998). Changing demographics in the American population: Implications for research on minority children and adolescents. In V. McLoyd & L. Steinberg (Eds.), *Studying minority adolescents: Conceptual, methodological, and theoretical issues* (pp. 3–28). Mahwah, NJ: Lawrence Erlbaum.

National Institute of Mental Health. (2000). *The Surgeon General's Conference on Children's Mental Health: Developing a national agenda.* Rockville, MD: U.S. Department of Health and Human Services.

National Institute of Mental Health National Advisory Mental Health Council, Work Group on Child and Adolescent Mental Health Intervention Development and Deployment. (2001a). *Blueprint for change: Research on child and adolescent mental health.* Rockville, MD: U.S. Department of Human Services.

National Institute of Mental Health. (2001b). *Draft strategic plan for reducing health disparities.* Rockville, MD: U.S. Department of Health and Human Services, National Institutes of Health.

Newacheck, P., Hung, Y., & Wright, K. (2002). Racial and ethnic disparities in access to care for children with special health care needs. *Ambulatory Pediatrics, 2*, 247–254.

Rumbaut, R., & Portes, A. (2001). Introduction-ethnogenesis: Coming of age in immigrant America. In R. Rumbaut & A. Portes (Eds.), *Ethnicities: Children of immigrants in America* (pp. 1–21). Los Angeles: University of California Press.

Samaan, R. A. (2000). The influences of race, ethnicity, and poverty on mental health of children. *Journal of Health Care for the Poor and Underserved, 11*(1), 100–110.

Siantz, de Leon, M. L. (1992). Directions in research of psychiatric nursing care of children and adolescents. In P. West & C. L. Sieloff Evans (Eds.), *Psychiatric and mental health nursing with children and adolescents* (pp. 391–405). Gaithersburg, MD: Aspen.

Siantz, de Leon, M. L. (1997). Factors that impact development outcomes of immigrant children. In A. Booth, A. C. Crouter, & N. Landale (Eds.), *Immigration and the family: Research and policy on U.S. immigrants* (pp. 149–161). Mahwah, NJ: Lawrence Erlbaum.

Siantz, de Leon, M. L. (2003). *Predictors of language, problem solving ability, and social competence of migrant Head Start children.* National and Seasonal Head Start Conference, Washington, DC.

Siantz, de Leon, M. L., & Smith, M. S. (1994). Parental factors correlated with developmental outcome in the Migrant Head Start Child. *Early Childhood Research Quarterly, 9*, 481–503.

Slaughter-Defoe, D. T., Nakagawa, K., Takanishi, R., & Johnson, D. J. (1990). Toward cultural/ecological perspectives on schooling and achievement in African and Asian American children. *Child Development, 61*, 363–383.

U.S. Census Bureau. (2001). *Profile of general demographic characteristics: 2000 Census of population and housing, United States.* Washington, DC: Author.

U.S. Department of Health and Human Services. (2001). *Mental health: Culture, race, and ethnicity. A supplement to mental health: A report of the Surgeon General.* Rockville, MD. U.S. Department of Health and Human Services, Public Health Service, Office of the Surgeon General.

USPHS. (1999). *Mental health: A report of the Surgeon General.* Rockville, MD: U.S. Department of Health and Human Services, Substance Abuse and Mental Health Services Administration, Center for Mental Health Services, National Institute of Health.

Wallen, J. (1992). Providing culturally appropriate mental health services for minorities. *Journal of the Mental Health Administration, 19,* 288–295.

Webster-Stratton, C. (1990). Stress: A potential disrupter of parent perceptions and family interactions. *Journal of Clinical Child Psychology, 19,* 302–312.

Webster-Stratton, C. (1998a). Parent training with low-income families. In J. R. Lutzker (Ed.), *Handbook of child abuse research and treatment* (pp. 183–210). New York: Plenum.

Webster-Stratton, C. (1998b). Preventing conduct problems in Head Start children: Strengthening parenting competencies. *Journal of Consulting and Clinical Psychology, 66,* 715–730.

PART IV

Intervention Approaches for Racial and Ethnic Minority Populations

Chapter 11

Utilization of Complementary and Alternative Medicine Among Racial and Ethnic Minority Populations: Implications for Reducing Health Disparities

ROXANNE STRUTHERS AND LEE ANNE NICHOLS

ABSTRACT

This chapter provides a review of research literature and describes the use of complementary and alternative medicine (CAM) among racial and ethnic minority populations. The relevance of CAM to health disparities is also discussed. *Complementary* and *alternative medicines* are terms used to describe methods of health care beyond the usual Western biomedical model. These treatments are prevalent and increasing in the United States. Many CAM therapies are ancient therapies among certain racial and ethnic minorities. Thus, it seems that complementary and alternative medicine is being used and/or could be used to decrease health disparities among these populations. A review of 26 research articles shows that we are at the beginning stages of examining this phenomenon and that CAM use by any population is only now being described. Of the reviewed studies, 19 studies documented use of CAM among racial and ethnic minorities; 7 revealed that CAM is not used more among ethnic groups than among White (non-Hispanic) populations. Although it is known that racial and ethnic people utilize CAM, the vast array of research questions and aims, CAM definitions, CAM practitioners, and diverse research methodologies result in mixed research findings and conclusions. In some instances, utilization of CAM modalities is stated to be a result of culture among particular groups. Even so, there is currently no evidence that scientifically supports the notion that CAM can be used to reduce health disparities within racial and ethnic minority populations.

Keywords: alternative medicine, complementary medicine, racial and ethnic minorities

Complementary or alternative medicine (CAM) is relatively new to Western biomedical health care. Research is currently being conducted related to CAM use, the effectiveness of CAM therapies, and how to incorporate CAM with other health care modalities and approaches. A topic that is of particular interest is the use of CAM to reduce health disparities among racial and ethnic minority populations in the United States. This chapter will critically review research that examines the use of CAM among these populations and discuss the implications of CAM in the reduction of health disparities.

Complementary and alternative medicines are a relatively new phenomenon to health care. Concern has been expressed by the biomedical field regarding the lack of scientific evidence related to these therapies. As a result, Congress established the National Center for Complementary and Alternative Medicine (NCCAM) in 1998 as an agency within the National Institute of Health. In 2001, NCCAM developed a 5-year strategic plan that identified four strategic areas for implementation: (a) investing in research, (b) training CAM investigators, (c) expanding outreach, and (d) facilitating integration. Each of these four areas includes objectives that address the special needs of America's most vulnerable populations, in particular, racial and ethnic minority groups. NCCAM regards America's diverse racial and ethnic minority groups as an invaluable resource for learning about systems of healing and health practices outside the mainstream. Many CAM practices have originated or are traditional in cultures and countries outside America and, except for the Native population, were brought here by the various populations that immigrated to the United States (NCCAM, 2003).

COMPLEMENTARY AND ALTERNATIVE MEDICINE

Complementary medicine and *alternative medicine* are commonly used terms to refer to the field of health care outside of or beyond traditional, allopathic, or Western medicine (Eisenberg et al., 1993). CAM includes treatments and health care practices not taught widely in medical schools, not generally used in hospitals (Eisenberg et al., 1993; Eisenberg, Davis, et al., 1998), and not usually reimbursed by medical insurance companies. People use CAM therapies in a variety of ways. CAM therapies used alone are often referred to as *alternative therapies*. When used in addition to conventional medicine, they are often referred to as *complementary*. More recently, the term *integrative medicine* has been introduced to describe the mingling of Western-based medicine and nontraditional CAM health care for which there is some high-quality scientific evidence of safety and effectiveness (NCCAM, 2002).

Western-based biomedicine has been the prevalent health model within the United States. For various reasons, people have returned to ancient holistic methodologies of healing. Use of complementary and alternative medicine among adults in the United States is prevalent and increasing (Eisenberg, Davis, et al., 1998; Kessler et al., 2001). Recent surveys indicate that 42% to 50% of adults use some type of alternative care (Astin, 1998; Eisenberg, Davis, et al., 1998), and Americans spend $27 billion out of pocket annually on complementary and alternative medicine (Eisenberg, Davis, et al., 1998). The typical CAM user is a younger woman of European descent with higher-than-average income and education (Drivdahl & Miser, 1998; Eisenberg et al., 1993; Lee, Lin, Wrensch, Adler, & Eisenberg, 2000; Leung, Dzankie, Manku, & Yuan, 2001). Thus, research to examine if, what, and how racial and ethnic minorities use CAM is important to determine the role of CAM in eliminating health disparities.

CAM covers a broad range of philosophies, approaches, therapies, and systems of care. Snyder and Lindquist (2002) state, "The scope of the field of complementary therapies is very broad and encompasses more than 1,800 therapies and systems of care" (p. xiii). Multiple websites list CAM therapies and are too numerous to mention. Wooten and Sparber (2001) have noted that difficulty and incongruence can occur when discussing and documenting complementary and alternative medicine because of the vastness of the topic area, differences of definition and therapies, and changing terminology.

CULTURE AND CAM

According to Fletcher (2000), illness and healing are not discrete phenomena that can be isolated and examined without considering social, cultural, and political contexts. When people seek care for health problems or other needs, they look for various options within these mentioned realms. Many people are literally going back to nature in their search for improved health and well-being. Some simply practice self-care and seek health care within their cultural group, and many CAM therapies are ancient methodologies with origins in certain cultures (Fontaine, 2000; Wooten & Sparber, 2001). Thus, while the mainstream is just discovering this approach to health and well-being, cultures like the Hispanic, American Indian, Tibetan, and Chinese cultures have used and integrated these approaches for centuries as part of their health care, and they continue their use today.

CAM RESEARCH AMONG RACIAL AND ETHNIC AND MINORITY POPULATIONS

In order to examine CAM research among racial and ethnic minority populations, a comprehensive literature review was conducted using the terms *alternative therapy, alternative medicine, alternative health care, complementary medicine, folk medicine, folk remedies, herbal remedies, health disparities, ethnic, ethnic minority, race, racial and ethnic groups, racial and ethnic differences, health promotion*, and *health*. Databases and dates included in the search included CINAHL (1982 to 2002); Allied and Complementary medicine (AMED) (1985 to 2002); Medline (1966 to 2002); PsychInfo (1972 to 2002); INSPEC (1969 to 2002); EBM Reviews-Cochrane Database of Systematic Reviews (1993 to 2003); Social Science: Article First (1990 to 2003); and Chicano Database (1967 to 2003).

During this literature search, the topic and its relevance to the discipline of nursing were considered, as well as its relevance to racial and ethnic minority populations in this country. The literature search resulted in 183 research studies that identified racial and ethnic minority populations using CAM. It is of interest to note that no research studies were found that examined the efficacy, efficiency, or cost of utilizing CAM in racial and ethnic populations. A total of 26 studies were included in this review, after eliminating duplicate articles, studies that were conducted outside the United States, and studies that did not identify or were not conducted with racial and ethnic minorities.

These 26 research studies included descriptions of CAM use among African American, Asian, Hispanic, and Native American groups, as well as among immigrant and underserved poor populations. Studies included multiple and diverse CAM therapies that have an effect on the physical, psychological, emotional, and spiritual elements of the person. Research reports included the use of CAM between adult males and females and different racial and ethnic minority populations for the purpose of managing illness as well as for health promotion and maintenance. There were six qualitative studies (ethnographic, anthropological qualitative, focus groups, semistructured interviews) and one study that used mixed qualitative and quantitative methods. Nineteen quantitative and descriptive studies were included that used different types of surveys, most self-designed. Organized thematically, this chapter summarizes research studies in the areas of (a) CAM use by ethnic and racial minority populations; (b) CAM use and special health issues: cancer and HIV; and (c) CAM use by specific racial and ethnic populations.

CAM USE BY ETHNIC AND RACIAL MINORITY POPULATIONS

Fourteen articles were concerned with CAM use by ethnic and racial populations. Racial and ethnic groups included in these studies were Hispanic, Native American, African American, Chinese, and Japanese (Asian). The majority of participants in the studies were both adult men and women. Most of the studies used surveys to identify CAM use among these different populations.

Frequency of Use

The frequency of CAM use varied in the populations being studied— anywhere from a high of 78% to a low of 21%. In the study by Ernst (1999), 68% of all participants used some form of CAM in the previous year; 78% of African Americans and 77% of Asians reported CAM use during this time. A study by Arcury, Quandt, Bell, and Vitolins (2002) found that African and Native American elders used home and folk remedies more often than European Americans. Cherniack, Senzel, and Pan (2001) reported that 58% of research participants used CAM. In contrast, Palinkas and Kabongo (2000) reported that only 21% of participants used one or more CAM therapy. Studies by Leung et al. (2001), Liu et al. (2000), and Rhee et al. (2002) found no relationship between race and CAM use.

General practitioners referred clients more frequently to CAM therapy when treating patients for pain, smoking cessation, and asthma. For example, a questionnaire and personal interviews using a semistructured survey were used to survey 300 patients attending hospital outpatient departments (Ernst, 1999). The aim of the study was to investigate patterns of herbal remedy use in the elderly urban population of Hispanic and non-Hispanic Whites in an ambulatory care clinic in New Mexico. A survey instrument was designed by the investigators and pilot-tested. No CAM definition was offered, but a list of herbs commonly used in this particular community was generated by reviewing the available literature and performing a pilot study using open-ended questions in a convenience sample of clinical patients. Sixty-eight percent had used some form of CAM in the previous year. These populations preferred herbal remedies, and half obtained herbal remedies from their country of origin. Half had tried CAM therapies before visiting a physician. Further, 86% of general practitioners referred patients for CAM therapy, mostly for pain, smoking cessation, depression, and asthma—mostly to acupuncturists (58%), osteopaths (58%), homeopaths (36%), and chiropractors (32%).

Arcury et al. (2002) examined ethnic and gender variation in CAM use among older adults. A site-based ethnographic approach was used to identify and recruit female and male African American, European American, and Native American elders, age 70 and older, from two North Carolina counties. One hundred and eight participants were surveyed using open-ended questions at the beginning and at the end of data collection. The definition of CAM was vague. For example, as part of a modified Block Food Frequency Questionnaire, participants were asked about their use of vitamins and minerals. Vitamins that were assessed included calcium, iron, zinc, folate, and Vitamins A, C, E, and B6. In the final interview, participants were asked a series of fixed questions about specific CAM use. Questions asked for information about (1) home remedies (those practices that an individual usually learns through an informal source, for example, traditional or folk remedies that are learned from parents and grandparents or novel remedies that are learned from friends and neighbors); (2) other remedies (turpentine, gasoline, kerosene, WD-40, or tobacco); and (3) the number of practices (chiropractic, biofeedback) used to treat illnesses or conditions or to maintain health. The qualitative data were categorized and analyzed using frequencies, cross-tabulations, and chi square. In this study, most participants used home and folk remedies, vitamins, and mineral supplements. African and Native Americans elders used home and folk remedies more than European Americans, whereas Europeans and Native Americans used vitamin and mineral supplements more than African Americans. Older Native Americans were from two to five times more likely than other ethnic groups to use home remedies.

Three other studies found no relationship between race/ethnicity and CAM use. A research study by Rhee et al. (2002) found that race was not a significant factor in determining use of CAM for 1,027 clients with glaucoma at two urban glaucoma practices. The nine following areas were defined as CAM for use with glaucoma: herbal remedies, acupuncture, homeopathy, faith healing, meditation, megavitamin therapy, therapeutic touch, exercise, and dietary modifications. Similarly, Leung et al. (2001) found that 39.2% of 2,560 patients awaiting elective noncardiac surgery at five San Francisco Bay hospitals admitted to using some form of alternative medicine supplements, of which herbal medicine was the most common type (67.6%). CAM was not clearly defined in the study. The tool was translated into Spanish, Russian, and Chinese. Caucasian race was a variable associated with the preoperative use of herbal medicine. Forty-four percent of participants did not consult with their primary physicians about taking alternative medicine supplements.

In another study conducted by Liu et al. (2000), race was not correlated with CAM use in 376 patients (70% response rate) undergoing preoperative or postoperative cardiothoracic surgical evaluations at an urban academic medical center. CAM, defined as health interventions not generally available at U.S. hospitals or taught widely in medical school, has gained greater acceptance by the general population as a means of maintaining health. The survey consisted of four parts, including demographic information, attitudes toward healing, patterns of use of complementary and alternative medicine, and willingness to discuss the topic with a physician. Only 48% discussed their use of CAM with their physicians, which may have serious safety implications in acute care situations.

Difference Between Majority and Minority Populations

Fourteen articles examined differences in CAM use between majority and racial and ethnic minority populations. Eight articles reported high CAM use among ethnic and racial populations (Arcury et al., 2002; Bair et al., 2002; Baldwin, Long, Kroesen, Brooks, & Bell, 2002; Dole et al., 2000; Ernst, 1999; Lundy, Morgan, Rhoads, & Curtis Bay, 2001; Palinkas &

Kabongo, 2000; Wolsko et al., 2000). Six articles demonstrated no significant differences in CAM use between ethnic and racial minority populations and mainstream populations (Cherniack et al., 2001; Factor-Litvak, Cushman, Kronenberg, Wade, & Kalmuss, 2001; Kroesen, Baldwin, Brooks, & Bell, 2002; Leung et al., 2001; Liu et al., 2000; Rhee et al., 2002). For example, Factor-Litvak et al. (2001) identified minimal differences in CAM use among Whites, African Americans, and Hispanics, whereas Rhee et al. (2002) did not find any significant differences among racial and ethnic groups in their study of participants with glaucoma.

Race was not a significant factor for predicting use of CAM in a study by Factor-Litvak et al. (2001). The purpose of this study was to document the use of complementary and alternative medicine in a cross-sectional, age-stratified telephone survey of 300 female residents living in New York City: 100 White, 100 African American, and 100 Hispanic/Latino women. A definition of CAM was provided, along with a discussion of the limitations and challenges of defining CAM. Three areas of CAM were explored in relation to women's health issues: (1) medicinal teas, homeopathic remedies, herbs, and vitamins, (2) yoga, meditation, spiritual practices, and (3) manual therapies, including chiropractor, massage, and acupressure. Focus groups with African American and Hispanic/Latina women were used to develop the survey questionnaire for this particular study.

Data analysis included descriptive statistics and chi square analysis. More than half the participants had used a CAM therapy, and 40% had visited a CAM practitioner. Most frequently used were medicinal teas, herbs, and vitamins, and practitioners most often visited were chiropractors (18%) and nutritionists (17%). Approximately one third of all treatments were rated as very effective by users. Racial and ethnic differences in CAM use as well as use of specific treatments and practitioners were minimal. The researchers speculated that this resulted from the broad categorization of ethnicity used in the study design.

In another study comparing CAM use among diverse groups, the presence of premenopausal symptoms was a major predictor of subsequent use of CAM in White, Japanese, and Chinese women. Bair et al. (2002) studied participants of the Study of Women's Health Across the Nation (SWAN) to examine self-reported use of herbal, spiritual, and physical manipulation for premenopausal symptoms and CAM use at midlife. Study purposes were to (1) estimate the prevalence and cross-sectional correlates of CAM use in a large, multiethnic sample of women enrolled in the

SWAN; and (2) examine the longitudinal correlates of CAM use in 486 White, Japanese, and Chinese women enrolled at the California SWAN study sites. Data were obtained at baseline and at one year following baseline.

The researchers assessed general use of complementary and alternative therapy use within the past 12 months. Items assessed the use of herbs or herbal remedies. This included homeopathy, Chinese herbs or teas, special diets or nutritional remedies (e.g., macrobiotic or vegetarian diets, vitamins or supplements), psychological methods (e.g., meditation, mental imagery, or relaxation), physical methods (e.g., massage, acupressure, or acupuncture), and folk medicine or traditional Chinese medicine. At a one-year follow-up visit, the participants completed a 105-item survey of CAM therapies. Individual therapies were grouped into the following categories: herbal remedies (16 items), spiritual methods (3 items about spiritual healing or prayer), and physical manipulation (6 items about reflexology, massage, acupressure, acupuncture, and chiropractic). All SWAN participants completed annual self-administered and interviewer-administered surveys eliciting detailed information on sociodemographic factors, lifestyle, and health-related behaviors, physical and mental health status, and menopausal symptoms. Cross-sectional and longitudinal analyses were used to analyze the data.

Almost half of the women had used CAM in the past year. Baseline psychological symptoms were associated with subsequent use of spiritual therapies among White and Chinese women. Conversely, baseline CAM use, rather than the presence of premenopausal symptoms, was a major predictor of subsequent use in White, Japanese, and Chinese women. Japanese women who reported anxiety symptoms and Chinese women who reported psychological symptoms at baseline were more likely to report herb use at the 1-year subsequent visit.

Lundy et al. (2001) also reported ethnic differences in CAM use. In this study, most Anglo and Hispanic patients surveyed in Phoenix, Arizona, reported using alternative medicine concurrently, but they used it in different ways. CAM was defined as "medical interventions not taught widely at U.S. medical schools or generally available at U.S. hospitals" (Eisenberg et al., 1993). English and Spanish versions of the survey instrument were piloted using a sample of 52 patients. The final survey had 22 questions addressing use of various alternative therapies and practitioners and four questions concerning whether or not patients had discussed their use of alternative medicine with their physicians. Demographic information was collected as well as a checklist of 12 chronic health problems. The self-administered questionnaire was administered to 516 low-income Anglo and Hispanic patients at eight community-based family practice clinics in Phoenix, Arizona. Forty-five percent of the participants completed the survey in English and 55% in Spanish. Chi square analysis and Fisher's exact tests were completed. Findings indicated a frequent lack of communication between physicians and their patients regarding use of alternative medicine. Further, Hispanics in the sample used alternative practitioners more frequently than Anglos, while Anglos used alternative therapies more frequently than Hispanics.

In contrast, there was no difference in ethnic use of CAM in a study by Kroesen et al. (2002). In this study, focus group methodology was used to examine issues surrounding CAM. Twelve focus groups were conducted with 100 veterans from this same facility regarding CAM. Recruitment of some of the participants occurred when making telephone calls to a random sample of veterans in a larger study. The ethnicity of only 95 participants was known—87% were non-Hispanic White, 7% were Hispanic, 4% were African American, and 2% were American Indian or Native Alaskan. CAM was defined as unconventional or unorthodox medicine in Western culture. The focus groups were audiotaped, and two authors analyzed the data by developing analytical categories based on project goals and new information provided by the focus group participants. Dissatisfaction with reliance on prescription medications and lack of holism (inadequate information regarding diet, nutrition, and exercise and ignorance of social and spiritual dimensions) were cited as important motivations for turning to CAM. No ethnic or racial difference regarding CAM use was reported.

In a subsequent study, CAM use among non-Hispanic Whites was described. Baldwin et al. (2002) surveyed CAM use among 508 military veterans in Tucson's Veterans Administration Health Care system using a telephone survey. CAM was defined using the categories outlined by the National Institutes of Health National Center on Complementary and Alternative Medicine (NCCAM): alternative medical systems (acupuncture and homeopathy), mind-body intervention (aromatherapy), biological-based therapies (herbal remedies), and manipulative and body-based therapies. A description of the questions asked was provided. Chi-square analysis was conducted. Of those surveyed, 252 or 49.6% reported CAM use. Ethnicity (non-Hispanic White), higher education, greater current daily stress, and overseas military experience were significant predictors of CAM use by the veterans surveyed.

Reasons and Predictors for Use

Reasons and predictors of CAM use varied for the therapies and conditions reported in the studies. For example, Dole at al. (2000) concluded that Hispanic culture may account for increased herb use, the choice and preferred form of herbs, and sources of knowledge (family members) about herbal remedies. Palinkas and Kabongo (2000) reported in a sample of Hispanic primary care patients that recommendations from friends or co-workers, a desire to avoid the side effects of conventional treatments, and the failure of conventional treatments to cure a problem were frequent reasons for using selected CAM therapies. Also, use of folk remedies was associated with Hispanic ethnicity.

In other studies, Wolsko et al. (2000) reported that female gender and lower self-rated health were significant predictors of the use of a CAM practitioner. Ernst (1999) found that Black and Asian populations preferred herbal remedies and that half obtained herbal remedies from their country of origin. Dissatisfaction with reliance on prescription medications and lack of holism (inadequate information regarding diet, nutrition, and exercise and ignorance of social and spiritual dimensions) were cited as important motivations for turning to CAM (Kroesen et al., 2002). Female gender and higher education were correlated with CAM use in a study with multiethnic elders by Cherniack et al. (2001). Leung et al. (2001) reported that Caucasian race was associated with the preoperative use of herbal medicine. Finally, Ernst (1999) found in his study that 86% of the general practitioners referred their clients for CAM therapy but did not describe predictors for how often participants used CAM.

In one study, ethnicity was a predictor for use of CAM therapy. Dole et al. (2000) compared the use of herbal remedies between 186 elderly Hispanic and non-Hispanic Whites attending a university-based ambulatory senior health center in a cross-sectional, interviewer-administered survey of elderly patients seeking care. The aim of the study was to characterize the herbs used in an elderly urban population of Hispanics and non-Hispanics. A definition of CAM was not provided. The survey instrument was developed by the researchers and pilot-tested. Chi-square and logistic regression was used to analyze the data. Overall, 61% of the participants had used a herbal remedy sometime in their life. A larger proportion of Hispanic subjects (77%) used herbal remedies than did non-Hispanic subjects (47%). Significantly more Hispanic subjects grew or gathered their own herbs and received their information from a family member than did the non-Hispanic subjects. Top perceived medical problems that herbs were utilized for included dyspepsia, upper respiratory infections, skin problems, and anxiety/nerves/insomnia.

The authors concluded that Hispanic culture might account for increased herb use, the choice and preferred form of herbs, and the source of knowledge (family members) of herbal remedies. Seventy-seven percent of Hispanic subjects used herbal remedies at some point in their lives, as compared to 47% of non-Hispanic Whites. Hispanics displayed more culturally traditional patterns of herbal use. Non-Hispanic Whites seemed to follow more recent trends in herbal use.

In a study by Palinkas and Kabongo (2000), participants cited several reasons for using CAM therapies. Patients ($N = 541$) 18 years and older attending 16 family practice clinics were recruited to determine their reasons for using CAM during a three-month period. Hispanics were included in the study, but the percentage of Hispanic participants was not reported. Patients were asked to complete a questionnaire administered by a survey worker in the waiting room before the scheduled visit with a family physician. Participants were asked if they used one or more of 16 CAM therapies or therapists for their principal medical condition. The list of CAM therapies was derived from previous studies. Univariate statistics and bivariate statistics, including chi square, paired sample t-test, and ANOVA, were used during data analysis.

Approximately 21% of the patients reported using one or more forms of CAM in conjunction with their most important health problems underlying their visit to the physician. The most common forms of therapies used were chiropractors (34.5%), herbal remedies and supplements (26.7%), and massage therapy (17.2%). Recommendation from friends or coworkers, a desire to avoid the side effects of conventional treatments, and failure of conventional treatments to cure a problem were the most frequently cited reasons for using these therapies. Use of folk remedies was associated with Hispanic ethnicity. Female gender and lower self-rated health were predictors of the use of a CAM practitioner.

In another study, participants were asked about their reasons for using CAM. Wolsko et al. (2000) surveyed 536 clinic attendees in three university hospital-affiliated general ambulatory clinics serving people of different socioeconomic status and racial origin. The objective of the study was to examine if there was a substantial use of a practitioner of alternative or complementary medicine by patients traditionally considered to be underserved. Participants were surveyed at three primary care practice sites and were given a self-administered questionnaire. They were asked about visits to medicine practitioners (acupuncture, chiropractic, herbal/ medicine, vitamin supplements, meditation/relaxation, and massage). No definition of CAM was provided. Findings suggested that CAM use is common in patients considered to be underserved and is not confined to higher socioeconomic groups. Female gender and lower self-rated health were significant predictors of the use of a CAM practitioner.

A cross-sectional survey to investigate the prevalence and predictors of CAM in urban multiethnic older adults was conducted in New York City (Cherniack et al., 2001). A pilot test of the survey questionnaire asked participants ($N = 20$) about their current use of CAM. CAM was not clearly defined in the article, but standard and uniform definitions of different types of alternative medicines were prepared to answer participants' questions about specific modalities. The questionnaire included questions about vitamins and minerals, herbal medicines, antiaging medicines, alternative care systems, and self-help or lifestyle methods. A convenience sample of 421 clients using a veteran's medical clinic and a university geriatrics primary care practice were asked if they had utilized CAM within the previous year. Results indicated that 58% used some form of CAM and 75% at the university practice alone. Female gender and a higher education were correlated with CAM use. Conversely, race, income, age, or self-perceived health status were not correlated with CAM use.

Summary

In summary, 14 articles were reviewed. Five studies discussed frequency of use among different populations. Frequency of use varied depending upon the population. There are no consistent findings that suggest which population uses CAM more frequently. Overall, the studies showed mixed results related to differences between majority and minority population and their use of CAM therapies. Eight articles showed that ethnic and racial minorities use CAM, and 6 demonstrated that CAM use is not different for ethnic and racial populations.

Qualitative focus groups and quantitative survey research methodologies were employed in different types of clinical settings and with diverse participants. Thirteen studies were descriptive, using a survey questionnaire to collect the data via telephone, in person, or through self-administration.

The challenge in documenting CAM use results from the differences in the operationalization of CAM. CAM was often defined by using the work done by Eisenberg et al. (1993). While CAM was defined in some studies, it was not well defined in most studies. Six of the studies developed their own questionnaires for use in the populations being studied, with few instruments being used across studies.

CAM USE AND SPECIAL HEALTH ISSUES: CANCER AND HIV

A major theme that emerged from the review was the use of CAM among racial and ethnic minority populations for specific illnesses—such as AIDS and cancer. Of the seven research studies reviewed, three studies were targeted at specific cancers: prostate, breast, and head and neck cancer. Two other studies examined CAM use among cancer patients listed on the Hawaii tumor registry that had various forms of cancer. Two studies examined CAM use among HIV-positive males. The study methodologies were diverse. One study used qualitative interviews, and the remaining six used quantitative surveys conducted over the telephone, via mail, and in person to examine CAM use in various geographic locations. The studies included adult men and women from the following populations: White, African American, Hispanic, Native Hawaiian, and Asian (specifically Indo-Asian, Chinese, Filipino, and Japanese). CAM was defined using the Eisenberg definition in two studies; one study revised the Alternative Medicine Checklist (AMC) developed by Rowlands and Powderly (1991), and four studies did not define CAM specifically but asked about selected CAM therapies.

Three studies examined use of CAM among patients that had specific types of cancers. Two studies were conducted in the San Francisco Bay area and selected their research sample from the Northern California Cancer Center tumor registry. Lee, Chang, Jacobs, and Wrensch (2002) conducted a 30-minute telephone survey of 543 men diagnosed in 1998 with prostate cancer to determine CAM use among four ethnic populations: White, Black, Hispanic, and Asian. CAM was not defined in the article. However, CAM therapies examined in the survey were described in another article and included dietary rules; herbal remedies; physical techniques like massage, acupuncture, and chiropractic; mental health remedies (including counseling or use of a support group); and homeopathy.

Overall, 30% of the men surveyed used at least one type of CAM. CAM users were younger, more likely to be a college graduate, and were influenced by friends and relatives with prostate cancer. Prevalence rates of CAM use and types of CAM use varied greatly according to ethnicity. The most widely used CAM therapy was herbal remedies, followed by mental health counseling or support group therapy. Black and White men in the sample reported more frequent use of mental health counseling. This study was the first to include significant numbers of non-English-speaking and Asian racial and ethnic minority men with prostate cancer. Upon examining racial groups separately, the researchers concluded that it is likely that CAM use is influenced by individual cultural norms and experiences. However, results may not be generalizable to men living in other areas of the country. Furthermore, the choice of specific CAM therapies used in this study was not clear.

Also, in San Francisco, some of the same researchers examined CAM use in a telephone survey among breast cancer patients using many of the same categories of CAM therapies as the study described above. Lee et al. (2000) studied the types and prevalence of conventional and alternative therapies used by Latino, White, Black, and Chinese women diagnosed with breast cancer from 1990 through 1992 in a 30-minute telephone survey. Participants were asked about dietary, herbal/homeopathy, mental, and physical methods of CAM defined in an appendix section of the article. Of the 379 interviewed subjects, one half of the women reported using at least one type of alternative therapy, and one third used at least two types after breast cancer diagnosis. Blacks most often used spiritual healing (36%); Chinese most often used herbal remedies (22%); and Latino women used dietary therapies (30%) and spiritual healing (26%). Among Whites, 35% used dietary methods and 21% used physical methods like massage and acupuncture. More than 90% of the subjects found the therapies helpful, and with the exception of homeopathy, would recommend them to their friend.

CAM use among patients with cancer of the head and neck was examined in two tertiary Toronto Centers. Warrick et al. (1999) researched 200 consecutive outpatients in a face-to-face cross-sectional survey study to determine the prevalence of alternative medicine use among this population. The National Institute of Health, Office of Alternative Medicine, classification was used to assess use of herbal remedies, manual healing methods, pharmaceutical treatments, traditional and folk remedies, mind-body techniques, and diet and nutrition. Results showed that, overall,

22.5% of patients with head and neck cancer used alternative therapies. Indo-Asian patients used alternative medicine more than other patients that participated in the study.

Two studies were conducted in Hawaii among patients recruited from the Hawaii tumor registry in 1995 and 1996. A self-report mailed survey to estimate the prevalence of CAM and its relation to quality of life (QOL) among 1,168 cancer patients was conducted by Maskarinec, Shumay, Kakai, and Gotay (2000). The ethnic composition of the participants mirrored that of Hawaiians diagnosed with cancer during 1995 and 1996. The survey, based upon another publication, examined these questions: (1) Since your diagnosis, have you tried any alternative therapies? (2) Are you currently using any alternative therapies? (3) What kind of alternative therapies for cancer have you tried? Twenty-one therapies were listed, including Hawaiian healing.

One in four research participants reported utilizing at least one CAM therapy since cancer diagnosis; nearly twice as many females as men reported using CAM. CAM use was highest among Filipino and Caucasian patients, intermediate for Native Hawaiians and Chinese, and lowest among Japanese. Some ethnic preferences for CAM followed along usual ethnic folk medicine traditions: for example—herbal medicines by Chinese, Hawaiian healing by Native Hawaiians, and religious healing or prayers by Filipinos. This study detected ethnic differences in CAM use and supports the importance of cultural factors in determining the frequency and type of CAM chosen.

Also, the same Hawaiian study recruited a subset of 143 persons to participate in qualitative interviews (Shumay, Maskarinec, Kakai, & Gotay, 2001). Of these, 14 multiethnic cancer survivors who declined partial or all recommended conventional cancer treatment took part in semistructured interviews. They were asked about their experience with conventional cancer treatment and providers, use of CAM, and beliefs about the disease. Analysis methodology was not identified. All participants used three or more types of CAM, most commonly herbal or nutritional supplements. All cited that the reason to decline conventional cancer treatment was to avoid damage or harm to the body. Some participants reported that their discovery of CAM contributed to their decision to decline usual medical cancer treatment. A limitation of the study is that the actual CAM therapies used by subjects to treat their cancer were not described.

Two studies examined CAM use among HIV-positive males. Risa et al. (2002) found that 38% (45) of 118 Veteran Medical Center male patients receiving highly active antiretroviral therapy (HAART) for HIV used alternative therapies. The males were predominantly Caucasian (45%) and African American (51%), but they also included Hispanic (2%) and other (2%). The self-administered survey included a question regarding the use of alternative therapies as proposed by Eisenberg, Davis, et al. (1998) and Burstein, Gelber, Gudagnoli, and Weeks (1999). Have you used any of the following therapies or treatments? Choices were contained in two categories: healing therapies and psychological therapies that involved primarily mental processes such as relaxation, self-help groups, spiritual methods, imagery, biofeedback, and hypnosis.

Interestingly, more than half (56%) began using CAM upon initiation of HAART. Although Caucasian patients were more likely to use alternative therapies, new users (or recent CAM discoverers) of alternative therapies were more likely to be African Americans. The main types of therapies used by the study participants included healing (multivitamins and massage) and psychological therapies (relaxation and spiritual healing). Patients who used alternative therapies were less likely to believe that HAART was beneficial. Alternative therapy users had greater psychological distress and were less satisfied with their emotional support.

Similarly, Suarez and Reese (1997) conducted self-administered surveys among 73 HIV-positive African American (n = 33) and Caucasian (n = 40) males on the relationship between CAM use, control over one's HIV, and coping and adjustment in Virginia. Five self-report instruments were used, including a revised Alternative Medicine Checklist (AMC) developed by Rowlands and Powderly that assesses CAM use in an HIV population. CAM use related to high perceptions of control and a high level of adaptive coping behaviors. Stress appraisals predicted a significant amount of variance in the use of CAM. Adjustment did not predict CAM use. This study points out that CAM use significantly helps with adaptive coping behavior.

Summary

The seven articles critiqued show that CAM is used for particular illnesses, specifically for various types of cancers and HIV, among racial and ethnic minority populations. The research studies point out that many times patients were utilizing CAM therapies before their illness diagnosis, while some patients start utilizing various CAM therapies upon diagnosis of cancer or HIV. For example, CAM therapies were commonly used among Hawaiian cancer patients who declined some or all recommended conventional cancer treatment, citing harm to the body as the reason for not utilizing conventional biomedical treatment. In another study, more than half the males from a Veterans Medical Center were likely to initiate CAM use with a diagnosis of HIV—perhaps in part because they were less likely to believe that HAART was beneficial

In one study, CAM therapies were cited as helpful, and 90% of women who had been diagnosed with breast cancer would, with the exception of homeopathy, recommend them to their friend. Two of the studies concluded that CAM use was a result of ethnic differences; they support the importance of cultural factors in determining the frequency and type of CAM chosen. Interestingly, Lee et al. (2002) and Maskarinec et al. (2000) found differences in CAM use related to gender and age. Further research related to CAM use for HIV and cancer treatment is warranted.

CAM USE BY SPECIFIC RACIAL AND ETHNIC POPULATIONS

Five articles were reviewed that describe CAM use by specific ethnic and racial populations. Hispanics, Mexican migrants, Dominican Republicans, caregivers of Puerto Rican children, and African Americans were the ethnic and racial groups studied. The majority of participants in the studies were adults; however, in a study by Pachter, Cloutier, and Bernstein (1995), mothers or caregivers were asked if they used CAM as children. Men and women were included in all the studies. The majority of the studies were surveys describing CAM use among specific populations.

The methodologies utilized in these studies were varied. Two research studies were conducted using participant observation and key informant methodology, and one used focus groups. Descriptive studies using a survey questionnaire were conducted in the remaining three studies; one study did not describe the questionnaire, and one questionnaire was developed for the study. CAM definitions were not consistent throughout the five studies. In three studies CAM was not clearly defined. However, Risser and Mazur (1995) operationalized CAM as "distinct ailments," and Pachter, Cloutier, and Bernstein (1995) defined CAM by interviewing key informants and observing store purchases.

These five articles demonstrated CAM use by ethnic and racial groups for various illnesses, even among children, and also for health maintenance.

Hispanics were the focus of the majority of articles reviewed. For example, African Americans and Hispanics were recruited in one study by Cushman, Wade, Factor-Litvale, Kronenberg, and Firester (1999). Findings indicated that the use of alternative practitioners was most common among older women in both groups. Younger Hispanic women reported the most skepticism toward CAM, especially when used by relatives as a substitute for conventional medical care. Few differences in CAM use emerged between the African Americans and Hispanics and between younger and older women.

In another study, Napolitano (2001) described CAM use among Hispanics in the San Francisco Bay Area. The demand for homeopathic care among the Spanish-speaking population was greater than the capacity to provide care because of the few Spanish-speaking practitioners in the area. Similarly, Risser and Mazur (1995) surveyed 51 Hispanic caregivers, mainly mothers, for their study. The majority of the caregivers believed in folk illnesses and used herbs and pharmaceuticals for the common childhood illnesses. The researchers found that CAM use for asthma was well known and commonly used.

Reasons for seeking, using, and not using CAM therapies varied among these populations. Mexican migrants told Napolitano (2001) that they sought homeopathic medicine because it did not harm them. Further, migrant women praised homeopaths for their ability to listen and understand their needs. Allen et al. (2000) found that Dominican CAM users were more likely to be female, longer-term residents of the United States who used religious practices for health problems. Risser and Mazur (1995) concluded that Hispanic study participants maintained cultural beliefs while relying on medical practitioners. Pachter, Cloutier, and Bernstein (1995) reported reasons for using ethnomedical therapies for asthma among Puerto Rican caregivers. These included attempts to maintain physical and emotional balance and harmony, religious practices, and ethnobotanical therapies. Interestingly, women in this study sought homeopathic medicine because they said it did not harm them.

As mentioned, Napolitano (2001) described the use of complementary medicine by Mexican migrants in the San Francisco Bay Area. The aim of this anthropological qualitative study, which used participant observation and interviews with key informants, was to describe the needs and attitudes of Mexican migrants seeking CAM treatments and the conditions required for CAM delivery to this specific cultural group. CAM was not clearly defined but was described briefly throughout the text as the medicine of CAM practitioners and self-help medicine (*medicina popular*): acupressure, reflexology, herbal remedies, Bach Flower remedies, massage, and basic homeopathic treatment. Methods used for data analysis were not described. Results point out that CAM was available in the Bay Area through organized health centers, Spanish-speaking practitioners, and *casa de salud* (herb stores). Because there was a lack of homeopathic practitioners in the area, some Mexican migrants maintained a telephone relationship with their homeopaths in their country of origin. When Mexican migrants were asked why they sought homeopathic medicine, they said it was because it did not harm them. Migrant women praised homeopaths for their ability to listen and understand their needs. The Mexican migrants in this study viewed CAM as part of a spectrum of possible treatment modalities.

In another study, CAM use in an emergency department that serviced Dominicans was examined. Allen et al. (2000) conducted a small pilot study among patients attending the emergency department of a large New York City urban hospital. CAM was not clearly defined but was operationalized as current use (within the past year) of any of a number of treatments or categories: vitamins and minerals, herbal medicines and other supplements, antiaging medicines, alternative systems, and self-help or lifestyle methods. This descriptive study used a questionnaire developed by faculty in the department of emergency medicine, the Center for Complementary and Alternative Medicine Research in Women's Health, and the School of Public Health. Bilingual personnel administered the questionnaire.

Most of the 50 participants were Dominican and of low socioeconomic status. Almost all had used CAM for their presenting complaint or for another health problem within the last year. Medicinal or herbal teas were the most frequent type of CAM used. CAM users were more likely to be female, longer-term residents of the United States and to have used religious practices for health problems (abdominal problems, accidents, rashes, respiratory problems, and dizziness).

In another study, focus groups were conducted among African American and Hispanic women to assess CAM use (Cushman et al., 1999). The purpose of this study was to obtain qualitative data that would aid in developing a structured questionnaire suitable for a telephone interview. Thirty-nine subjects participated in the focus groups—two groups of African-American women and two groups of Hispanic women. The participants were also asked to fill out a sociodemographic questionnaire and a checklist of CAM modalities. A description of CAM was not included in the report.

Questions asked of the focus groups were not presented. The research team analyzed the data by categorizing it into three areas: most important health concern, CAM remedies used, and CAM practitioners seen. Use of alternative practitioners was most common among older women in both groups. Younger Hispanic women reported the most skepticism toward CAM, especially when used by relatives as a substitute for conventional medical care. Overall, few racial and ethnic differences emerged in patterns of CAM use between these two ethnic groups in relation to self-care or treatment by practitioners.

Hispanic caregivers were surveyed to determine their use of CAM therapies with their children. Risser and Mazur (1995) surveyed 51 Hispanic caregivers, mostly mothers, attending a pediatric primary care facility in an urban Hispanic neighborhood in Houston, Texas. The purpose of this study was to explore Hispanic traditional folk beliefs and remedies. A folk illness was defined as a distinctive ailment belonging to a particular cultural group and for Hispanics was operationalized as *Mal ojo, empacho, mollera caida, and susto*. The interview contained questions about immigration status, use of home remedies for the child's illness(es), familiarity with four folk illnesses (*Mal ojo, empacho, mollera caida, and susto*), use of *curanderos* (traditional healers), and ideas about differences between *curanderos* and medical doctors. Data analysis methodology was not reported. Results indicated that participants used a combination of herbs and pharmaceuticals for many illnesses. Belief in folk illness was common: 36% or 70% had experience with *mal ojo* (evil eye), 33% or 64% with *empacho* (blocked intestine), 27% or 52% with *caida de mollera* (fallen fontanelle), and 19% or 37% with *susto* (fright). Twenty percent had taken their children to *curanderos* for treatment of folk illnesses. Twenty (39%) of the participants believed that a medical practitioner's medicine was more reliable and effective, while 16 (31%) believed that a *curanderos*'s medicine was more effective in treatment of folk illnesses. This article indicates that the use of alternative therapies, the use of folk healers, and the use of medical practitioners are not mutually exclusive.

CAM use in specific populations was described in several studies. In one study, caretakers of Puerto Rican children ($N = 118$) were interviewed in their Hartford Connecticut homes (Pachter, Cloutier, & Bernstein, 1995). Subjects were selected from two community health clinics in an inner city in the eastern United States. The goal of this study was to describe the various ethnomedical practices and therapies for childhood asthma in a mainland Puerto Rican community. Bilingual community health educators conducted the interviews. The therapies described in this study were based on items developed from prior open-ended interviews with key informants. In addition, observations were made of purchasing in *botanicas* (stores commonly found in Puerto Rico communities where religious items and folk remedies are sold), and the owner of the *botanica* was asked to describe remedies for asthma. Descriptions of the remedies were included in the study. Descriptive analysis found that ethnomedical therapies for asthma in this population were well known and commonly used. These practices included attempts to maintain physical and emotional balance and harmony, religious practices, and ethnobotanical and other therapies. The authors indicated that some of the traditional therapies are not discordant with biomedical therapy.

Summary

In summary, the five articles reviewed demonstrate CAM use by ethnic and racial minority populations. However, CAM definitions were not consistent throughout the five studies. In three studies CAM was not clearly defined. Qualitative and quantitative measures were used in these five studies. Hispanic populations were most frequently studied. Reasons for seeking, using, and not using CAM therapies varied but included distrust or negative experiences with the dominant health system. CAM use was consistent with cultural beliefs and practices.

SUMMARY

Several different peer-reviewed journals from multiple disciplines discussed the topic of CAM and racial and ethnic minority populations, indicating that this is an area of interest and importance. However, research to date reveals mixed findings. Of the selected 26 qualitative and quantitative research studies that discussed CAM use among this population, seven did not find a difference between CAM use among racial and ethnic minority populations and the mainstream population. Nineteen studies documented that CAM use was high among these racial and ethnic minority populations.

Overall, several difficulties were noted among the research studies. The definitions of CAM and of CAM practitioners remain indistinct. At times, CAM was not defined. Other studies defined CAM through qualifiers or lists of therapies, discussed CAM in general terms, derived a definition from previous studies, or followed Eisenberg's CAM definition (Eisenberg et al., 1993; Eisenberg, Davis, et al., 1998). A limitation of Eisenberg's definition for CAM is that it is a mainstream definition based on what is usual and customary in Western biomedical schools, hospitals, and insurance companies. CAM practitioners in the studies reviewed included lay and folk practitioners, such as *curanderos*; people who pass cultural knowledge from generation to generation, including family and friends; and mainstream professionals like chiropractors and nutritionists. Clearly, these definitions limit racial or ethnic minority cultural perspectives or approaches related to traditional healing methods, therapies, and practitioners. Thus, in most instances, *culture* is not included in the mainstream definition of CAM because these groups used ancient health care practices since time immemorial, before language was written.

In view of that, it may be that racial and ethnic minorities have a different definition (other than CAM) of healing methods that are typically used as part of their culture. Keywords used to find articles in literature searches might include *traditional healing, indigenous healing, faith healing*, and *cultural healing*. In this way, racial and ethnic populations may use their customary healing approaches to health care as alternative medicine, which is defined as those therapies or methods used alone and apart from Western biomedical medicine. Consequently, a discrepancy may exist regarding the definition of CAM and CAM usage among racial and ethnic populations and mainstream populations. As well, these populations obtain their alternative health information from sources outside the formal education system, such as relatives, friends, and other persons within their culture. Many times, these teachings are oral and are not documented in writing.

Various research questions and goals were included in this review. Some goals were to describe CAM use among selected populations or groups, or to describe CAM use for certain illnesses. Bair et al. (2002) were interested in CAM use for premenopausal symptoms at midlife; Dole et al. (2000) examined herb use in an elderly population of Hispanics and non-Hispanics that health care providers encountered; and Lee, Chang, et al. (2002) and Lee, Lin, et al. (2000) studied CAM use among racial and ethnic minority patients with a specific type of cancer.

Different methodologies were used: qualitative methodologies (ethnography, focus groups, qualitative interviews, and anthropological qualitative methods); descriptive quantitative methodologies; and mixed survey and semistructured interviews conducted in person, in groups, over the telephone, through the mail, or by self-administered questionnaires, some of which were translated into various languages or collected by a bilingual research team member. Accordingly, diverse research findings were noted in relation to the research question and methodology. In view of that, it is not clear if there has been sufficient descriptive research to provide a clear understanding of what comprises CAM. This is clearly a barrier to producing reliable research results.

Emerging themes from the articles regarding the utilization of complementary and alternative medicine among racial and ethnic minority populations were as follows: (1) both genders, of all ages, use CAM; (2) CAM use among racial and ethnic minority populations is comparable to use reported by recent surveys showing that 42% to 50% of adults used some type of alternative care in the past year (Astin, 1998; Eisenberg, Davis, et al., 1998); and (3) some researchers demonstrated that CAM use was part of broader cultural beliefs. Culture is an integral component of life. Thus CAM therapies have and are being used by racial and ethnic minority populations for health and well-being. Perhaps all populations, including the mainstream, use CAM therapies that reflect past practices and traditions. If so, CAM is not new, but is an older method of health care than is generally realized.

However, CAM is purportedly a new field in today's health care system. Based upon this research review, CAM presently comprises a wide variation of therapies, vastly different terminology and definitions, broad dissimilarities in the surveys and methods used to collect research data, and extensive disparate investigative research questions and goals. As a result, limitations loom large as to what CAM is, how it is defined, and how it is measured.

To illustrate this point, the following example is offered. Becerra and Iglehart (1995), in a comprehensive literature review, described folk medicine practices among African Americans, Mexican Americans, Chinese Americans, and White non-Hispanic urban dwellers. Although there are a wide variety of definitions for folk medicine (specific practices, use of medical practitioners outside biomedical health care, "good" remedies), a summative review of the literature showed that folk and home remedies are widely used among all groups and in both rural and urban settings. Findings suggest that folk medicine is used in addition to, rather than in place of, formal biomedical health care. It is used primarily to treat minor illnesses and prevent serious illness.

The congruence of CAM with cultural beliefs and practices has not been well explored. This may be a result of inadequate knowledge or lack of experience among researchers in examining the use of CAM within a cultural context. Of the reviewed studies, only a few were cited in which the researcher was of the same cultural group. Such researchers hold promise in describing culturally specific healing practices.

CAM AND HEALTH DISPARITIES

Health disparities are complex and multifaceted, and a search continues for approaches and methods to reduce them. One potential means is by using complementary and alternative medicine. This seems like a natural approach. As noted above, certain cultures have utilized and continue to use complementary and alternative medicine for health. However, the question continues to loom: What is the relevancy or efficacy of CAM use among racial and ethnic populations? Can CAM be utilized to reduce health disparities?

There is little research that explores how CAM can be used to assist with the reduction of health disparities within racial and ethnic minority populations. These populations do utilize CAM at high rates, often as a part of their cultural beliefs. However, according to the reviewed research, other factors are also related to CAM use: frequent lack of communication between physicians and patients, failure of conventional medicine to cure an illness, the desire to avoid the side effects of conventional treatments, dissatisfaction with reliance on prescription drugs, and avoidance of damage or harm to the body.

CAM use is also influenced by recommendations from friends or coworkers and the availability of herbs from the user's country of origin. Findings suggest that some prefer CAM instead of conventional treatment. Some believe in folk illnesses and thus choose CAM therapies for the treatment of such conditions. Some use CAM practitioners because they can speak the patient's native language, or because of a lack of holism (inadequate information regarding diet, nutrition, and exercise and ignorance of social and spiritual dimensions) within the conventional medical system. Others choose CAM as a means of maintaining physical and emotional balance and harmony. Thus, CAM is used for multiple reasons, not always specifically cited as cultural, by racial and ethnic minority populations. Conceivably, the question may be: How can we integrate

CAM to build trust and provide culturally appropriate health care, while maintaining the desires and beliefs of racial and ethnic minority populations?

FUTURE RESEARCH DIRECTIONS

This research review on complementary and alternative medicine use among racial and ethnic minority populations points out that additional work related to CAM is needed. While the articles reviewed are an important first effort in describing CAM, the vast majority lacked sufficient detail about methodology, thus making replication of studies difficult.

The holistic foundation of nursing has a tradition of using complementary therapies, and thus nurses are poised to be future leaders in this research area (Snyder & Lindquist, 2002). To create a scientific research base for the area of CAM, research fundamentals such as consistency in the definition of CAM, uniformity in what constitutes a CAM therapy and practitioner, standardization of tools and measurements, reliability and validity of measurements used, and replication of studies among diverse research samples are necessary. The broadness of the topic of CAM presents a challenge. Employing qualitative research studies that clearly and soundly define CAM, its uses, and its practitioners is a first step. Then, descriptive studies that use the same tools and measurements are needed so that reliability and validity can be established among diverse research samples. In the future, efficacy studies are also needed to examine CAM within specific populations and for both health promotion and illness management.

The studies presented in this chapter indicate that CAM is used among racial and minority ethnic populations. However, new research data are needed on how CAM influences the overall health of this population and, furthermore, on how it might be integrated into current biomedical practices as a means to reduce health disparities. Racial and ethnic groups use CAM because it is part of their culture. It has been used in the past and present and will continue to be used in the future. Thus, constructing a solid research base in the area of CAM is an initial step to subsequent studies that could determine the cultural underpinnings of CAM practices as well as the safety, efficacy, and cost of CAM therapies and approaches. These studies could add a new dimension to a health care system that is currently trying to find ways to address the inequities in health care experienced by racial and ethnic minority populations.

REFERENCES

Allen, R., Cushman, L. F., Morris, S., Feldman, J., Wade, C., McMahon, D., Moses, M., & Kronenberg, F. (2000). Use of complementary and alternative medicine among Dominican emergency department patients. *American Journal of Emergency Medicine, 18*(1), 51–54.

Arcury, T. A., Quandt, S. A., Bell, R. A., & Vitolins, M. Z. (2002). Complementary and alternative medicine use among rural older adults. *Alternative Health Practitioner: The Journal of Complementary and Natural Care, 7,* 167–186.

Astin, J. A. (1998). Why patients use alternative medicine: Results of a national study. *Journal of the American Medical Association, 279,* 1548–1553.

Bair, Y. A., Gold, E. B., Greendale, G. A., Sternfeld, B., Adler, S. R., Azari, R., & Harkey, M. (2002). Ethnic differences in use of complementary and alternative medicine at midlife: Longitudinal results from SWAN participants. *American Journal of Public Health, 92,* 1832–1840.

Baldwin, C. M., Long, K., Kroesen, K., Brooks, A. J., & Bell, I. R. (2002). A profile of military veterans in the Southwestern United States who use complementary and alternative medicine: Implications for integrated care. *Archives of Internal Medicine, 162,* 1697–1704.

Becerra, R. M., & Iglehart, A. P. (1995). Folk medicine use: Diverse populations in a metropolitan area. *Social Work in Health Care, 21,* 37–58.

Burstein, H. J., Gelber, S., Gudagnoli, E., & Weeks, J. C. (1999). Use of alternative medicine by women with early stage breast cancer. *New England Journal of Medicine, 340,* 1733–1739.

Cherniack, E. P., Senzel, R. S., & Pan, C. X. (2001). Correlates of use of alternative medicine by elderly in an urban population. *Journal of Alternative and Complementary Medicine, 7,* 277–280.

Cushman, L. F., Wade, C., Factor-Litvak, P., Kronenberg, F., & Firester, L. (1999). Use of complementary and alternative medicine among African-American and Hispanic women in New York City: A pilot study. *Journal of the American Medical Womens Association, 54,* 193–195.

Dole, E. J., Rhyne, R. L., Zeilmann, C. A., Skipper, B. J., Mc Cabe, M. L., & Dog, T. L. (2000). The influence of ethnicity on use of herbal remedies in elderly Hispanics and non-Hispanics Whites. *Journal of American Pharmaceutical Association, 40,* 359–365.

Drivdahl, C. E., & Miser, W. F. (1998). The use of alternative health care by family practice population. *Journal of American Board of Family Practice, 11,* 193–199.

Eisenberg, D. M., Davis, R. B., Ettner, S. L., Apple, S., Wilkey, S., Van Rompay, M., & Kessler, R. C. (1998). Trends in alternative medicine use in the United States, 1990–1997: Results of a follow-up national survey. *Journal of the American Medical Association, 280,* 1569–1575.

Eisenberg, D. M., Kessler, R. C., Foster, C., Norlock, F. E., Calkins, D. R., & Delbanco, T. L. (1993). Unconventional medicine in the United States: Prevalence, costs, and patterns of use. *New England Journal of Medicine, 328,* 246–252.

Ernst, E. (1999). Ethnic differences in complementary medicine use. *Focus on Alternative and Complementary Therapies, 4*(1), 9–10.

Factor-Litvak, P., Cushman, L. F., Kronenberg, F., Wade, C., & Kalmuss, D. (2001). Use of complementary and alternative medicine among women in New York City: A pilot study. *Journal of Alternative and Complementary Medicine, 7*, 659–666.

Fletcher, A. B. (2000). African American folk medicine: A form of alternative therapy. *ABNF Journal, 11*(1), 18–20.

Fontaine, K. L. (2000). *Healing practices: Alternative therapies for nursing.* Upper Saddle River, NJ: Prentice Hall.

Kessler, R. C., Davis, R. B., Foster, D. F., et al. (2001). Long-term trends in the use of complementary and alternative medical therapies in the United States. *Annals of Internal Medicine, 135*, 262–268.

Kroesen, K., Baldwin, C. M., Brooks, A. J., & Bell, I. R. (2002). US military veterans' perceptions of the conventional medical care system and their use of complementary and alternative medicine. *Family Practice, 19*(1), 57–64.

Lee, M. M., Chang, J. S., Jacobs, B., & Wrensch, M. R. (2002). Complementary and alternative medicine use among men with prostate cancer in 4 ethnic populations. *American Journal of Public Health, 92*, 1606–1609.

Lee, M. M., Lin, S. S., Wrensch, M. R., Adler, S. R., & Eisenberg, D. (2000). Alternative therapies used by women with breast cancer in four ethnic populations. *Journal of the National Cancer Institute, 92*(1), 42–47.

Leung, J. M., Dzankie, S., Manku, K., & Yuan, S. (2001). The prevalence and predictors of the use of alternative medicine in presurgical patients in five California hospitals. *Anesthesia and Analgesia, 93*, 1062–1068.

Liu, E. H., Turner, L. M., Lin, S. X., Klaus, L., Choi, L. Y., Whitworth, J., Ting, W., & Oz, M. C. (2000). Use of alternative medicine by patients undergoing cardiac surgery. *Journal of Thoracic and Cardiovascular Surgery, 120*, 335–341.

Lundy, M. B., Morgan, L. L., Rhoads, K. V. L., & Curtis Bay, R. (2001). Hispanic and Anglo patients' reported use of alternative medicine in the medical clinic context. *Alternative Health Practitioner: The Journal of Complementary and Natural Care, 6*, 205–217.

Maskarinec, G., Shumay, D. M., Kakai, H., & Gotay, C. C. (2000). Ethnic differences in complementary and alternative medicine use among cancer patients. *Journal of Alternative and Complementary Medicine, 6*, 531–538.

Napolitano, V. (2001). Complementary medicine use by Mexican migrants in the San Francisco Bay Area. *Western Journal of Medicine, 174*, 203–206.

National Center for Complementary and Alternative Medicine. (2002). *What is complementary and alternative medicine (CAM)?* National Institute of Health. NCCAM Publication No. D156. Retrieved May 28, 2003, from http://nccam.nci.nih.gov/health/whatiscam/#3

National Center for Complementary and Alternative Medicine. (2003). *About the National Center for Complementary and Alternative Medicine.* Retrieved February 6, 2003, from www.nccam.nih.gov

Pachter, L. M., Cloutier, M. M., & Bernstein, B. A. (1995). Ethnomedical (folk) remedies for childhood asthma in a mainland Puerto Rican community. *Archives of Pediatric and Adolescent Medicine, 149*, 982–988.

Palinkas, L. A., & Kabongo, M. L. (2000). The use of complementary and alternative medicine by primary care patients: A SURF*NET study. *Journal of Family Practice, 49*, 1121–1130.

Rhee, D. J., Spaeth, G. L., Myers, J. S., Steinmann, W. C., Augsburger, J. J., Shatz, L. J., Terebuh, A. K., Ritner, J. A., & Katz, L. J. (2002). Prevalence of the use of complementary and alternative medicine for glaucoma. *Ophthalmology, 109*, 438–443.

Risa, K. J., Nepon, L., Justis, J. C., Panwalker, A., Berman, S. M., Cinti, S., Wagener, M. M., & Singh, N. (2002). Alternative therapy use in HIV-infected patients receiving highly active antiretroviral therapy. *International Journal of STD and AIDS, 13*, 706–713.

Risser, A. L., & Mazur, L. J. (1995). Use of folk remedies in a Hispanic population. *Archives of Pediatric and Adolescent Medicine, 149*, 978–981.

Rowlands, C., & Powderly, W. G. (1991). The use of alternative therapies by HIV-positive patients attending the St. Louis AIDS Clinical Trials Unit. *Missouri Medicine, 88*, 807–810.

Shumay, D. M., Maskarinec, G., Kakai, H., & Gotay, C. C. (2001). Why some cancer patients choose complementary and alternative medicine instead of conventional medicine. *Journal of Family Practice, 50*, 1067.

Snyder, M., & Lindquist, R. (2002). *Complementary/alternative therapies in nursing* (4th ed.). New York: Springer Publishing Co.

Suarez, T., & Reese, F. L. (1997). Alternative medicine use, perceived control, coping, and adjustment in African American and Caucasian males living with HIV and AIDS. *International Journal of Rehabilitation and Health, 3*, 107–118.

Warrick, P. D., Irish, J. C., Morningstar, M., Gilbert, R., Brown, D., & Gullane, P. (1999). Use of alternative medicine among patients with head and neck cancer. *Archives of Otolaryngology—Head and Neck Surgery, 125*, 573–579.

Wolsko, P., Ware, L., Kutner, J., Lin, C., Albertson, G., Cyran, L., Schilling, L., & Anderson, R. J. (2000). Alternative/complementary medicine: Wider usage than generally appreciated. *Journal of Alternative and Complementary Medicine, 6*, 321–326.

Wooten, J. C., & Sparber, A. (2001). Surveys of complementary and alternative medicine: Part 1. General trends and demographic groups. *Journal of Alternative and Complementary Medicine, 7*, 195–208.

Chapter 12

Community Partnerships: The Cornerstone of Community Health Research

CARMEN J. PORTILLO AND CATHERINE WATERS

ABSTRACT

Community partnerships have been recognized as the cornerstone of community research. The recent Institute of Medicine report, *Unequal Treatment*, puts forth the idea of creating community partnerships as a strategy to address racial and ethnic disparities in health care. Community-based research is frequently reported in the literature as a study conducted in the community versus with the community. The objective of this review is to examine models of community partnerships, to consider their implications for community-based research, and to identify directions for future nursing research.

Keywords: community-based research, community health, racial and ethnic minorities

Efforts of nurses in the United States to improve the quality of lives of communities can be traced to the nursing care provided to immigrant families and their women and children: Lillian Wald's work among the poor in the Henry Street Settlement, which is typically considered the first American community health program, Mary Breckenridge's community work in the rural hills of Kentucky, and Margaret Sanger's efforts to help women control their fertility. Since the late 1800s community health nursing interventions have continued to evolve. In 1978 the Declaration of the Alma-Ata brought fresh attention to bringing health care "as close as possible to where people live and work." The Declaration of the Alma-Ata also engaged multidisciplinary efforts in improving the quality of health for communities, particularly for racial and ethnic minority communities. Although our singular and collective efforts to improve the quality of health for communities has grown, our ability to effectively work with communities to reduce health disparities through community-centered prevention efforts has been slower.

Unhealthful behaviors, such as physical inactivity, excessive eating and obesity, improper nutrition, tobacco use, and excessive alcohol consumption, account for half of the leading causes of death in the United States. These are modifiable lifestyle choices that are disproportionately higher among underrepresented populations (McGinnis & Foege, 1993). The positive health outcomes of effective risk reduction mechanisms to prevent disease and control illness are well known, but they remain difficult to attain for all populations. Effective efforts to eliminate health disparities require both individual- and community-level participation.

Copious discourse pertaining to community health nursing, public health nursing, community-based nursing, community health nursing interventions, and population-focused care exists in the nursing literature. This, in and of itself, created a challenge in the review of this body of literature.

METHOD

A systematic approach was used to identify and retrieve literature on community health nursing and relevant concepts. Nursing research literature was first identified via a computerized search of the Cumulative Index of Nursing and Allied Health Literature (CINAHL) citations from 1982 to August 2003 and of PubMed, a service of the National Library of Medicine that includes MEDLINE citations from 1976 to 2003. *Community health nursing* was used for a keyword search in the CINAHL search. This first iteration resulted in 10,129 citations. No citations resulted from PubMed. Next we used the term *community health nursing interventions* in both databases. The CINAHL search produced 5,917 citations with abstracts. Using PubMed, 296 citations with abstracts resulted. The last term used was *community-based health interventions*. CINAHL produced 2,220 citations with abstracts, and PubMed produced 1,698 citations. Further winnowing included cross-referencing citations from both databases, examining those with abstracts, including citations published only in nursing journals, and reducing the time frame from 1990 to 2003. Further, only those that focused on community-based research as opposed to "conducting research in a community" were included. The final sample totaled 30 citations; articles were those that primarily focused on interventions conducted in the United States. Article titles and abstracts were reviewed for the identified words and phrases. The work of nonnurse investigators was included when needed to enrich and elaborate on the method of conducting community-based research.

Community participation has been recognized as a cornerstone of community health nursing and for improving the health of a community. The concept of community varies from passive participation to active participation, with diverse types of representation and varying numbers of community members (Aguirre-Molina & Parra, 1995; Courtney, 1995; Courtney, Ballard, Fauver, Gariota, & Holland, 1996; Meleis, 1992; Ramos, May, & Ramos, 2001). The main characteristics of partnership are captured by the following three adjectives: *informed, flexible*, and *negotiated* (Eng, Parker, & Harlan, 1997).

IMPLEMENTING COMMUNITY HEALTH INTERVENTIONS WITH COMMUNITY AS PARTNER

Current prevailing thought on intervening with communities to improve health and eliminate health disparities focuses on active community involvement, and shared control of decision making and resources between the community and interventionists (Bruhn, 2001; Israel, Schulz, Parker, & Becker, 1998; Israel et al., 2003; Marcus, 2000; McElmurry & Keeney, 1999; Meleis, 1992; Moyer, Coristine, Jamault, Roberge, & O'Hagan, 1999; Moyer, Coristine, MacLean, & Meyer, 1999; Nuñez, Armbruster, Phillips, & Gale, 2003; Rothman, Lourie, Gaughan, & White, 1999; Rowley, Dixon, & Sheldon, 2002; Wallerstein & Duran, 2003). Academics, researchers, health departments, hospitals, and community agencies and organizations are shifting away from the notions of "autonomy, individualism, and universality" and "passive recipient, beneficiary, or research subject" toward "community and cultural relevance," "social responsibility and common good," and "citizen participation and constituency building and advocacy" (Institute of Medicine, 2003a, b). Israel, in an early article (2000) and subsequently with a group of colleagues (Israel et al., 2003), speaks cogently for the value of community-based participatory research, for both practical and ethical reasons—for creating partnerships in interventions and in the research that guides these interventions. On a practical level, engaging the community in public health research can be facilitative in dealing with complicated issues such as defining research priorities or interpreting results. On an ethical level, it is important to involve the community that is being studied beyond the individual consent process.

Effective models that enhance community participation are gaining more attention (Green & Kreuter, 1999; Israel, 2000). Community-based participatory research enhances limited community participation in traditional population-based health research; builds and strengthens the capacity of community residents to address health risks; sustains effective culturally relevant community-based health programs; broadens the dissemination of research findings and community health intervention outcomes; and affects national policies (Israel, 2000). In a three-year community-based participatory project, public health nurses collaborated with an elderly population in a francophone urban area of Canada (Moyer, Coristine, Jamault, et al., 1999; Moyer, Coristine, MacLean, et al., 1999). The Elderly in Need Project (EIN) employed a case study design embedded within an action research study. A four-stage model of capacity building was used to engage elderly communities to establish a community-based health program, while at the same time increase future collaboration. The four stages were: (1) identifying common ground, (2) establishing self as a community player, (3) working on a common project, and (4) working with multiagency/multisectoral partners. The study demonstrated how public health nurses gained access to three communities of older adults at risk of losing their independence and became instrumental in developing culturally relevant preventive interventions for these communities. The premise of the four-stage capacity-building community model is resonant with a number of other community models in the literature (Green & Krueter, 1999; Eng, Salmon, & Mullan, 1992; Rothman & Tropman, 1987).

A conceptual model that has been widely adopted in nursing is the PRECEDE-PROCEED program planning model (Green & Kreuter, 1999). Hecker (2000) employed the model to implement and evaluate a communitywide health fair in Mexico. A health fair was held in a suburban community located 20 kilometers outside of Mexico City, where approximately 200 individuals participated. The outcome of the fair resulted in process-type outcomes. While the focus of the model was on planning and evaluating community health education programs, a major advantage of this planning model is that it is useful in helping communities change their behaviors. It begins by assessing the environment in which the group lives and considering the social factors that influence health behaviors. Next, the model examines both the internal and environmental factors of the group that predispose it to certain behaviors or health problems (PRE-CEDE). The model then calls for the identification of factors that will help the group to adopt healthy actions. Priorities are set. The program is developed, implemented, and evaluated (PROCEED).

Many community health nursing interventions have been designed and focused on certain health conditions or populations at risk as identified in *Healthy People 2010* (USDHHS, 2001) (Chalmers et al., 2001; Hecker, 2000; May, McLaughlin, & Penner, 1991). A frequent area of focus has been in the development of community partnerships to improve access to prenatal care (Mahon, McFarlane, & Golden, 1991; May, McLaughlin, & Penner, 1991). May et al. (1991) organized public health nurses to effectively mobilize neighborhood outreach volunteers using a social marketing framework. The partnership, called the Pregnancy Outreach Program of the Arizona Department of Health Services, sought to assess the needs of women at risk for inadequate health care and develop an outreach model aimed at increasing early entry into prenatal care. Outreach workers assisted in case finding and coordination by working as liaisons between high-risk women and appropriate services. Public health nurses provided core leadership in program development; established community networks; intervened through case management of prenatal clients; and recruited, trained, and supervised community outreach workers. The time frame of this project precluded measuring outcome data associated with the program's impact on low birth weight, prematurity, or infant mortality. Process outcomes in community-based nursing interventions were a common finding in the literature, and also a limitation of the research.

Similarly, Mahon et al. (1991) utilized Hispanic volunteer mothers to visit 2,000 Hispanic pregnant women in the De Madres a Madres program in a Texas community. This program very successfully developed and has sustained to date a partnership between the business community, the general public, and, particularly volunteer mothers, which has been the "heart and soul" of this program. A more recent report chronicles from the perspectives of the women how the women formed partnerships with the community, business, churches, and health and social service agencies. The steps these women took in coalition building has been based on feminist theory (McFarlane, Kelly, Rodriguez, & Fehir, 1994).

The significance and effectiveness of partnership in improving community health has been supported by a growing body of literature. Community health interventions have long included lay community members, referred to as community health workers (CHWs) or *promotoras,* as the key to the "bridge" between the intervention and interventionist, particularly in working with populations at greatest social risk (McElmurry & Keeney, 1999; PEW, 1994; Ramos, May, & Ramos, 2001). Hill, Bone, and Butz (1996) highlight the importance of CHWs in meeting the needs of the underserved communities. However, the authors state that CHWs have remained overlooked since the federal government first endorsed their use for expanded health access to the underserved in the 1960s. CHWs can communicate basic health information and help the interventionist understand the local culture, values, and practices. In addition, communities and individuals are more likely to accept new information from people they know and trust (Eng & Young, 1992; Hill et al., 1996). The national demand to eliminate health disparities and recent socioeconomic pressures have focused attention on the use of CHWs to improve community health. Still underutilization occurs.

A useful review of evaluation research and the use of community health workers is Nembcek and Sabatier's (2003) article. Eighteen CHW programs are summarized, including the type of setting (urban or rural), the population, the program components, and CHW duties: outcome evaluation and process evaluation interventions. Of the 18 programs, all but 1 appeared to target an ethnic group. The authors conclude by suggesting three major areas as quality indicators to further evaluate best practices of CHW programs in the future: (1) a therapeutic relationship that is supported by health beliefs and provider-patient trust, which can improve health care utilization; (2) appropriate health care utilization that involves improving access to care and use of services; and (3) risk reduction, accomplished through culturally competent prevention and health promotion.

Similarly, Swider (2002) provides an integrative literature review on the outcome effectiveness of community health workers. She reviewed 19 database articles on CHWs effectiveness in increasing access to care, particularly in underserved populations. Swider concludes by saying that further work is needed to understand the cost of services provided by CHWs and to determine whether the CHW effect on access to care is cost-effective. She provides a note of caution by indicating that the role of the CHW has the potential of failing because of overly high expectations, lack of a clear focus, and lack of documentation.

Hildebrandt (1996) illustrates a collaborative model that guided activities for community empowerment through deliberate transfer of information and expertise from the public health nurses to members of the community. The model was applied over a 2-year period in a Black township in South Africa, where unemployment was over 50%, fewer than 10% of the homes had electricity, and only one third had access to the sewage removal system. Although this model was applied internationally, the principles are also valid in the United States and have implications for racial and ethnic communities.

The foremost advantage of a community's participation in a partnership is the opportunity to inform action that will affect the health of the community. Other advantages are being a part of a collaborative effort that values and respects the community's views; feeling visible, empowered, and important; being a part of a solution that focuses on the community's assets rather than its deficits; and gaining knowledge about health, research, and job training and skills (Meleis, 1992). Most important is probably the advantage of having an impact on how data about the community are collected, analyzed, interpreted, and disseminated (Kelly & Van Vlaenderen, 1996). Several methods and tools have been designed to evaluate the community as partner or the level of participation (Bichmann, Rifkin, & Shrestha, 1989; Kelly & Van Vlaenderen, 1996; LaForgia, 1985; Ugalde, 1985). A 14-item tool developed by Kroutil and Eng (1989) assesses the incorporation of community participation. This instruments builds on the work of Bichmann, Rifkin, and Shrestha (1989), which focuses on three primary dimensions for participation: (1) who, (2) what, and (3) how.

Another tool of evaluation is Narayan's (1996) description of water and sanitation community health projects. Community-based participation projects were implemented throughout different parts of world based on principles of capacity development, multiple methods, and the notion of capturing the use of the nonexperts in the community. Included are innovative data collection methods that work in the field and information on the training of lay field workers. Narayan's reference is a useful evaluation handbook for community-based researchers.

Community-Based Organizations as Partners

A major advantage of collaboration for community-based organizations is the potential access to more resources to implement community health programs that are not duplicative. Another advantage for these organizations is the opportunity for staff development funded by pooled resources of the partnership. Because these organizations are close to the population they serve, they are a crucial part of the public health system, and thus are sources for identifying needs and responses and evaluating the results of community health interventions. For example, community-based groups that represent particularly hard-to-reach populations and the interests of ethnic communities (e.g., National Council of La Raza, Congress of National Black Churches, National Coalition of Ethnic Minority Nurse Associations, Inc.) are advocacy groups that are instrumental in mobilizing and educating communities and advocating for policy change to safeguard their health.

The burden of environmental problems is frequently borne by ethnic and minority populations. The Lead Awareness: North Philly Style project (Rothman et al., 1999) is an example of how a grassroots community-based relationship between a community-based organization and faculty of the Department of Nursing, College of Allied Health Professions, at Temple University evolved. Both parties recognized that in order for a collaborative project to be successful, the community would need to be the lead in implementing and evaluating the project. The target population was a poor African American urban community in north central Philadelphia. Culturally appropriate prevention strategies were developed with community residents in alliance with other agencies that had a demonstrated history of grassroots activism in the community. The focus of the project was twofold: (1) to test community-developed, community-based prevention/intervention strategies that increase knowledge of the environmental health risk of childhood lead poisoning; and (2) to test community-developed, community-based prevention/intervention strategies that will increase hazard, exposure, and outcome surveillance for lead as an environmental agent. The authors reported that community-developed intervention strategies were the key to the project. They further illustrate how the strategies used were based on classic tenets of community health: the health of the community, the vulnerability of the community, the capability of the community, and the likelihood that the community would act.

Church-based health programs, another form of a community-based health program, have been largely administered within the African American community (Castro et al., 1995; Lasater, Becker, Hill, & Gans, 1997; Lasater, Carleton, & Wells, 1991; Voorhees et al., 1996; Weinrich et al., 1998). Successful community-based health programs have been found to have seven key elements: (1) partnerships, (2), positive health values, (3) availability of services, (4) access to facilities, (5) community-focused interventions, (6) health behavior change, and (7) supportive social relationships (Peterson, Atwood, & Yates, 2002).

Major challenges of collaboration for community-based organizations are concerns about being used only as research recruitment agencies; "turf" issues related to their target clients and communities; and conflicts over funding, goals, objectives, deliverables, the work plan, leadership, time commitment, and involvement of staff. Many community-based organizations already have limited resources. Lending resources to participate in a partnership further taxes the organization's already limited resources of time, people, and money. In addition, a budget to absorb the costs to sustain community health programs initiated from the partnership after funding ceases is almost nonexistent.

Academic Researchers as Partners

There are a number of advantages for academic researchers when there is active community involvement in all phases of the research process. The advantages include improved content, quality, validity, and relevance of data; more efficient recruitment, retention, and outreach to community residents, especially underrepresented populations; and a socially, culturally, and environmentally sensitive, scientifically sound intervention design and implementation. Because there is community involvement, and thus implied rapport, a collaborative effort potentially decreases the community's suspicion of researchers and "their" science agenda, which is perceived as having little to do with the community. This type of partnership has the potential to translate research findings into practice and policy that address the realities, priorities, and constraints of people's lives and their communities.

For Marcus (2000), the collaboration between the community and academic setting resulted in five specific preventive outcomes and additional benefits that were not expected. For example, faculty increased their community scholarship and community awareness, sustained interventions on substance abuse, and expanded their collaborations with other community-based organizations.

Two major challenges for academic researchers as partners in community-based participatory efforts are the need to be flexible and in rhythm with community life, and the need to meet the time demands associated with the partnership in addition to the time demands of university responsibilities. The community must perceive that the researcher is making meaningful connections with the community by seeing the researcher participating in community events on a regular basis. Compared to laboratory settings, such as a hospital or clinic, the community's milieu cannot be controlled by the researcher. Often a community's social environment can be unwieldy and unyielding, resulting in a considerable loss of control for the researcher, which can jeopardize the validity and reliability of the research. Community partners are not necessarily interested and are often impatient with the details of the research process.

SUMMARY

There are two primary reasons for including community as partner: it is practical and ethical. But there are also challenges to including the community as a partner, such as the extensive time it involves and the internal "politics" among community residents. The partnership must offer more than empty rhetoric and incentives, for many communities have been overly "coalitioned, advocated, and empowered" without realizing any significant benefits. From a research perspective, challenges for the community are understanding the methodological, controlled, and often lengthy nature of research; trusting that the community will not be exploited and that there is a genuine interest in improving the health of the community; feeling comfortable that community residents are regarded as sentient human beings, not just a statistic; and knowing that community values and standards will not be violated.

Community-based research serves as a model that can be effective with ethnic and racial communities. This type of research seeks to overcome some of the criticisms and distrust of academic research by emphasizing the participation and influence of nonacademic researchers in the process of creating knowledge (Israel et al., 1998).

Conceptually related is the PRECEDE-PROCEED model, which is an effective program planning and evaluative model and one that has broad implications for ethnic minority communities. For instance, from the very beginning the researcher/interventionist is forced to include the community in the planning and identification of the problem.

Virtually all of the studies reviewed considered inclusion of community health workers or *promotoras* as part of the research team. Roles and responsibilities varied from study to study, although the project De Madres a Madres appeared to have the most success with a wider scope of work for the *promotoras* (McFarlane et al., 1994). In the process of learning to work with community lay workers, it appears that roles and responsibilities evolve as the relationship builds, which only leads to greater successes. If this is commonly recognized in the literature, why do we fail to use community health workers in community health interventions more often? What are the cost implications of this type of study?

Overall, most of the researchers did not provide sufficient detail about an intervention. In the literature presented, it was very difficult to discern why the intervention worked. In the literature reviewed, we did not come across any reports of a failed intervention and the reasons why. Bruhn (2001) states that we know less than we should about unsuccessful interventions because reports about them are not published, or if they are, they provide insufficient information about what went wrong (and what went right) to help the reader know what to avoid (or do) in a replication. Therefore, it is not surprising that few interventions are replicated. Given the complicated nature of working with ethnic and racial minority communities and developing partnerships, it is important that researchers and clinicians are encouraged to publish their successes and failures, without judgment.

FUTURE DIRECTIONS

Community health interventions cannot be understood by analyzing the research conducted by one discipline such as nursing. Community health research *requires* the involvement of multidisciplinary participants working in collaboration with members of the community.

There is a greater need for community-based research with direct involvement of the community. This type of research is an effective way of truly providing culture-specific interventions that may better sustain outcomes in affecting health disparities. Although community-based research is costly in financial resources and energy, the positive results outweigh the costs. It is time that we move beyond "quick and dirty" research conducted in the community with very little long-term impact. Researchers need to move to more multisite intervention studies. Further, it is important to be honest with our communities and community of scholars about successes and failures.

At the same time, nursing needs to prepare more culturally competent nurses and faculty. The lack of ethnic minority nurses entering nursing is a problem in itself. But increasing the number of ethnic minority nurses within nursing cannot be considered the only solution. A multifaceted approach to developing and promoting cultural competence among all students and faculty is needed.

Currently, much of the community-based health research in nursing is being published in Canada, Australia, or the United Kingdom. The majority of the research being reported is descriptive or experimental at the level of the client as the community. Although this research is necessary, more balance in developing population- or community-based research is needed.

Nursing has the potential of providing conceptual direction and research in community health interventions. However, community health is a conceptual arena for practice and research that continues to develop within the discipline.

Community health interventions do not occur independently of social, cultural, religious, political, and economical factors. Using a community-based participatory model for community health research and practice interventions shows promise for promoting long-term positive health outcomes in ethnic-minority communities. There are facilitating factors as well as challenges for using this approach. Community representation in decision making requires strategies for inclusion, accountability and responsibility, tenacity and patience, clear communication, negotiation skills, and valuing the community's perceptions regardless of the interventionist's feeling that the community is misguided.

A final area of reflection that needs to be considered by researchers conducting community-based research is developing criteria that are of concern in the specified research and determining what types of evaluation designs are the best means of tying the focus and criteria together. This would provide a discussion guide for the community health intervention research. While this topic was not fully covered in this chapter, this may be a suggestion for future consideration.

Above all, community health research *requires* that nurses shift their thinking to concern for health care that includes the community.

REFERENCES

Aguirre-Molina, M., & Parra, P. A. (1995). Latino youth and families as active participants in planning change: A community-university partnership. In R. E. Zambrana

(Ed.), *Understanding Latino families: Scholarship, policy, and practice*. Thousand Oaks, CA: Sage.

Bichmann, W., Rifkin, S. B., & Shrestha, M. (1989). Towards the measurement of community participation. *World Health Forum, 10*, 467–472.

Bruhn, J. G. (2001). Ethical issues in intervention outcomes. *Family and Community Health, 23*(4), 24–35.

Castro, F., Elder, J., Coe, K., Tafoya-Barraza, H., Moratto, S., Campbell, N., & Talavera, G. (1995). Mobilizing churches for health promotion in Latino communities: Compañeros en la salud. *Journal of the National Cancer Institute Monographs, 18*, 127–135.

Chalmers, K., Bramadat, I. J., Cantin, B., Nurnaghan, D., Shuttleworth, E., Scott-Findlay, S., & Tataryn, D. (2001). A smoking reduction and cessation program with registered nurses: Findings and implications for community health nursing. *Journal of Community Health Nursing, 18*, 115–134.

Courtney, R. (1995). Community partnership primary care: A new paradigm for primary care. *Public Health Nurse, 12*, 366–373.

Courtney, R., Ballard, E., Fauver, S., Gariota, M., & Holland, L. (1996). The partnership model: Working with individuals, families, and communities toward a new vision of health. *Public Health Nurse, 13*, 177–186.

Eng, E., Parker, E. A., & Harlan, C. (1997). Lay health advisor intervention strategies: A continuum from natural helping to paraprofessional helping. *Health Education Behavior, 24*, 413–417.

Eng, E., Salmon, M. E., & Mullan, F. (1997). Community empowerment: The critical base for primary health care. *Family Community Health, 15*, 1.

Eng, E., & Young, R. (1992). Lay health advisors as community change agents. *Family & Community Health, 15*, 24–40.

Green, L. W., & Kreuter, M. W. (1999). *Health promotion planning* (3rd ed.). New York: McGraw-Hill.

Hecker, E. J. (2000). Feria de Salud: Implementation and evaluation of a community-wide health fair. *Public Health Nursing, 17*, 247–256.

Hildebrandt, E. (1996). Building community participation in health care: A model and example from South Africa. *Image: Journal of Nursing Scholarship, 28*, 155–159.

Hill, M. N., Bone, L. R., & Butz, A. M. (1996). Enhancing the role of community health workers in research. *Image: Journal of Nursing Scholarship, 28*, 221–226.

Institute of Medicine. (2003a). *The future of public's health in the 21st century*. Washington, DC: National Academy Press.

Institute of Medicine. (2003b). *Unequal treatment. Confronting racial and ethnic disparities in healthcare*. Washington, DC: National Academy Press.

Israel, B. A. (2000). *Community-based participatory research principles, rationale and policy recommendations*. Research Triangle Park, NC: National Institute of Environmental Health Sciences.

Israel, B. A., Schulz, A. J., Parker, E. A., & Becker, A. B. (1998). Review of community-based research: Assessing partnership approaches to improve public health. *Annual Review of Public Health, 19*, 173–202.

Israel, B. A., Schulz, A. J., Parker, E. A., Becker, A. B., Allen, A. J., & Guzman, J. R. (2003). Critical issues in developing and following community based participatory research principles. In M. Minkler & N. Wallerstein (Eds.), *Community-based participatory research for health* (pp. 53–76). San Francisco: Jossey-Bass.

Kelly, K., & Van Vlaenderen, H. (1995). Evaluation participation processes in community development. *Evaluation and Program Planning, 18*, 371–383.

Kelly, K. J., & Van Vlaenderen, H. (1996). Dynamics of participation in a community health project. *Social Science & Medicine, 42*, 1235–1246.

Kroutil, L. A., & Eng, E. (1989). Conceptualizing and assessing potential for community participation: A planning method. *Health Education Research, 4*, 305–319.

La Forgia, G. M. (1985). 15 years of community organizing for health in Panama. *Social Science and Medicine, 21*, 55–65.

Lasater, T., Becker, D., Hill, M., & Gans, K. (1997). Synthesis of findings and issues from religious-based cardiovascular disease prevention trials. *Annals of Epidemiology, 7*(Suppl. 7), S46–S53.

Lasater, T., Carleton, R., & Wells, B. (1991). Religious organizations and large-scale health related lifestyle change programs. *Journal of Health Education, 22*, 233–239.

McElmurry, B. J., & Keeney, G. B. (1999). Primary health care. In J. J. Fitzpatrick (Ed.), *Annual Review of Nursing Research* (Vol. 17, pp. 241–268). New York: Springer Publishing Co.

McFarlane, J., Kelly, E., Rodriguez, R., & Fehir, J. (1994). De Madres a Madres: Women building community coalitions for health. *Health Care Women International, 15*, 465–476.

McGinnis, J. M., & Foege, W. H. (1993). Actual causes of death in the United States. *Journal of the American Medical Association, 270*, 2207–2212.

Mahon, J., McFarlane, J., & Golden, K. (1991). De Madres a Madres: A community partnership for health. *Public Health Nursing, 8*, 15–19.

Marcus, M. T. (2000). An interdisciplinary team model for substance abuse prevention in communities. *Journal of Professional Nursing, 16*, 158–168.

May, K., McLaughlin, F., & Penner, M. (1991). Preventing low birth weight: Marketing and volunteer outreach. *Public Health Nursing, 8*, 97–104.

Meleis, A. I. (1992). Community participation and involvement: Theoretical and empirical issues. *Health Services Management, 5*, 5–16.

Moyer, A., Coristine, M., Jamault, M., Roberge, G., & O'Hagan, M. (1999). Identifying older people in need using action research. *Journal of Clinical Nursing, 8*, 103–111.

Moyer, A., Coristine, M., MacLean, L., & Meyer, M. (1999). A model for building collective capacity in community-based programs: The elderly in need project. *Public Health Nursing, 16*, 205–214.

Narayan, D. (1996). *Toward participatory research* (World Bank Technical Paper Number 307). Washington, DC: World Bank.

Nemcek, M. A., & Sabatier, R. (2003). State of evaluation: Community health workers. *Public Health Nursing, 20*, 260–270.

Nuñez, D. E., Armbruster, C., Phillips, W. T., & Gale, B. J. (2003). Community-based senior health promotion program using a collaborative practice model: The Escalante health partnership. *Public Health Nursing, 20*, 25–32.

Peterson, J., Atwood, J. R., & Yates, B. (2002). Key elements for church-based health promotion programs: Outcome-based literature review. *Public Health Nursing, 19*, 401–411.

PEW Health Professions Commission. (1994). *Community health workers: Integral yet often overlooked members of the health care workforce.* San Francisco: UCSF Center for Health Professions.

Ramos, I. N., May, M., & Ramos, K. S. (2001). Environmental health training of promotoras in colonias along the Texas-Mexico border. *American Journal of Public Health, 91*(4), 568–570.

Rothman, N. L., Lourie, R., Gaughan, J., & White, N. (1999). A community-developed, community-based lead poisoning prevention program: Lead awareness North Philly style. *Holistic Nursing Practice, 14*(1), 47–58.

Rothman, J., & Tropman, J. E. (1987). Models of community organization and macro practice perspectives: Their mixing and phasing. In F. M. Cox, J. L. Erlich, J. Rothman, & J. E. Tropman (Eds.), *Strategies of community organization: Macro practice* (pp. 3–25). Itasca, IL: Peacock.

Rowley, C., Dixon, L., & Sheldon, J. (2002). Focusing on local health needs and promoting new partnerships. *British Journal in Community Nursing, 7*(1), 47–51.

Swider, S. M. (2002). Outcome effectiveness of community health workers: An integrative literature review. *Public Health Nursing, 19*(1), 11–20.

Ugalde, A. (1985). Ideological dimensions of community participation in Latin American health programs. *Social Science and Medicine, 21*, 41–53.

U.S. Department of Health and Human Services. (2001). *Healthy people in healthy communities.* Washington, DC: U.S. Government Printing Office.

Voorhees, C., Stillman, F., Swank, R., Heagerty, P., Levine, D., & Becker, D. (1996). Heart, body, and soul: Impact of church-based smoking cessation intervention on readiness to quit. *Preventive Medicine, 25*, 277–285.

Wallerstein, N., & Duran, B. (2003). The conceptual, historical, and practice roots of community based participatory research and related participatory traditions. In M. Minkler & N. Wallerstein (Eds.), *Community-based participatory research for health* (pp. 27–52). San Francisco: Jossey-Bass.

Weinrich, S., Holdford, D., Boyd, M., Creanga, D., Cover, K., Johnson, A., Frank-Stromberg, M., & Weinrich, M. (1998). Prostate cancer education in African American churches. *Public Health Nursing, 15*, 188–195.

Index

Contents of Previous 10 Volumes

VOLUME XIV

Joyce Fitzpatrick and Jane Norbeck, Editors

VOLUME XV

Joyce Fitzpatrick and Jane Norbeck, Editors

VOLUME XVIII: Research on Chronic Illness

Joyce Fitzpatrick, Series Editor; Jean Goeppinger, Volume Editor

VOLUME XXI: Research on Child Health and Pediatric Issues

Joyce Fitzpatrick, Series Editor; Margaret Shandor Miles and Diane Holditch-Davis, Volume Editors